ELECTROCARDIOGRAPHY AND CARDIAC DRUG THERAPY

Developments in
Cardiovascular Medicine

VOLUME 92

ELECTROCARDIOGRAPHY AND CARDIAC DRUG THERAPY

edited by

V. HOMBACH
Department of Cardiology-Angiology-Pneumology,
University Hospital Ulm,
Ulm, F.R.G.

H.H. HILGER
Department of Cardiology – Angiology – Pneumology
University of Cologne,
Cologne, F.R.G.

and

H.L. KENNEDY
Division of Cardiology,
St. Louis University, School of Medicine,
St. Louis, Missouri, U.S.A.

KLUWER ACADEMIC PUBLISHERS
DORDRECHT / BOSTON / LONDON

Electrocardiography and cardiac drug therapy.

   (Developments in cardiovascular medicine ; 92)
   Includes bibliographies.
   1. Electrocardiography. 2. Electrocardiography,
Ambulatory. 3. Heart--Diseases--Chemotherapy.
4. Cardiovascular agents. I. Hombach, V. (Vinzenz)
II. Hilger, H. H. III. Kennedy, Harold L. IV. Series:
Developments in cardiovascular medicine ; v. 92.
[DNLM: 1. Cardiovascular Diseases--drug therapy.
2. Electrocardiography. W1 DE997VME v.92 /
WG 140 E374]
RC683.5.E5E38 1988   616.1'061   88-13046
ISBN-13:978-94-010-6976-2   e-ISBN-13:978-94-009-1081-2
DOI: 10.1007/978-94-009-1081-2

Published by Kluwer Academic Publishers,
P.O. Box 17, 3300 AA Dordrecht, The Netherlands.

Kluwer Academic Publishers incorporates
the publishing programmes of
D. Reidel, Martinus Nijhoff, Dr W. Junk and MTP Press.

Sold and distributed in the U.S.A. and Canada
by Kluwer Academic Publishers,
101 Philip Drive, Norwell, MA 02061, U.S.A.

In all other countries, sold and distributed
by Kluwer Academic Publishers Group,
P.O. Box 322, 3300 AH Dordrecht, The Netherlands.

printed on acid free paper

Table of Contents

V

PART IV: DRUG THERAPY

Preface

This book is a comprehensive overview of electrocardiography and the major effects of current cardiac pharmacological therapy on electrocardiography. The text is based on work presented at the International Symposium on Non-invasive Cardiovascular Diagnosis and Therapy, held in May, 1987 at the University of Cologne. The theme of the book is to review, in broad clinical perspective the current state-of-the-art of electrocardiography as it pertains to standard electrocardiograms, exercise testing, ambulatory electrocardiography, electrocardiographic telemetry, and high resolution electrocardiography. Furthermore, advances in cardiac drug therapy in relation to diuretics, beta blocking drugs, antiarrhythmic agents and thrombolytic agents are reviewed. The emphasis of the conference and this book is to review the clinical state-of-the-art information and applications in this regard.

In the initial section on electrocardiography, Dr. *Spodick* reviews our present day physiologic and pathophysiologic understanding of systolic time intervals, and how they are affected by a variety of cardiac disease states and pharmacologic agents. Dr. *Ellestad* examines problems and provides pragmatic tips on exercise testing in the diagnosis of coronary artery disease, and advances in exercise scores and computer analysis. Dr. *Graboys* reviews the value of exercise testing in the diagnosis and management of patients with serious ventricular arrhythmias. Dr. *Kellermann* presents the complimentary role that exercise testing plays in comprehensive follow-up therapy of the cardiac patient, and the use of exercise for work and physical training. Detailed information concerning the interaction of cardiac rehabilitation and ventricular arrhythmias are examined.

The second section on ambulatory electrocardiography begins with the use of the Holter ECG and the evaluation of patient symptoms by Dr. *Weber*. Limitations, sensitivity and predictability of ambulatory electrocardiography for this clinical application are thoroughly reviewed. Doctors *Kennedy* and *Wiens* present a review of current state-of-the-art Holter technology, and a review of the literature with regards to ambulatory electrocardiography applications in the diagnosis, prognosis and assessment of therapeutic interventions in patients with cardiac arrhythmias.

Doctors *Stern* and *Tzivoni* detail a state-of-the-art review of ambulatory electrocardiography in the detection, characteristics, and significance of silent myocardial ischemia. Dr. *Höher* reviews the applications of ambulatory electrocardiography in the evaluation of the pacemaker patient. A lucid discussion of the problems encountered in the emerging bichamber pacing era are addressed. Dr. *Wenger's* cogent discussion of ECG telemetry and ambulatory electrocardiography in cardiac rehabilitation, and Dr. *Schmidt's* presentation of the variability of ventricular arrhythmia over chronic durations of time present a comprehensive review of these diverse aspects of ambulatory electrocardiography. Dr. *Raftery* reviews the rationale, methodology, and knowledge of ambulatory blood pressure, and its utilization and specific diagnostic applications. Furthermore, the unique prognostic value of this measurement is discussed. Lastly but not least, the emergence of using ambulatory electrocardiography to assess sleep apnea syndrome in patients with cardiorespiratory disorders are addressed by Doctors *Peter* and *von Wichert*.

The third section on high resolution electrocardiography begins with a discussion of the merit of amplified surface electrocardiographic activity to detect His-bundle potentials by Dr. *Vincent*, and detection of late potentials with signal averaging by Dr. *Berbari*. Basic and clinical aspects of high resolutional electrocardiography are extensively discussed and illustrated by Dr. *El-Sherif* in a most comprehensive manner which compliments the aforegoing discussion. The effects of fibrinolytic therapy on the frequency and pattern of these micro-potentials by *Goedel–Meinen* et al, and their clinical and prognostic significance by *Breithardt* et al provides a current state-of-the-art knowledge of late potential and signal averaging electrocardiography. Dr. *Hombach* discusses the dynamic changing behavior of these micro-potentials, particularly when examined on a beat by beat basis, and reports from Doctors *Fenici* and *Siltanen* add new information of the recording of the magnetic field (magnetocardiography) and how it relates to high resolution electrocardiography.

The final section of the book reviews for the clinician a state-of-the-art presentation of diuretics by Dr. *Sieberth*, and beta adrenoceptor blocking drugs by Dr. *Prichard*. The emergence of new antiarrhythmic agents in 1987 by Doctors *Camm* and *Linker*, and thrombolytic agents by Doctors *Ostermann* and *Schmitz-Huebner* timely discuss the plethora of new emerging pharmaceutical agents and their promising applications in patients with ischemic heart disease. Finally, the appreciation of the importance of low density lipoprotein as a contributor to familial hypocholesterolemia was discussed as a provocative stimulus to the appreciation of familial hypercholesterolemia by Dr. *Borberg*.

The reader may find some overlap in the presentations in this volume, but rather than detracting, this adds additional information and perspective to the interpretation of the reported literature. The book is strongly recommended to students of electrocardiography as a resource text.

Harold L. Kennedy, M.D., M.P.H.

List of Contributors

E.J. Berbari, VA Medical Center, 921 Northeast 13th Street, Oklahoma City, OK 73104, USA.
Co-authors: B.J. Scherlag, R. Lazzara

H. Borberg, Haemapheresis Unit, Department of Medicine, University of Cologne, Joseph-Stelzmannstrasse 9, 5000 Cologne 41, FRG
Co-authors: A. Gaczkowski, V. Hombach, K. Oette, W. Stoffel

G. Breithart, Department of Cardiology, Pneumology and Angiology, University Hospital, University of Münster, Albert Schweitzer-Strasse 33, 4400 Münster, FRG
Co-authors: M. Borggrefe, A. Podczeck, K. Haerten, A. Martinez-Rubio

A.J. Camm, Department of Cardiological Sciences, St. George's Hospital Medical School, Cranmer Terrace, London SW17 0RE, England
Co-author: N.J. Linker

M.H. Ellestad, Memorial Heart Institute, Memorial Medical Center, P.O. Box 1428, Long Beach, CA 90801, USA

N. El-Sherif, Cardiology Division, SUNY, Health Science Center, 450 Clarkson Avenue, Box 1199, Brooklyn, NY 11203, USA
Co-authors: M. Restivo, W. Craelius, R. Henkin, G. Kelen, J.M. Fontaine, S.N. Ursell, G. Turitto

R.R. Fenici, Cardiovascular Biomagnetism Unit, CNR, Catholic University of S. Heart, Largo Agostino Gemelli 8, I-00168 Rome, Italy
Co-authors: M. Masselli, L. Lopez, G. Melillo

L. Goedel-Meinen, 1st Department of Internal Medicine, Technical University Munich, Ismaningerstrasse 22, 8000 Munich 80, FRG
Co-authors: M. Hofmann, G. Schmidt, G. Jahns, G. Klein, W. Baedeker

T.B. Graboys, Cardiovascular division, Department of Medicine, Brigham and Women's Hospital, 75 Francis Street, Boston, MA 02115, USA

M. Höher, Department of Cardiology – Angiology – Pneumology, University of Ulm, Robert-Koch-Strasse, D-7900, Ulm, FRG

XI

Co-authors: E. Vonderbank, H.W. Verhoeven, T. Eggeling, M. Kochs, V. Hombach, H.H. Kilger

V. Hombach, Department of Cardiology – Angiology – Pneumology, University Hospital of Ulm, Robert-Koch-Strasse, D-7900, Ulm, FRG
Co-authors: M. Kochs, H.W. Höpp, H. Kebbel, T. Eggeling, A. Oster- spey, H. Hirche, H.H. Hilger

J.J. Kellermann, Herman Mayer Cardiac Rehabilitation Institute, Chaim Sheba Medical Center, Sackler School of Medicine, Tel Aviv University, Tel Aviv, Israel
Co-authors: E. Ben-Ari, M. Hayet, E.Z. Fisman

H.L. Kennedy, Division of Cardiology, Department of Internal Medicine, St. Louis University School of Medicine, St. Louis, MO 63104, USA

H. Ostermann, Department of Internal Medicine, Wilhelms University of Westphalia, Albert Schweitzer-Strasse 33, 4400 Münster, FRG
Co-author: U. Schmitz-Huebner

J.H. Peter, Medical Polyclinic, Baldingerstrasse, D-3550 Marburg, FRG
Co-author: P. von Wichert

B.N.C. Prichard, Department of Clinical Pharmacology, University Col- lege London, 5 University Street, London WC1E 6JJ, England

E.B. Raftery, Cardiology Department, Northwick Park Hospital and Clinical Research Center, Watford Road, Harrow, Middlesex, HA1 3UJ, United Kingdom

G. Schmidt, Department of Cardiology, 1st Department of Internal Medi- cine, Technical University Munich, Ismaningerstrasse 22, 8000 Munich 80, FRG
Co-authors: K. Ulm, L. Goedel-Meinen, G. Jahns, P. Barthel, B. Stief, U. Schaudig

H.G. Sieberth, Departmenr of Internal Medicine II, Technical University of Aachen, Pauwelsstrasse, 5100 Aachen, FRG

P. Siltanen, Cardiovascular Laboratory, Helsinki University Central Hos- pital, 00290 Helsinki, Finland
Co-authors: T. Katila, M. Mäkijärvi, M. Leinio, J. Nenonen, J. Mon- tonen, S. Madekivi

D.H. Spodick, Cardiology Division, Saint Vincent Hospital, Worchester, MA 01604, USA

Stern, S., The Heiden Department of Cardiology, Bikur Cholim Hospital, Jerusalem, 5 Strauss Street, P.O. Box 492, Israel
Co-author: D. Tzivoni

R. Vincent, Department of Cardiology, Royal Sussex County Hospital, Eastern Road, Brighton BN2 5BE, United Kingdom

H. Weber, Department of Cardiology, University Clinic Vienna, Gar- nisongasse 13, A-1090 Vienna, Austria

Co-authors: H. Schmidinger, Ch. Auinger, J. Wolfram, T. Rimpfl, Y. Norman, R. Schmidt

N. Wenger, Department of Cardiology, Emory University School of Medicine, 69 Butler Street, Atlanta, Georgia 30303, USA

Part I: Electrocardiography

1. Systolic time intervals: basis and application

DAVID H. SPODICK

Clinical Cardiology, Saint Vincent Hospital; University of Mass. Medical School; Tufts University School of Medicine; Boston University School of Medicine, U.S.A.

Introduction

Systole, like diastole, can be divided into physiologically (and ultimately clinically) significant intervals. They have been explicitly or intuitively measured for more than a century, but the modern application of systolic time intervals (STI) results from the work of Blumberger; all subsequent work has been variations on the remarkable range of his physiologic, clinical and pharmacologic investigations, though perhaps with more sophisticated statistical analyses. More recent interest in STI was stimulated by the many contributions of Weissler.

Identification and measurement

The principal systolic intervals can be measured from catheterization curves as long as a central aortic trace is recorded [1]. In all cases, the *q* wave of the electrocardiogram (ECG) is used as 'zero time' from which all other points are measured on the aortic pressure pulse curve. The aortic pulse upstroke corresponds to the onset of ventricular ejection, therefore the time from the ECG *q* wave to the onset of the upstroke is the 'pre-ejection period' (PEP). The period of ejection of blood from the left ventricle begins with the aortic upstroke and ends at its incisura, yielding the left ventricular ejection time, abbreviated LVET [2]. The combination, PEP + LVET is considered to represent electromechanical systole (EMS) [3]. There are other systolic intervals; however, PEP, LVET, EMS and the ratio PEP/LVET account for almost one hundred percent of the practical work in the field. This discussion will be restricted to these left ventricular intervals. The question is, how to obtain them noninvasively?

Systolic intervals can be obtained noninvasively from numerous types of tracing. For example, the M-mode echocardiogram, when technically

V. Hombach, H. H. Hilger and H. L. Kennedy (eds), Electrocardiography and Cardiac Drug Therapy. ISBN 978-94-010-6976-2
© 1989, Kluwer Academic Publishers, Dordrecht –

excellent, displays the aortic valve opening and closing ('aortic box'), the duration of which is the LVET, exactly as on the aortic pulse trace. The time from the ECG q wave to the opening of the 'aortic box' is thus the PEP. Doppler tracings of the aortic velocity profile can be used in the same way as the aortic pulse curve. However, the most common method used, which is applicable in many more patients due to technical difficulties in some patients in whom good Doppler traces or 'aortic box' are not recordable (notably in aortic valve disease and emphysemal), is the 'triple trace': ECG (conventionally, lead II), phonocardiogram (PCG) displaying a good aortic component of the second heart sound and a peripheral arterial displacement pulse—usually the carotid pulse (CAR), although any arterial pulse with a good incisura will suffice [4]. The LVET on peripheral pulses is identical to the aortic LVET [1], permitting its direct use from noninvasive displacement traces. How, then, to calculate the PEP? Fortunately, the incisura of the aortic pulse coincides with the aortic component of the second heart sound [II_A]. Therefore, II_A is a noninvasive marker of the aortic pulse incisura which can be obtained noninvasively using the PCG [3]. Moreover, the time between the carotid incisura and the aortic component of the second heart sound, designated the pulse transmission time (PTT), represents the time taken for the pulse wave to travel from the central aorta to the carotid artery [5]. This time is therefore subtracted from the timing of the carotid upstroke, to yield the timing of the onset of the aortic upstroke—the PEP. Thus, we have the following time relationships: ($q = 0$):

1. II_A to carotid incisura = PTT;
2. q to carotid upstroke *minus* PTT = PEP;
3. carotid upstroke to carotid incisura = LVET;
4. PEP + LVET = EMS.

In practice, therefore, one measures three points from the ECG q wave: the time periods to the carotid upstroke, to its incisura, and to II_A. From these three points PEP, LVET, EMS ($q - II_A$) and PEP/LVET are calculated.

Heart-rate effects

LVET and EMS are heart rate (HR) related, whereas the PEP is not (despite much erroneous information on the PEP [3, 6]). During atrial pacing (i.e. "pure rate" changes) the PEP is stable, in contrast to situations where circulating catecholamines give a spurious PEP-heart rate (HR) relationship. During pacing and all other HR changes LVET and EMS change inversely with HR. Regression equations against HR permit calculation of indexes: LVETI and EMSI [2].

Pulsus alternans: a model for STI relationships

Pulsus alternans, a condition in which there is perfect alternation of strong and weak heart beats, illustrates, through its effects on STI, the implications of changes in STI and their responses to challenges [7, 8]. Though many mechanisms have been proposed for pulsus alternans, it is agreed that, by any measurement, alternate beats are 'strong' and 'weak'. The PEP is always shorter in the stronger beats and longer in the weak beats; the LVET varies reciprocally: it is shorter in the weak beats and longer in the strong beats. PEP/LVET behaves more like the PEP itself—smaller in the strong beats and larger in the weak beats. Thus, any *weak beat* would be characterized by longer PEP and PEP/LVET and a shorter LVET [7, 8].

Physiologic and pharmacologic effects on STI (Table 1)

Positive inotropic stimuli tend to shorten both the PEP and the LVET (and, consequently, also to shorten the EMS). *Stroke volume changes* are equally important for the duration of LVET so that, at a constant inotropic level,

Table 1. Effects of interventions on systolic time intervals

PEP/LVET	Interventions	PEP	LVET	EMS

↓	Positive inotropic
	  Digitalis
	  Adrenergic Stimulation
	  Isoproterenol
		↓	↓	↓

↑	At constant inotropic level– ↑ Afterload	↑	↑	↑
↓	↑ Stroke Volume	↓	↑	0
↑	↑ Heart Rate	0	↓	↓
↑	↑ Heart Rate Atrial Pacing	0	↓	↓
↑	Vagal Block	0	↓	↓
↓	Adrenergic Stimulation	↓	↓	↓
↓	↑ Ejection Fraction	↓	↑	

an increased stroke volume will increase LVET while, due to Starling effect (i.e. increased preload), it will shorten PEP [9]. At a constant inotropic level, *increased heart rate* (as by atrial pacing) will not affect PEP, but will shorten LVET and consequently EMS, whereas *increased heart rate from adrenergic stimulation* will decrease PEP and LVET [9]. In this connection, PEP/LVET is a convenient overall indicator of left ventricular function. For example, in our studies, PEP/LVET was inversely related to velocity of contractile fibers (Vcf): $r = -0.65$, $P < 0.001$ [6]. The relation between PEP/LVET and ejection fraction was also inverse: $r = -0.85$, $p < 0.001$ [6].

An example of a strong inotropic stimulus is the injection of *glucagon* into both animals and human beings [10]. This is followed by a sharp immediate rise in pressure rate product (PRP) and LVETI, the ejection time index (i.e. LVET corrected for heart rate); at the same time, LVET itself (uncorrected) falls as does pre-ejection period and PEP/LVET—typical inotropic effects [10]. Another, more complex, inotropic stimulus, *dynamic exercise*, gives characteristic changes in systolic intervals with a fall in pre-ejection period and PEP/LVET as well as LVET (reflecting the reduced stroke volume), and a rise in ejection time index [11]. In recovery from exercise, these changes are progressively reversed over time [12].

Another, common physiologic state is ordinary quiet *respiration*. This shows changes in STI, which are consistent with what is known from the changes in cardiac function during the respiratory cycle. Accordingly, during inspiration LVET falls, PEP rises (as does PEP/LVET), and this is reversed in expiration [13]. During pericardial effusion, even without cardiac tamponade [14], these respiratory changes in STI are significantly exaggerated, and particularly so during tamponade with pulsus paradoxus [15], recognized clinically by measuring arterial blood pressure.

STI changes in disease

In *coronary artery disease* the use of systolic intervals is limited when applied epidemiologically since many patients will have normal LV function. Over large numbers of patients, compared to age- and sex-matched normal control subjects, the patients with coronary disease *as a group* will have small but significant changes in the direction of impaired cardiac function (even when the absolute mean figures are close to normal). Accordingly, the ejection time index (LVETI) is shorter, while the pre-ejection period and PEP/LVET are longer in *groups of patients* with stable coronary disease [16]. However, the *individual* overlap is so great that this is of limited diagnostic use, although in patients hospitalized for coronary angiography it has been shown that there is a progressive rise in PEP and PEP/LVET and a concomitant fall in LVETI with increasing (1, 2, or 3) coronary vessel disease.

Dilated cardiomyopathy often produces the largest changes in the PEP—so large that there are almost diagnostic of this condition (in the absence of left bundle branch block) [17]. The PEP is greatly prolonged from its normal range of approximately 85–105 milliseconds: it is often in excess of 140 milliseconds. The LVETI is variably shortened, while PEP/LVET often doubles (normal range: 0.28 to 0.41). In a blinded study of non-cardiac alcoholics compared with age- and sex-matched normals and with patients with dilated alcoholic cardiomyopathy, we showed that the cardiomyopathic alcoholics were at the extreme of a pathologic continuum. This was because the results for the systolic time intervals in the group of alcoholics without cardiac disease were between the STIs of normal controls and the STIs of cardiomyopathic alcoholics [17].

Pharmacologic challenge

Systolic time intervals lend themselves easily to pharmacologic studies because they are obtained totally noninvasively and inexpensively, with complete safety, and can be repeated as often as necessary. Thus, for example, a typical *nitrate* effect on the PEP/LVET shows increases to degrees and durations depending on the dose and the agent. Erythrityl tetranitrate 5 mgs., for example, will increase PEP/LVET for six hours (as usual, due mainly to prolongation of PEP [18].) This effect can be dramatically cancelled if the patient eats a meal, presumably owing to the adrenergic effects of food [19].

Valvular heart disease

In valvular heart disease, patients with *aortic stenosis* often have normal systolic time intervals, but with progression of disease the LV ejection time becomes greatly prolonged in the absence of heart failure. In fact, with advanced disease, normalization of the LVET (LVETI) suggests that the left ventricle is failing.

In acute and chronic *mitral regurgitation* (MR) the PEP/LVET correlates well with the ejection fraction ($r = 0.84$, $p < 0.001$) [20]. Valve replacement with various kinds of artificial heart valve tends to correct both the MR and the prolonged PEP/LVET [21].

8

Other conditions

In a number of 'non-mechanical' pathologic conditions STI will not only reflect metabolic effects on the heart, but also the success or failure of treatment. Thus, the increased PEP/LVET of *hypothyroidism* is reduced dramatically with effective treatment [22].

Conclusions

In conclusion, STIs are precise, perfectly safe, infinitely repeatable, totally noninvasive measures of net ventricular function. They have practical limitations inherent in any 'net' indices with mixed dependency on pre- and afterload, among other factors. However, they are frequently sensitive reflectors of pathologic and physiologic conditions. With experience, the STIs are very useful to estimate ventricular status, responses to physiologic and pharmacologic challenges and to document and monitor pathologic changes.

Summary

The systolic time intervals (STI) were introduced in modern form by Blumberger. They have stood the test of time as easily and inexpensively as well as safely obtained indices of cardiac function. The STI represent divisions of cardiac systole which can be obtained in many ways, both invasively and noninvasively, but the standard method is the 'triple trace'—electrocardiogram, phonocardiogram and carotid displacement pulse. Cardiac electromechanical systole is measured from the Q wave of the electrocardiogram to the aortic component of the second heart sound (Q–S2) in milliseconds. This is further divided into the pre-ejection period (PEP) and left ventricular ejection time (LVET). LVET is measured from the rapid upstroke of the carotid pulse to its incisura. PEP is measured by subtracting LVET from Q–S2 or by first calculating the central pulse transmission time (PTT), the time between the aortic component of the second sound and the carotid incisura. The pre-isovolumic period is sometimes measured from the Q wave to the mitral component of the first heart sound, but this has much less utility under most circumstances. STIs have a wide range of application. They can be used to measure cardiac function during acute myocardial infarction and arrhythmias, in valve disease (particularly aortic valve disease) and hypertrophic and other cardiomyopathies, as well as during chronic and acute congestive heart failure. The

STI respond sensitively to physiologic and pharmacologic interventions, including during and after exercise.

References

1. Shaver JA, Kroetz FW, Leonard JJ, Paley HW (1968) The effect of steady-state increases in systemic arterial pressure on the duration of left ventricular ejection time. J Clin Invest 47:217–222

2. Spodick DH, Kumar S (1968) Left ventricular ejection period: Measurement by atraumatic techniques: Results in normal young men and comparison of methods of calculation. Am Heart J 76:70–73

3. Kumar S, Spodick DH (1970) Study of the mechanical events of the left ventricle by atraumatic techniques: Comparison of methods of measurement and their significance. Am Heart J 80:401–413

4. Chirife R, Pigott VM, Spodick DH (1971) Measurement of the left ventricular ejection time by digital plethysmography. Am Heart J 82:222–227

5. Spodick DH, Lance VQ (1976) Noninvasive stress testing: Methodology for elimination of the phonocardiogram. Circulation 53:673–676

6. Spodick DH, Doi YL, Bishop RL, Hashimoto T (1984) Systolic time intervals reconsidered: Reevaluation of the pre-ejection period: Absence of relation to heart rate. Am J Cardiol 53:1667–1670

7. Spodick DH, St. Pierre JR (1970) Pulsus alternans: Physiologic study by noninvasive techniques. Am Heart J 80:766–777

8. Spodick DH, Khan AH, Pigott VM (1974) Systolic and diastolic time intervals in pulsus alternans: Significance of alternating isovolumic relaxation. Am Heart J 87:5–10

9. Spodick DH (1974) Investigation of cardiac dynamics by mechanocardiography (Systolic Time Intervals), Zoneraich S. (Ed.): Noninvasive Methods in Cardiology, Springfield, IL, Charles C Thomas, pp 296–319

10. Byrne MJ, Pigott VM, Spodick DH (1972) Cardiovascular responses to glucagon in normal man: Physiologic measurement by external recordings. Amer Heart J 83:635–643

11. Lance VQ, Spodick DH (1975) Constant load versus rate targeted exercise: Responses of systolic intervals. J Appl Physiol 38:794–800

12. Nandi PS, Spodick DH (1977) Recovery from exercise at varying work loads: Timecourse of responses of heart rate and systolic intervals. Br Heart J 39:958–966

13. Pigott VM, Spodick DH (1971) Effects of normal breathing and expiratory apnea on duration of the phases of cardiac systole. Am Heart J 82:786–793

14. Spodick DH, Paladino D, Flessas AP (1983) Respiratory effects on systolic time intervals during pericardial effusion. Am J Cardiol 51:1033–1035

15. Spodick DH, Paladino DM (1983) Exaggerated respiratory variation in left ventricular ejection time during lax pericardial effusion. Cardiology 70:1–5

16. Spodick DH (1982) Systolic time intervals: Prognostic value and exercise responses. Advances in Cardiol 31:35–37

17. Spodick DH, Pigott VM, Chirife R (1972) Preclinical cardiac malfunction in chronic alcoholism. Comparison with matched normal controls and with alcoholic cardiomyopathy. NEJM 287:678–680

18. de la Paz LR, Kerigan AT, Koch GG, Kolman WA, Spodick DH (1979) Erythrityl tetranitrate: Sustained effects on systolic time intervals. Changes consistent with sustained preload reduction. Am J Med Sci 277:173–177

10

19. Haffty BG, Nakamura Y, Long RA, Hull JH, Spodick DH (1982) Bioavailability of organic nitrates: A comparison of methods for evaluating plethysmographic responses. J. Clin Pharmacol 22:117–124
20. Boudoulas H, Lewis RP, Dervenagas S, Fontana ME, Vasko JS (1979) Abbreviation of systolic time intervals in acute mitral regurgitation: Effect of prosthetic mitral valve replacement. Am J Cardiol 44:595–600
21. Saito K (1979) Systolic time intervals before and after mitral valve replacement with different prostheses. J Cardiogr 9:143–147
22. Plotnick GD, Vassar DL, Parisi AF, Hamilton BP, Carliner NH, Fisher MD (1979) Systolic time intervals in hypothyroidism. Am J Med Sci 277:263–268

2. Exercise testing problems in the diagnosis of coronary artery disease

MYRVIN H. ELLESTAD

Memorial Heart Institute, Memorial Medical Center of Long Beach; University of California at Irvine, U.S.A.

Key words: myocardial ischemia, exercise testing, ST segments, heart rate, blood pressure response, computer processing

Abstract

Problems associated with exercise testing will always require special consideration. Disease prevalence, analysis of multiple variables, lead selection and many factors influence the diagnostic power of the method. New information indicates that septal Q waves, R wave amplitude, and possibly QT intervals are of importance in the diagnosis of ischemia. The analysis of blood pressure and heart rate response also contribute to the predictive power. At times, the response to nitroglycerin and beta blockers will help in the analysis of ST changes. Also, the time of ST onset and offset are helpful. Although computer analysis of the ECG is becoming more common, special attention to the fiduciary points, especially the baseline, will help identify errors introduced by these machines.

Introduction

Although exercise induced ST depression has been recognized as a marker of myocardial ischemia for almost 70 years, there are still uncertainties in the application of the technique when attempting to diagnose and quantitate the severity of coronary artery disease. This paper will discuss some of these problems and suggest some coping mechanisms.

When we correlate exercise test findings with coronary angiograms, it is important to realize that reduction in coronary flow does not correlate well with estimates of anatomical reduction in lumen diameter, especially if the apparent narrowing is less than 80 or 90 percent. Thus, we should search for signs that correlate with follow-up studies as well as coronary anatomies to validate their significance.

V. Hombach, H. H. Hilger and H. L. Kennedy (eds), Electrocardiography and Cardiac Drug Therapy. ISBN 978-94-010-6976-2
© 1989, Kluwer Academic Publishers, Dordrecht –

Prevalence of disease

The appreciation that a low disease prevalence in the population under study will reduce the specificity of the ST depression has explained the high false-positive rate found in younger, asymptomatic men and possibly in women. This is explained by Bayes Theorem which is a mathematical rule that relates past experiences to our present observations in order to predict the reliability of the final result, or the 'post-test probability' or uncertainty. It describes the information content which pertains to how much we know about the presence or absence of disease before the test, and its effect on the reliability of the diagnosis of the test.

Diamond [1] and others have proposed that the pre-test information content, or pre-test probability, can be predicted from the patients symptoms. Typical angina, for example, almost assures the presence of coronary artery disease (nearly 90 percent) so that a test that increased the probability by 50 percent would only increase the post-test probability to 95 percent. On the other hand, Diamond found non-anginal chest pain to be associated with an intermediate pre-test probability of about 35 percent, thus, when exercise induced ST depression increased the probability 50 percent, it added much more information and, thus, making a greater contribution to the diagnosis. We know, of course, that the symptoms are only one of the determinants of coronary disease probability. Some of the others being sex, age, family history, smoking, etc.

Because the prevalence of coronary artery disease is very low in certain population groups such as young asymptomatic men or women, an abnormal response (such as ST segment depression) has little likelihood of indicating disease. Thus, in this setting, most of the abnormal responders are likely to be 'false-positive'. The recognition that depressed ST segments should be used as a risk factor, rather than an absolute diagnostic sign, becomes easier to understand when the above is kept in mind.

ST configuration. Upsloping ST depression

For many years horizontal and downsloping configurations were the only ones accepted as being 'positive'. Epidemiological studies in our laboratory [2] demonstrated that subjects with this configuration had the same prevalence of cardiac events during follow-up as those with a horizontal ST response. When correlated with coronary angiography [3], they are reported to have a slightly lower specificity than horizontal depression but should still be regarded as a useful marker for ischemia in most subjects.

Horizontal and downsloping ST response

These patterns have long been recognized to be predictive of coronary disease when correlated with coronary angios and also with events in a follow-up study. We have found a downsloping pattern to predict a higher prevalence of subsequent coronary events than the horizontal pattern and also found that when horizontal ST depression evolves into a downsloping pattern during recovery, it indicates an increased probability of subsequent coronary problems.

Septal Q waves, magnitude of ST and R waves

If the septal Q wave increases with exercise, this provides strong evidence against the presence of ischemia, particularly in the left anterior descending coronary [4]. Patients with non-specific cardiomyopathies often have ST depression and increasing septal Q waves with exercise, thus suggesting the diagnosis of coronary artery disease. Unfortunately, less than 50% of the usual population tested have resting septal Q waves. If the septal Q waves are present at rest and reduced during exercise, this provides very good evidence of ischemia due to narrowing of the left anterior descending coronary artery. The magnitude of the ST depression generally believed to quantitate ischemia, probably only does this when it appears at low work loads and in subjects without left ventricular hypertrophy. When the R wave is very tall, ST magnitude tends to increase and when the R wave is short (less than 9 mm), ischemia may not result in significant ST depression.

Time course

ST depression that improves even as exercise load increases, or that which disappears immediately after exercise is terminated, may not be due to coronary artery disease; while ST changes that persist during recovery have an increase in specificity and more reliably indicates severe ischemia [5]. Rapid dissolution of ST depression is most common when it occurs only at high work loads.

Hyperventilation

ST depression following hyperventilation prior to the test has been believed to be a negative predictor for significant disease. Recent work, however, has shown that alkalosis from prolonged hyperventilation may result in severe coronary spasm and actually produce ischemia [6]. Thus it may be an important indication of spasm even in subjects with significant coronary disease.

Exercise protocol

A very rapid increase in work load is believed to produce ST depression in some subjects without coronary disease. Therefore, a 2 to 3 minute warmup with moderate exercise is standard practice. Other variations of the protocol are of less importance. The amount of work applied should be the maximum the patient can do safely. Horizontal or recumbent exercise results in less total body work but at near maximum increases the cardiac work load because of the increased ventricular filling. Upright exercise on a bicycle or treadmill remains the most practical and most popular. The use of isometric handgrip results in less total body work as does most arm ergometry. Isometric work while exercising on a treadmill, however, may delay the onset of ischemia [7].

Endurance

Short exercise times have been shown to be good predictors of increased mortality in coronary patients. It may, however, only indicate poor conditioning in older subjects or in those who by habit are poorly conditioned. Thus, its significance must be correlated with the general information known about the patient.

Heart rate and blood pressure

A reduction in the expected response in either of these modalities may predict coronary pathology but it is important to realize that these findings have a low specificity. A recent report that a sustained systolic blood pressure during recovery signals coronary narrowing needs further confirmation [8]. We have seen numerous subjects with normal coronary vessels exhibit blood pressure elevation for several minutes after exercise. Also, a dropping blood pressure during exercise is normal after the patient exceeds his anerobic threshold, so only early onset changes have importance in diagnoses.

ST changes with drugs

Nitroglycerine preparations, beta blockers, and calcium blockers have all been demonstrated to reduce the magnitude of ST depression during exercise. It would appear, however, that only rarely will these agents completely eliminate ST depression if exercise is pushed to the maximum. We have also found that ST depression completely eliminated by beta blockers strongly suggests that they are not due to coronary narrowing. There is also some evidence that failure to improve ST depression with nitro provides evidence that the changes are not due to ischemia [9]. Persantine in large oral or moderate i.v. doses may aggravate ischemia and increase the sensitivity of the test.

Lead systems

A problem with the number and placement of the ECG leads still exists. Three lead monitoring has come to be the standard, probably because of equipment design. Advocates of 14 leads and 16 lead maps have still not established their clear superiority, although they may provide a slightly greater sensitivity.

Testing in women

Women as always are a vexing problem. The prevalence of ST depression with exercise prior to menopause is higher than afterward, tending to confirm other data that these changes in premenopausal women are not due to coronary disease [10]. After menopause, ST depression becomes almost as specific as it is in men if it is associated with one or two conventional risk factors.

Testing after myocardial infarction

Those subjects who have exercise induced ST segment depression after myocardial infarction are most likely to have additional ischemic areas of myocardium at risk. Other findings such as recurrent pain, persistent tachycardia, and failure to increase blood pressure during exercise may be almost as useful. Although it has been accepted for some years that ST depression 10–14 days after infarction helps identify patients at increased risk [11], we should remember that those who have had a complicated course and, thus, are not suitable for testing are at greater risk.

Therapeutic interventions

Although the ST segment seems to loose some of its specificity after bypass surgery and possibly angioplasty, the recurrence of this finding after the intervention is likely to be associated with disease progression.

Ryan [12] has recently reported that when used prior to surgery, those with a short exercise time have been shown to do better with surgery than if they are treated medically. When surgery or angioplasty results in reversion of pre-operative ST depression to normal after surgery, one can predict with considerable likelihood that the ischemia has been improved. Although patients with improved perfusion usually increase their exercise tolerance, the same thing can be said for a fair number of patients who have all of their grafts closed. This may be due to the fact that angina is often abolished after bypass surgery even when there are no patent grafts. Thus, the reason for stopping the exercise test preoperatively may be eliminated post operatively, even though myocardial perfusion does not seem to be improved.

The most reliable predictor of improved perfusion is elimination of ST segment depression or a delay in onset of ST depression so that it comes on at a higher double product (heart rate times blood pressure).

When a post operative patient has been without ST depression or pain for a time and then these changes return during an exercise test, it is a highly reliable indicator of progressive ischemia, either due to graft closure or progression in the native circulation.

Exercise scores and computer analysis

Many ways to manipulate data and make ECG measurements have become relatively easy to do with present computer technology. Also, printouts and calculations become very efficient. Computer measurements may, however, contain errors and methods to check the accuracy must be utilized continually. It is all too easy to accept computer measurements without question. On the other hand, the lack of agreement between several observers in the measurement of ST depression and the failure of experts to agree with themselves upon repeat examination of tracings is well known. Crow [13] tested a commercially available system (Quinton) and found the measurements of ST depression to be accurate within a ±0.1 mm, 79% of the time on repeat analysis. Heart rate and ST slope were also highly repeatable measurements. This type of consistency is far in excess of that possible by visual analysis.

Useful measurements not easily done visually

Not only is it possible to measure ST depression more accurately but the ST slope and the ST integral (area subtended by the ST depression) can be easily and accurately measured and recorded. The slope and integral have been reported to be useful adjuncts in the analysis of exercise tracings [14] but it still remains to be determined if they are superior to ST segment displacement. Other measurements such as R wave amplitude and QT interval can also be done. The problem with these devices is that a large body of data from multiple centers has not been accumulated to evaluate the various programs being implemented. Extravagant claims being made for some of them [15, 16] are not substantiated by other workers. Much work needs to be done in this important area before we can depend on the various manipulations being proposed. A few more years should clear the air in this area.

Conclusion

This paper obviously does not deal with all the problems inherent in exercise testing but is presented to some perspective for those using this valuable method in the clinical setting.

References

1. Diamond GA, Hirsch M, Forrester JS, Staniloff HM, Vas R, Halpern SW, Swan HJC (1981) Application of information theory to clinical diagnostic testing. Circulation 63(4):915–921
2. Stuart RJ, Ellestad MH (1976) Upsloping ST segments in exercise testing: Six-year follow-up of 438 patients and correlation with 248 angiograms. Am J Cardiol 37:19–22
3. Goldschlager N, Selzer A, Cohn K (1976) Treadmill stress tests as indicators of presence and severity of coronary artery disease. Ann Intern Med 85:277
4. Morales-Ballejo H, Greenberg PS, Ellestad MH (1981) The septal Q wave in exercise testing. Am J Cardiol 48:247–251
5. Barlow JB (1985) The 'false-positive' exercise electrocardiogram: Value of time course patterns in assessment of depressed ST segments and inverted T waves. Am Heart J 110(6):1328–1336

6. Case RB, Felix A, Wechter M, Kyriakidis G, Castellana F (1978) Relative effect of CO_2 on canine coronary vascular resistance. Circ Res 42:410
7. Kerber RE, Miller RA, Najjar SM (1975) Myocardial ischemic effects of isometric dynamic and combined exercise in coronary artery disease. Chest 67:388–394
8. Amon KW, Crawford MH, Petra MA, O'Rourke RA (1983) Value of post exercise systolic blood pressure in diagnosing coronary disease. (Abstr) Circ II, 6B:36
9. Zoman LR, Carroll LR (1981) The nitroglycerin exercise test. Cardiology (Suppl 2) 68:169
10. Wu SC, Secchi MB, Radice M, Giagnoi G, Iachero A, Altrona L, Morosini PL, Folli G (1981) Sex differences in the prevalence of ischemic heart disease and in the response to a stress test in a working population. Eur Heart J 2:461–465
11. Theroux P, Waters DD, Halphen C, Debaisieux JC, Mizgala HF (1979) Prognostic value of exercise testing soon after myocardial infarction. N Engl J Med 301:342–345.
12. Ryan TJ, CASS Principal Investigators & Associates (1984) The role of exercise testing in the randomized cohort of CASS (Abstr) Circulation II: 20:78
13. Crow SR, Campbell S (1978) Accurate automatic measurement of ST segment response in the exercise electrocardiogram. Comput Biomed Res 11:243
14. Sheffield LT, Holt JH, Lester FM, Conroy DV, Reeves TJ (1969) On-line analysis of the exercise electrocardiogram. Circulation 40:935
15. Elamin MS, Boyle R, Kardesh MM, Smith DR, Stoker JB, Whitaker W, Manny DA, Linden RJ (1982) Accurate detection of coronary heart disease by new exercise test. Br Heart J 48:311–320
16. Hollenberg M, Budge WR, Wisneski JA, Gertz, EW (1980) Treadmill score quantifies electrocardiographic response to exercise and improves test accuracy and reproducibility. Circulation 61:276–285

3. The current role of exercise testing in the diagnosis and management of patients with cardiac dysrhythmias

THOMAS B. GRABOYS

Cardiovascular Division, Department of Medicine, Brigham; Women's Hospital and the Department of Nutrition, Harvard School of Public Health, Boston, MA, U.S.A.

Key words: exercise testing, arrhythmias

Abstract

The utility of exercise stress testing, both for the evocation and management of cardiac arrhythmias has emerged in the past decade and complements ambulatory electrocardiographic monitoring. Exercise provokes arrhythmia in the normal individual primarily through sympathetic neural and endogenous catecholamine release. Among patients with structural heart disease, particularly ischemic heart disease, changes in cellular automaticity may occur as a function of increasing ischemia, changes in ventricular wall contractility, and metabolic, specifically potassium abnormalities. Precipitation of sustained supraventricular arrhythmias are uncommon (1%) with reentrant supraventricular tachycardia being the most common sustained arrhythmia provoked. The prevalance of ventricular ectopic activity is a function of the population being studied. Thus, while 2–4% of patients free of structural heart disease will exhibit repetitive forms during exercise testing, approximately 75% of individuals undergoing exercise testing for management of malignant ventricular arrhythmia will have such forms of ectopic depolarizations. The utility of exercise testing in the management of patients with malignant ventricular arrhythmia is as an adjunct to ambulatory ECG monitoring. Importantly this procedure defines either drug inefficacy or a 'pro-arrhythmic' effect seen only during exercise, underscoring the need for exercise studies in patients being treated with antiarrhythmic drugs.

Exercise stress testing has been utilized for over five decades in the evaluation of cardiac disorders. However, it has only been in the last decade or so that usefulness of this procedure to disclose dysrhythmias has

V. Hombach, H. H. Hilger and H. L. Kennedy (eds), Electrocardiography and Cardiac Drug Therapy. ISBN 978-94-010-6976-2
© 1989, Kluwer Academic Publishers, Dordrecht –

achieved acceptability. Bourne [1] was one of the first to note the relationship of ventricular premature beats during exercise among individuals with coronary artery disease. However, this relationship was neglected for several decades until more recently when the technique was applied systematically for exposing cardiac arrhythmias [2] and for defining antiarrhythmic drug efficacy [3].

The purpose of this chapter is to present an overview of exercise-induced supraventricular and ventricular arrhythmias, implications for management of patients with and without organic heart disease and how to best utilize the technique among individuals receiving chronic antiarrhythmic therapy.

Pathophysiologic basis of arrhythmia

There are a host of physiologic changes, which occur with exercise, which may serve as triggers for arrhythmia. In the individual free of structural heart disease, an increase in sympathetic neural activity with or without endogenous catecholamine release may enhance cellular automaticity resulting in dysrhythmia. This occurs simultaneously with withdrawal of vagal tone. Circulating catecholamines may also have a direct effect by increasing the rate of spontaneous discharge of normal pacemaker tissue within the atrium, His purkinje area, or ventricular tissue. In addition, increased sympathetic activity promotes flux of calcium from the extracellular to the intracellular space, further increasing so-called triggered automaticity or effecting delayed after potentials [4]. Paradoxically, any increase in heart rate may reduce the frequency of arrhythmia as the result of overdrive suppression. This is frequently encountered in the normal heart when arrhythmia may be completely suppressed at a particular threshold heart rate. However, overdrive suppression does not exclude the presence of underlying coronary atherosclerosis.

With an increase in sympathetic tone, circulating catecholamines, elevated blood pressure and heart rate, there is an increase in myocardial oxygen consumption. In the presence of coronary artery disease, myocardial ischemia may occur as well as a number of secondary metabolic events. These include changes in myocardial pH and electrolyte balance, particularly movement of the potassium to the intracellular space, which may result in increased automaticity and the provocation of, in particular, ventricular arrhythmia [5].

In addition to the direct effects on the ischemic ventricle of catecholamine and electrolyte shifts, there are mechanical effects which may also be arrhythmogenic. Thus, contraction abnormalities occurring with ischemia, changes in ventricular compliance or intramyocardial tension, and elevated ventricular filling pressure may enhance the likelihood of ventricular arrhythmia. These effects may also alter left atrial pressure or left atrial size facilitating the induction of atrial arrhythmia, including atrial fibrillation.

Exercise may provoke changes in intraventricular conduction that occurs during acute ischemia, but may be facilitated during antiarrhythmic therapy, particularly in the setting of left ventricular dysfunction [6].

Prevalance of arrhythmias during exercise

In order to document arrhythmia with exercise some form of continuous on-line recording is necessary [7]. Our experience with trendscription monitoring, which is a continuous recording of all electrical activity during the control, exercise, and recovery period has provided information substantiating the increased yield during this type of monitoring. Thus, there was an eightfold higher yield of repetitive ventricular arrhythmia when trendscription recordings were compared to so-called intermittent sampling that is frequently carried out during exercise stress testing [7].

Supraventricular arrhythmias

It is difficult to assess the actual incidence and frequency of these arrhythmias during exercise. In our experience, among 625 patients undergoing a thousand studies, 17% exhibited atrial premature beats (2). More recently, we assessed the prevalence of sustained supraventricular arrhythmias and found that 29 of the 3000 patients (1%) exhibited either supraventricular (N. 24), atrial fibrillation (N. 4), or atrial flutter (N. 1) (Figure 1).

In general, the significance of exercise-induced supraventricular arrhythmias is minimal. Occasionally individuals who have experienced paroxysms of atrial fibrillation occurring during exercise will reproducibly exhibit this rhythm disturbance. Management thus is facilitated by pretreating the patient with a particular agent, i.e. beta blockers or membrane active antiarrhythmic drug prior to exercise. In our experience supraventricular arrhythmias pose no particular problem during exercise testing and even among individuals with compromised ventricular function, one is more likely to encounter ventricular than supraventricular arrhythmias [8].

22

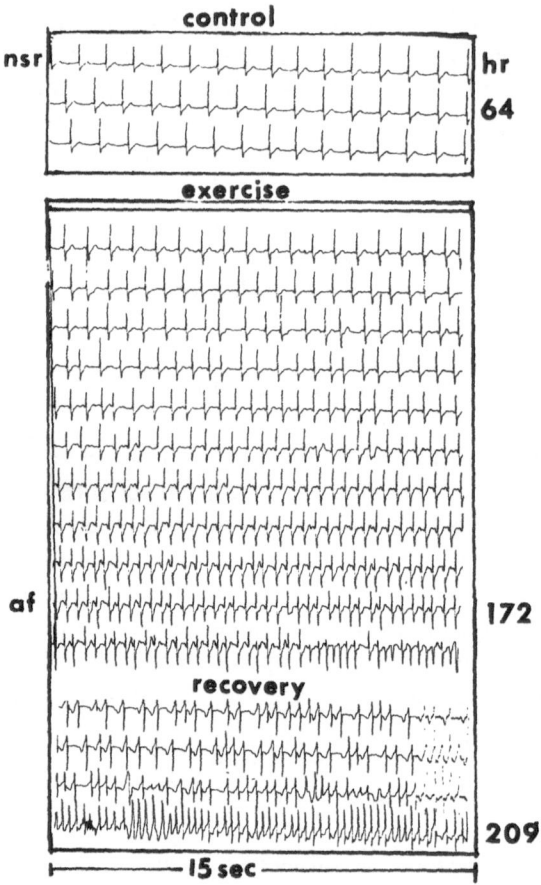

Figure 1. Provocation of atrial fibrillation (af) during Bruce protocol treadmill testing.

Prevalence of ventricular arrhythmias

Ventricular ectopic activity occurring during exercise remains a function of the population of patients studied (Table 1). Among individuals without evidence of structural heart disease, the documentation of simple ventricular premature beats during exercise ranges from 5 to 35%, while among individuals with ischemic heart disease, approximately 65–70% will exhibit some ventricular ectopic activity. Complex forms of VPBs, specifically repetitive forms are documented in approximately 2% of individuals free of structural heart disease while among patients with coronary artery disease, approximately 20% will exhibit repetitive VPBs [9]. Patients who have experienced an episode of sustained malignant

Table 1. Incidence of ventricular arrhythmia during exercise as a function of population studied

	VPBs %	Repetitive forms*
Normal	20	2
Ischemic heart disease	60	20
Malignant ventricular arrhythmia	90	75

* Couplets, salvos of ventricular tachycardia.

ventricular tachyarrhythmia as a subgroup generally have a high density of ventricular ectopic activity. Our experience among some 275 patients referred for management of these arrhythmias indicate that approximately 75% will have complex or repetitive forms [6, 10].

The significance of exercise-induced arrhythmias

Because ventricular premature beats are so common in the general population and the fact that both density and complexity of these forms increase with age, common sense dictates that the sensitivity and the specificity of these events for sudden cardiac death are a function of the population in which they occur. While epidemiologic studies have documented the association of ventricular ectopic activity, particularly repetitive forms with subsequent cardiac demise, the specific augmentation of risk among individuals experiencing exercise-induced ventricular arrhythmia is more difficult to define. Earlier work by Udell and Ellestad [11] demonstrated an increased risk for cardiac mortality among coronary patients exhibiting both exercise-induced ventricular arrhythmia and ST segment depression, ventricular arrhythmia was an independent predictor and further augmented the risk of ischemic changes with exercise. Califf et al. [12] reported on a three-year follow-up among individuals exhibiting exercise-induced arrhythmia, among nearly 1300 nonsurgically treated patients undergoing exercise testing within six weeks of cardiac catheterization, the mortality for patients exhibiting exercise-induced repetitive forms was 25% as compared to 17% for those with simple ventricular premature beats and 10% for individuals without any exercise-induced arrhythmia. Our own experience among individuals experiencing malignant ventricular arrhythmia has been that patients continuing to exhibit repetitive forms during exercise despite suppression of such arrhythmia on ambulatory monitoring continued to be at risk for sudden cardiac death [13].

24

Perhaps the most salient aspect of exercise-induced arrhythmia may be in the patient who is receiving antiarrhythmic therapy. Hence, it has been our practice to carry out control (off-drug) exercise testing prior to initiation of antiarrhythmic therapy and then repeat the study once antiarrhythmic drugs have been initiated. This practice is based on earlier experience indicating that all antiarrhythmic drugs have the potential for aggravating the very arrhythmia we would hope to suppress [14]. One cannot assume that a sustained ventricular dysrhythmia provoked during exercise on an antiarrhythmic drug is a drug failure. If this arrhythmia was not provoked prior to initiation of therapy, changes in ventricular function, intraventricular conduction, the refractory period and cellular automaticity may all be occasioned by antiarrhythmic drugs and exaggerated during exercise, culminating in a so-called pro-arrhythmic effect (Figure 2).

Unfortunately there is no specific profile of the patient, who will experience an aggravation of arrhythmia. That is, the underlying heart disease, electrocardiographic intervals, changes in the QT interval on therapy, and a host of other factors are not helpful in defining propensity

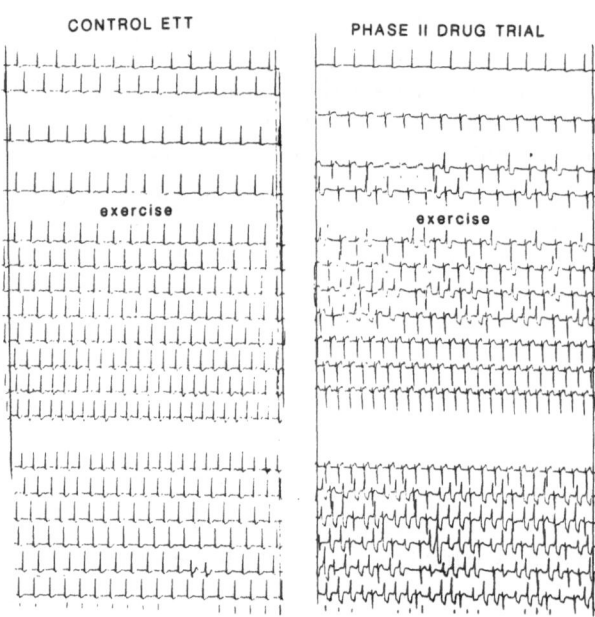

Figure 2. Example of aggravation of ventricular arrhythmia exposed by exercise testing during antiarrhythmic drug trial. Control (off drug) exercise treadmill test (ETT) (left panel) is free of significant arrhythmia. Four days after initiation of flecainide (Phase II Trial), emergence of frequent VPBs and salvos of ventricular tachycardia during exercise and in recovery. Note orthostatic change in QRS axis during drug trial (right panel).

for pro-arrhythmia. The only two features which have proved helpful are firstly the clinical presenting arrhythmia, and secondly the ejection fraction. Thus, patients whose clinical arrhythmia is either sustained ventricular tachycardia or ventricular fibrillation have a nearly three-fold higher risk for drug aggravation than patients whose presenting arrhythmia is non-sustained VT or simple ventricular premature beats. Similarly individuals whose ejection fraction is less than 35% have a two-fold higher risk for drug aggravation than individuals with preserved ventricular function [15].

Safety of maximal exercise testing for exposure of arrhythmia

It is acknowledged that exercise testing is a generally safe procedure for individuals with and without heart disease. We recently evaluated the safety of this procedure among individuals who have presented with so-called malignant ventricular arrhythmia. Thus, among 263 patients who under-went 1377 maximal exercise tests, we encountered a significant dysrhyth-mia complication in 32 of the 1377 tests [6]. Ventricular fibrillation occurred in 9 patients and sustained ventricular tachycardia requiring intervention in 22 patients, and one individual experienced a symptomatic bradycardiac event. No deaths, myocardial infarctions, or significant mor-bidity were recorded. One might expect a higher complication rate among individuals who were presenting with serious or life-threatening arrhythmia. The risk for cardiac arrest during routine exercise test is quite low. Thus, among 3444 patients undergoing 8221 Bruce protocol treadmill tests we encountered 4 episodes of ventricular fibrillation (0.05%).

Conclusions

Exercise-induced arrhythmias are a commonplace occurrence and as a rule are of no particular significance in the general population. The relevance of these events, the subsequent cardiac morbidity or mortality is a function of the population being evaluated. The only absolute indication for treatment of exercise-induced arrhythmia would be among individuals, who are experiencing symptomatic exercise-related events. Even among individuals with ischemic heart disease or a recent myocardial infarction exhibiting complex or repetitive ventricular arrhythmia there is no conclusive evi-dence to date, which documents improved survival with antiarrhythmic therapy. Nonetheless it has been our practice to incorporate this technique as an important adjunct to ambulatory ECG monitoring for the manage-ment of patients deemed in need of chronic antiarrhythmic therapy. If there is little else to be gained by exercise testing of the patient it may be that a potentially life-threatening pro-arrhythmic effect would be divulged.

Acknowledgements

Supported by the Rappaport International Program in Cardiology, Geneva, Switzerland.

References

1. Bourne G (1923) An attempt at the clinical classification of premature ventricular beats. Q J Med 20:219–223
2. Jelinek MV, Lown B (1974) Exercise stress testing for exposure of cardiac arrhythmia. Prog Cardiovasc Dis 26:497–510
3. Grossman LA, Grossman M (1955) Myocardial infarction precipitated by a Master step-test. JAMA 158:179–183
5. Wit AL, Cranfield PF (1976) Triggered activity in cardiac muscle fibers with a Simian mitral valve. Circ Res 38:85–92
5. Podrid PJ, Graboys TB (1984) Exercise stress testing in the management of cardiac rhythm disorders. Med Clinics of North America 68:1139–1152
6. Young D, Lampert S, Graboys TB, Lown B (1984) Safety of maximal exercise testing in patients at high risk for ventricular arrhythmia. Circulation 70:184–190
7. Antman ES, Graboys TB, Lown B (1979) Comparison of continuous to intermittent electrocardiographic monitoring during exercise testing for exposure of cardiac arrhythmias. JAMA 241:2802–2805
8. Graboys TB, Wright RF (1980) Provocation of supraventricular tachycardia during exercise testing. Cardiovasc Rev & Rep 1:57–59
9. Ryan M, Horn HR, Lown B (1975) Comparison of ventricular ectopic activity during 24 hour monitoring and exercise testing in patients with coronary heart disease. N Engl J Med 292:224–229
10. Graboys T, Lampert S, Lown B (1982) Yield of ventricular arrhythmia during exercise testing in patients with prior cardiac arrest (abstract). Circulation 66:11–27
11. Udall JA, Ellestad MJ (1977) Predictive implications of ventricular premature contractions associated with treadmill stress testing. Circulation 56:985–989
12. Califf RM, McKinnis RA, McNeer F, Harrell FE, Lee KL, Pryor DB, Waugh RB, Harris PJ, Rosat RA, Wagner GS (1983) Prognostic value of ventricular arrhythmias associated with treadmill exercise testing in patients studied with cardiac catheterization for suspected ischemic heart disease. J Am Coll Cardiol 12:1060–1067
13. Graboys TB, Lown B, Podrid PJ, DeSilva RA (1982) Long-term survival of patients with malignant ventricular arrhythmia. Am J Cardiol 50:427–433
14. Velebit V, Podrid PJ, Lown B, Cohen B, Graboys TB (1982) Aggravation and provocation of ventricular arrhythmias by antiarrhythmic drugs. Circulation 65:886–894
15. Podrid PJ, Lampert S, Graboys TB, Blatt CB, Lown B: Aggravation of arrhythmia by antiarrhythmic drugs—incidence and predictors of occurrence. Am J Cardiol (in press, 1987)

4. The use of exercise testing in Comprehensive Coronary Care (C.C.C.)

J.J. KELLERMANN, E. BEN-ARI, M. HAYET & E.Z. FISMAN

Hermann Mayer Cardiac Rehabilitation Institute; Joseph and Krystyna Kasierer Center for Preventive Cardiology; Chaim Sheba Medical Center, Sackler School of Medicine, Tel Aviv University, Tel Aviv, Israel

Introduction

For some mysterious reasons, which remain unclear, the rehabilitation of cardiac patients has been considered for decades as equal to physiotherapy and as a kind of psychological intervention. Clinical cardiology has shown an unfounded dogmatic aversion against rehabilitation and it has often been stated that there is a lack of scientific proof to show that cardiac rehabilitation influences longevity and prevents reinfarction. Despite the fact that a number of randomized trials have been undertaken in the past decade, only the so-called historically controlled, but not randomized studies, have demonstrated that there is a decreased mortality in the intervention groups. Randomized studies also had a beneficial effect, at least in the short term (up to 4 years), but it has proven almost impossible to continue these studies for the last few years due to various problems concerning compliance, drop-outs, drop-ins and contaminations [1]. It was also impossible to avoid a number of other biases which would influence the studies outcome and the approach fact that cardiac rehabilitation is identical to comprehensive multifactorial therapeutic approach has been neglected.

In our own experience [2] the intervention groups who were undergoing a physical training program, with different methodology, were also treated by antianginal antiarrhythmic and/or antihypertensive drugs and a major proportion of them underwent C.A.B.G. (See Table 1 and Table 2).

Before elaborating on the use of exercise testing in rehabilitation of cardiac patients we feel it is necessary to explain that cardiac rehabilitation is an integrative part of comprehensive coronary care and that exercise testing procedures cannot be based on a rigid protocol, but must be adapted to the individual needs and to the specific aims of testing together with the clinical and practical validity of a laboratory procedure [3].

There are an enormous number of papers and books, which have been

V. Hombach, H. H. Hilger and H. L. Kennedy (eds), Electrocardiography and Cardiac Drug Therapy. ISBN 978-94-010-6976-2
© 1989, Kluwer Academic Publishers, Dordrecht –

Table 1. Comprehensive coronary care mode of intervention* (percentage)

	Study 1 1981/2 $N = 152$	Study 2 1985/86 $N = 253$
Exercise only	19.3	13.04
Exercise + CABG	3.6	0.4
Exercise + Drugs	69.0	52.9
Exercise + CABG + Drugs	8.1	33.6

* Risk factor modifications included.

Table 2. Comprehensive coronary care drug distribution (percentage)

	Study 1 $N = 152$	Study 2 $N = 232$ – 21 non treated
Beta blockers	51.9	35.3
Calcium antagonists	27.6	35.3
Antiarrhythmics	19.7	17.2
Nitrates	25.6	25.0
Digoxin	3.3	3.0

published during the last two decades, dealing with the importance of exercise testing (E.T.) as a diagnostic technique, especially in the diagnosis of coronary heart disease [4, 5, 6]. We do not want to repeat, once again, what has already been established namely, the indications, contraindications, limitations, i.e. specificity and sensitivity of various testing protocols, intercenter variabilities and problems concerning the patients selection and end-point criteria, [7, 8]. Therefore, we would like to limit our discussion to the indications for E.T. within the framework of C.C.C.

Exercise prescription for work and physical training

Work prescription

For many years we have used a near maximal spiroergometric test for a work and training prescription. To adapt the results of the tests we used the recommendations of Brody [9], namely 'Machines are not usually run at more than 50% of their capacity and a similar safety margin should perhaps be allowed to men and animals, so as to avoid injury and untimely death'.

We have therefore taken the 50% safety margin as a basis for our prescription, e.g. if the highest workload achieved during exercise testing was 100 Watt, representing a caloric expenditure of 7.5 cal/min, we recommended occupations that require 3.5 to maximum 4 cal/min.

We found that the 50% safety load enables full-time occupation without complaints or with insignificant symptoms in almost 90% of patients, who needed prescription for work. It may be argued that a 50% load is too low and that at least some patients could have been involved in occupations requiring higher caloric expenditures. Despite this argument, it was and remains our policy, to maintain a 50% safety margin to prevent death, reinfarction or deterioration of the clinical condition of the patient, that might be linked to occupational activities [10].

Training prescription

1. Patients eligible to undergo a physical training program are assigned to either the patient group with angina pectoris or to the asymptomatic group of patients after myocardial infarction. To achieve maximal patient safety, we have measured the caloric requirements of all exercises in the program [3].

2. In patients with angina pectoris in whom high intensity training is applied, it is of paramount importance to establish the angina pectoris threshold heart rate. Training in these patients is based initially on a 55% threshold workload and later on a 90% heart rate threshold. In this group of patients, work prescription is based entirely on the outcome of two subjective maximal E.T. procedures. The training of these patients requires high intensity in order to achieve a therapeutic effect.

3. We have also recently introduced ergometric arm training, especially for patients with impaired ventricular function (EF less than 40%). As a guideline we use the outcome of spiroergometric testing, with special attention to the achieved VO_2 max/min/kg body weight (see Table 3).

Table 3. Comparison between NYHA classification and spiroergometry testing

NYHA class	Submaximal PWC % of normal*	Caloric expenditure/min	VO_2 max/min ml/kg.b.w.
I	60	5.0–7.5	15–21
II	40–59	3.5–4.5	10–13
III	18–39	2.0–3.00	6–9
IV	0–17	1.5	<6

* As established in healthy individuals of the same sex and age.

Physical training as a placebo

The effect of different training programs on various physiological parameters and the role of a possible placebo effect was investigated in 33 patients after myocardial infarction who suffered from angina pectoris.

During the first 40 weeks, all patients practiced together in a slow rate low intensity training program. Then patients were divided according to the severity of pain during stress testing and daily activities into two groups: (1) those with severe pain ($n = 18$) started intensive (90% of pain threshold heart rate), prolonged (continuous 30 min) ergometric training, and (2) patients ($n = 15$) with lesser complaints who continued with the calisthenics program. The results of the latter group, after 18 months of training, did not reveal a significant change in submaximal heart rate (HR), systolic blood pressure (SBP), O_2 pulse, double or triple product (DP, TP).

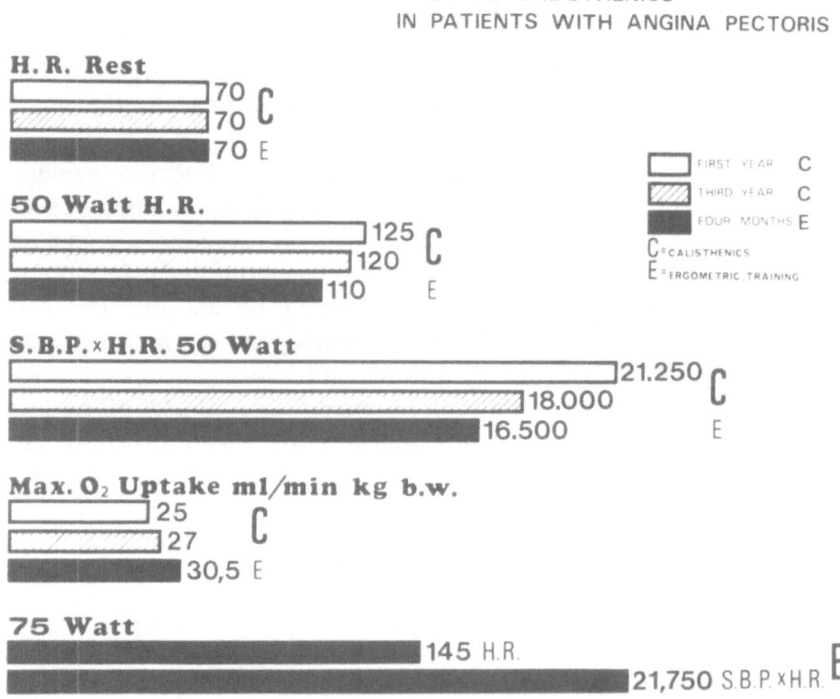

Figure 1. Shows the comparison between calisthenics and leg training in a group of patients with angina pectoris. Both training periods were of 10 months duration. It became clear that leg training is much more effective as can be seen from the heart rate, double product, total performance and maximal O_2 update obtained in both training modalities. The figure is reproduced from Ref. 11 by permission from the publisher and editor of Cardiology.

However, in 20% of the patients a higher pain threshold HR was tolerated and the higher DP reached before the onset of anginal pain.

Ergometric training caused a significant change in all the circulatory parameters mentioned above. In addition, four patients increased their pain threshold of both HR and DR. It is clear that 20% of the patients increased their maximal HR and DP, regardless of exercise intensity. The following conclusions are suggested: (1) Favorable changes in physiological parameters are responsible for the improved work performance. (2) Training intensity plays the most important role in achieving the benefit of the exercise program with anginal patients and (3) Psychological response can be achieved whether or not physiological improvements are demonstrated [11] (see Figure 1).

Comparison of arm and leg training

In another study [12] we compared the cardiocirculatory responses to arm and leg training in patients with angina pectoris. A subjective maximal exercise protocol has been used, the results of which can be seen in Table 4, and showed that:
1. The angina pectoris threshold heart rate (ATHR) of arm exercise is significantly higher than the ATHR of leg exercise.
2. Intensive arm training also effects the central parameters at subjective maximal work levels.
3. Intensive arm training can be considered an effective therapeutic modality in decreasing anginal complaints during exercise.

The findings obtained in this latter study were especially applied in patients with severe coronary artery disease, who also suffer from impaired

Table 4. Comparison of Arm vs. Leg work capacity, ATHR, SBP, DP, and anginal complaints before (T1) and after Leg (T2) and Arm (T3) training

	T1		T2		T3	
	Arm	Leg	Arm	Leg	Arm	Leg
Watts	55 ± 7	$80 \pm 15^*$	55 ± 8	$90 \pm 10^*$	73 ± 15	$90 \pm 14^*$
ATHR	130 ± 12	$117 \pm 10^*$	130 ± 10	$117 \pm 9^*$	135 ± 15	$124 \pm 12^*$
SBP	155 ± 23	$160 \pm 18\dagger$	155 ± 21	$155 \pm 20\dagger$	145 ± 17	$165 \pm 22^*$
RPP	200 ± 30	$195 \pm 21\dagger$	200 ± 25	$181 \pm 15^{**}$	195 ± 20	$207 \pm 32\dagger$
Angina	3	19	3	16	1	5
No angina	16	–	16	3	18	14

* $P = 0.01$; ** $P = 0.05$; † Not significant: $RPP = ATHR \times SBP$.

Table 5. 24 months of arm training in patients with impaired ventricular function

Age	PWC	THR	RPP	EF%
56.2	41.8 ± 14.1	115.2 ± 10.8	176.9 ± 20.4	30.9 ± 8.8
± 6.1	53.3 ± 12.5*	122.7 ± 17.7	223.0 ± 46.4**	36.2 ± 10.2***

* $P < 0.001$; ** $P < 0.01$; *** NS

ventricular function. In order to prove our hypothesis that arm training will further increase the physical capabilities of these severely ill group of patients, we introduced more than two years ago, an intensive ergometric arm training in a group of patients with severe C.A.D. and resting ejection fractions ranging from 13% to 40% [13]. Symptom limited testing was used and the table shows that there is a significant increase in the total work performance and in the target rate pressure product, while the increase in E.F. proved not to be significant (see Table 5). The importance of this study lies in the fact that despite the introduction of systematic physical training in severely diseased patients, no deteriorating effect has been found during the 24 months training period. Furthermore, almost none of the patients complained of anginal pains during repeated E.T. even after a seven months training period [14].

Different training intensities

As a further step we have compared the effects of different leg training intensities on the untrained arm exercise response in angina pectoris. 58 patients with angina pectoris were randomized to either an intensive (at least 85% of the symptom-limited E.T. $n = 28$) or a moderate (70 to 85% of symptom-E.T. exercise $n = 30$) training group. Patients trained for 6 months twice a week for 30 minutes. Results of the 2 groups after training showed (1) similar significant ($p = 0.001$) decreases in heart rate (HR), systolic blood pressure (BP) and HR × BP product for trained legs and untrained arms at matched subanginal workloads and (2) significant ($p = 0.01$ to 0.001) increases in anginal threshold HR and HR × BP for the onset of 1 mm or more ST horizontal depression during testing of trained legs as well as of untrained arms. The improvement in exercise capacity at subanginal workloads results from decreased HR × BP product. In contrast, the significant increase in HR × BP product for the onset of ST-segment displacement and precipitation of anginal pain for both the trained and untrained limbs may imply an increase in myocardial blood flow. Thus, prolonged intensive or moderate training may significantly improve coronary blood flow in selected patients with angina pectoris. Patients with the highest anginal threshold HR and HR × BP product before training showed the most improvement 6 months after training [15].

Prognostic value of exercise testing in patients with angina pectoris

Hayet and Kellermann [16] investigated the prognostic value of angina threshold heart rate (ATHR) in 330 patients with a typical anginal syndrome, who have been treated and followed at our Institute. 330 patients aged 27–65 years, after myocardial infarction with a typical anginal syndrome, under follow-up at our Institute, were included in the present study. All patients were eligible to undergo exercise testing; none had unstable angina, congestive heart failure, a history of ventricular tachycardia or multifocal ventricular ectopic beats or coupled ventricular contractions at rest. A few patients who proved to have chronotropic incompetence or an inappropriate heart rate response were excluded from the study. An examination has been done at least once per year during a 5 year follow-up, and a multistage subjective maximal exercise protocol was used.

Results

330 patients were divided into two groups according to an empiric parameter. Group I consisted of all those whose ATHR was 120 beats/min and above, and group II with ATHR below 120 beats/min. The mean age of group I was 48.3 + 4.8 years and group II was 53.9 + 4.9 years.

Group I with ATHR and above 120 consisted of 189 patients, 51.8% had no change in their ATHR within a 5 year follow-up. 20.6% decreased their ATHR during follow-up. Infarction occurred in 13.2%, coronary bypass surgery was performed in 6.3% and 7.9% died of a cardiac cause.

Group II with ATHR below 120 consisted of 141 patients within a 5-year follow-up, 53.9% had no change in their ATHR, 4.3% decreased their ATHR. Infarction occurred in 5.7%. Coronary bypass surgery was performed in 15.6% and 21.3% died of a cardiac cause.

Comparison of the symptom-limited workloads in 300 of the 330 patients based on a 5-year follow-up showed the following (see Table 6): (a) 83 patients with a mean age of 51 + 3.2 years performed less than 50 Watt of work. During a 5 year follow-up, 47% had an unchanged ATHR. In 3.6% there was a decrease in ATHR, 9.6% suffered myocardial infarction.

34

Table 6. Physical working capacity—symptom limited (5-year prognosis, $n = 300$)

| | Workload, W | | |
	50	50–100	100
Number	83	160	57
Mean age, years	51 ± 3.2	49.7 ± 2.3	49.7 ± 3.4
Unchanged ATHR, %	47.0	53.1	54.3
Decreased ATHR, %	3.6	18.4	19.2
Myocardial infarction, %	9.6	11.8	17.5
Coronary bypass surgery, %	13.3	5.6	–
Cardiac death, %	26.5	10.0	8.8

13.3% underwent coronary bypass surgery and 26.5% died of a cardiac cause (b) 160 patients with a mean age of 49.7 + 3.2 years performed between 50 Watt and 100 Watt of work. The ATHR was unchanged during follow-up in 53.1%. ATHR decreased in 18.4%. 11.8% suffered myocardial infarction, 5.6% underwent coronary bypass surgery and 10% died of a cardiac cause. (c) The group who performed 100 Watt or more consisted of 57 patients with a mean age of 49.7 + 3.4 years. 54.3% had an unchanged ATHR during the 5 year follow up, 19.2% decreased their ATHR, 17.5% suffered myocardial infarction, no patients had coronary bypass surgery and 8.8% died of a cardiac cause.

In order to examine the five year follow-up of patients with angina pectoris who underwent a continuous comprehensive rehabilitation program, a group of 124 patients were compared with 159 outpatients who did not participate in any supervised or advised systematic rehabilitation program. The protocol was based on a symptom limited test and the following results were obtained (see Table 7) [17].

Table 7. Outpatients without rehabilitation and continuous supervised rehabilitation

N	Outpatients without rehabilitation 159	Continuous supervised rehabilitation 124
Unchanged	44.6%	64.5%
Reinfarction	11.3%	7.2%
Surgery	12.6%	11.5%
Died	17.6%	4.8%

Summary

1. The sensitivity, specificity, predictive value and thus the power of exercise test data as a prognostic tool are dependent on a number of variables.
2. There is definite correlation between the ATHR and prognosis, especially mortality.
3. In most of our patients, significant horizontal ST deflections were recorded during or following the appearance of pain, but there was no correlation of the prognostic value of the exercise test, whether the coronary disease was only symptomatic or also signomatic (ST abnormality).
4. A small number of patients with chronotropic incompetence or with a lack of increase of systolic blood pressure during work performance were excluded, but these patients represent a special group with a poor prognosis as a consequence of impaired left ventricular function.
5. The time of appearance of symptoms and the level of exercise performance represent at least the same criteria for the severity of coronary obstruction as the ECG findings alone.

Exercise testing in patients with impaired ventricular function

In discussing the value of exercise testing, the importance of the blood pressure responses to exercise is especially important in patients with established heart disease. In a 21 year follow-up, 67 out of 363 patients died of a cardiac cause. Of these 67 patients, 45% had a flat or hypotensive blood pressure response during exercise testing, while among the survivors this abnormal blood pressure response was observed in 4.3% (Kellermann, unpubl. observations). The last examination of patients who died was done between 3 months and 3 years prior to death. The prognostic importance of a flat blood pressure response has also been observed by others [4]. To examine the hemodynamic consequences of this abnormal blood pressure response, we will describe the results of a study done by Fisman et al. [18] at our Institute.

The significance of exertional hypotension (EH) after submaximal exercise was studied in 13 asymptomatic healthy males. EH was defined as either a drop in systolic blood pressure (SBP) below resting values or a failure to increase SBP at least 10 mm Hg above resting values at the end of a submaximal workload. All patients underwent an echocardiographic assessment of left ventricular function (LVF) at rest and after a supine ergometric test, at the same workload that was performed in the standard upright cycloergometric test. LVF was analyzed before the test and 2–4 min after the completion of exercise. Identical tests were performed in a control group of 11 age-matched healthy individuals with a normal SBP response to exercise. The EH group showed a significantly lower end systolic volume (ESV) and end diastolic volume (EDV) than the control group at rest ($p = 0.01$ and 0.001, respectively). In most EH patients, the ESV increased after exercise, whereas EDV, ejection fraction (EF), fractional shortening (FS), stroke volume (SV) and left ventricular posterior wall excursion (LVPWE) decreased. Interventricular septum excursion (IVSE) increases slightly and cardiac output (CO) and cardiac index (CI) did not significantly change. In the control group, myocardial contractility was enhanced after exercise, with an increase in LVPWE, IVSE, SV, EF, FS, CO and CI. ESV diminished and EDV did not change significantly. We conclude that: (1) immediate postexercise echocardiography is a feasible technique to evaluate left ventricular response to exercise. (2) EH was reproducible, irrespective of positional changes (appearing both in the supine and upright positions) and in our opinion this seems to be of intrinsic myocardial origin. (3) Most parameters examined presented an opposite trend in the EH patients when compared to the control group, showing that EH was associated with an underlying abnormal hemodynamic response to exercise.

We found that in symptom limited exercise testing applied, to patients with severe left ventricular impairment, a 'physiological' cardiocirculatory response to exercise is obtained. In these patients the exercise electrocardiogram does not contribute to the detection of patients with impaired ventricular function [14]. A subgroup of patients who have chronotropic incompetence, a flat or hypotensive systolic blood pressure response and who do not rise their stroke volume even at low to moderate work loads, represent a minority of severely diseased patients. There is a poor correlation between exercise performance and impaired ventricular function.

Exercise stress testing and continuous Holter monitoring [19]

It is generally accepted that one of the major risk factors in patients suffering from C.A.D. are personality traits and environmental emotional stress. In following up our patients for more than two decades it is our experience that routine clinical assessment including E.T., echocardiography, scintigraphy and also Holter monitoring, will enable an early detection of a deterioration and eventually, as a consequence, a timely initiation of therapy. This concept can, in our opinion, be seen as one of the most important objectives of supervised systematic rehabilitation programs. In order to illustrate our observations the following three figures are presented.

As pointed out initially the testing protocol utilized in C.C.C. must be flexible and should be adapted to the individual needs. We have found that the detection of silent ischemia as well as of arrhythmias is significantly higher by using 24 hours of Holter monitoring, when compared to exercise testing. In a group of 75 patients, with C.H.D., a symptom limited exercise testing was performed.

The target heart rate (HR) obtained was $131.9 + 20$ beats/min (b/m). The patients with angina pectoris (A.P.) (38 patients) had a mean exercise HR of 130 b/m and the group without A.P. (36 patients) a mean HR of 138 b/m. (One patient with myocardial infarction by history, was excluded from further assessments). The mean physical work capacity (PWC) for the angina group was 85.8 Watt which represents 68% of the norm of healthy male individuals as standardized at our Institute according to age. The group without A.P. had a mean PWC of 95 Watt which represents 76% of

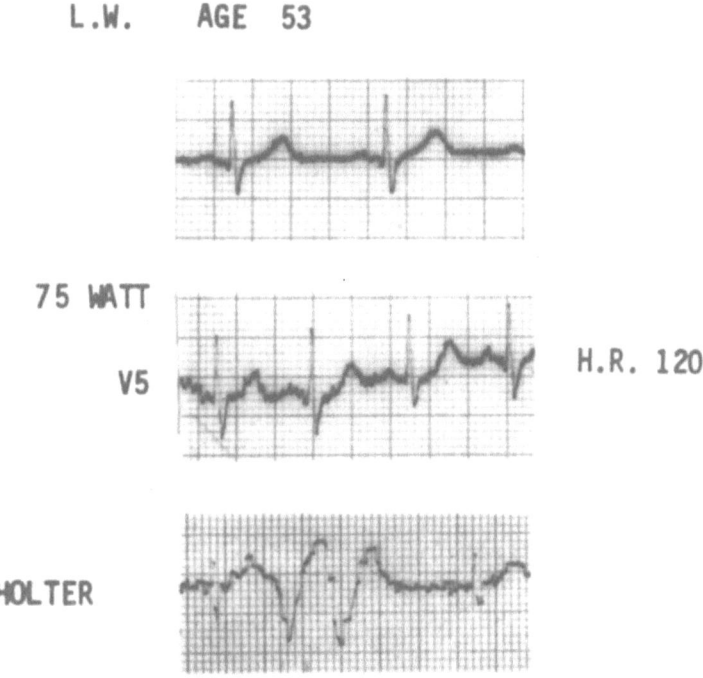

Figure 2. A 53 year old man, past transmural diaphragmatic lateral M.I. with residual angina, at heart rate 120/min (75 Watts) had no ventricular ectopy during exercise, but during driving he developed ventricular ectopy (couplets) some of them quite close to the vulnerable phase.

N.Z.   AGE 38

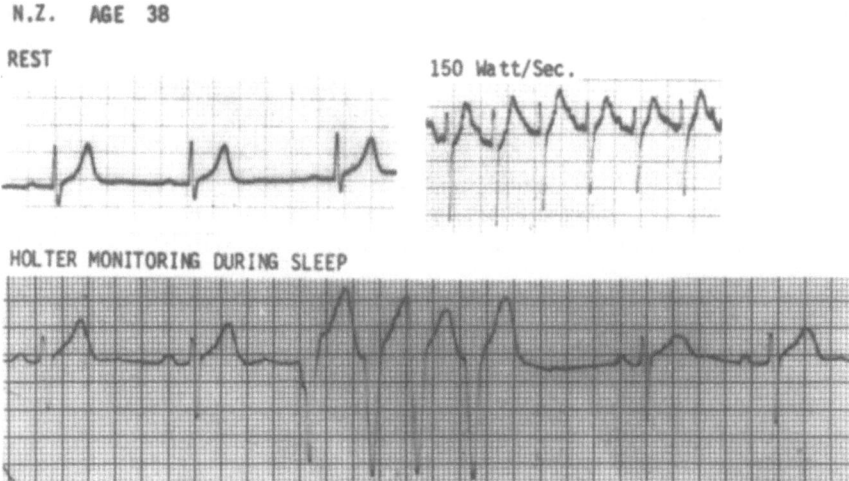

Figure 3. A 38 year old patient after sub endocardial infarction could perform 150 Watt without angina or any other symptoms and without ECG pathology. During sleep (dreaming) he developed V.T. at a rate of about 200/min.

R.A. AGE 44

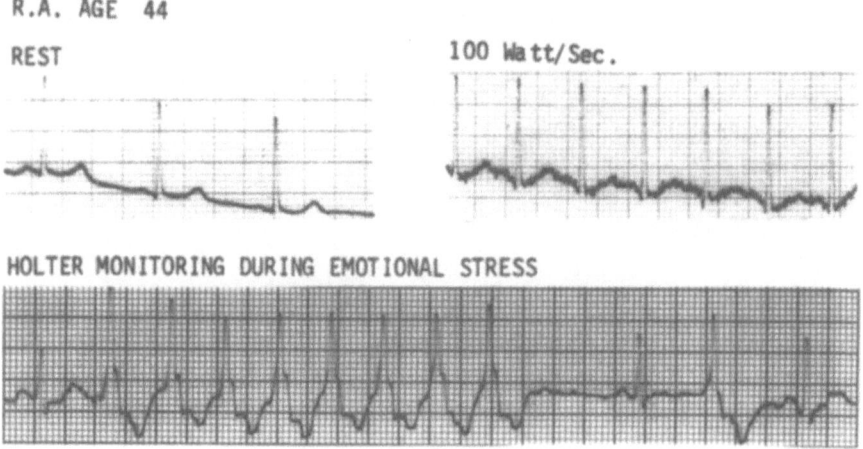

Figure 4. Shows the electrocardiogram at rest and during 100 Watt in a patient without documented C.A.D., but in a high risk group, facing a sudden emotional situation.

the norm. The double product was 21 900 for the angina group and 24 300 for the non-angina group. These results point to the fact that the physical capabilities of both groups were more than satisfactory and demonstrate a fairly high PWC.

Table 8. Ventricular Ectopic Activity

Patients with AP	18.4%	21.1%	
			67.7%
Patients without AP	22.2%	27.7%	

Ventricular Ectopic Activity (VEA)

(i) 18.4% of the angina group and 22.2% without angina experience VEA at rest (recorded in a 3 minutes, 12 leads, resting EKG);

(ii) During exercise, in 21.1% of the patients with A.P. VEA was found whereas in 27.7% of patients without A.P.;

(iii) In 67.7% of the whole group VEA was disclosed during Holter monitoring (see Table 8).

a) In 40 patients recorded during driving, 52.5% developed VEA, while in the same patients only 20% had VEA during ergometry. 27.5% experienced VEA in both situations.

b) In the 29 patients recorded during sex activity, VEA was experienced in 34.5%, while in stress testing it was experienced by 55.1%, in 10.3% VEA was recorded during both situations.

c) In 32 patients recorded during daily work activities, 90.6% developed VEA, while only 9.4% had ventricular premature contractions during stress testing.

d) 22 patients were recorded during leisure time (TV). 86.3% had VEA while watching crime films, only 4.3% of these patients had VEA during stress testing and 9.1% had VEA in both situations, (see Table 9).

e) In a group of 8 patients who had tachycardias and/or tachyarrhythmia, during the majority of daily activities, beta blocking compounds such as Propranolol and Oxyprenolol in relatively low dosage were administered for several weeks.

Table 9. Detection of VEA during stress and Holter recording (percent)

Variable event	N	VEA	VEA during ergometry	VEA during event ergometry
Driving	40	52.5	20.0	27.5
Sex	29	34.5	55.1	10.3
Desk work	32	90.6	9.4	–
Leisure	22	86.3	4.5	9.1

Holter recording was repeated during treatment and a significant decrease in HR and VEA was found. (Because of the smaller number of patients involved statistical assessment was not possible).

In another study we compared exercise testing and Holter monitoring in 93 patients who underwent a continuous supervised physical training program and who were divided into two groups according to symptoms (angina pectoris).

Results

A. *42 patients were asymptomatic with a mean age of 52.9 + 5 years*

1. Submaximal Ergometric Test.
The submaximal H.R. obtained in 42 asymptomatic patients was 135.4 + 26.5 b/m. The mean PWC for the group was 88.2 Watt + 23.77% of the norm of healthy male individuals. The mean target double product was 24 000.

VEA was present during the exercise test in 14.6% but only 9.7% of the patients had VEA also during one of the daily activity events.

2. Heart Rate Holter Recording.
a) During driving under heavy traffic conditions the mean HR was 90.8 + 10.2 b/m.
b) During physical exertion such as calisthenics, walking, climbing stairs, etc. the mean HR was 105.3 + 22.8 b/m.
c) 34 out of the 42 patients were recorded during desk work. The mean HR reached was 85.6 + 24.6 b/m.
d) 26 out of the 42 patients were recorded during leisure time activity, mostly watching TV. The mean HR was 82 + 14.7 b/m.
e) During sleeping the mean HR was 56 + 8.7 b/min.

3. Ventricular Ectopic Activity.
a) 54.0% of the group experienced VEA at rest and in 10.2% VEA was present also at ergometry.
b) During driving 52.9% had VEA and 11.7% had VEA during driving and ergometry.
c) 21.2% had VEA during physical exertion and 6.7% had VEA during both physical exertion and ergometry.
d) 52.9% experienced VEA while working at their office, 8.8% during both, desk work and ergometry.
e) At leisure 46.2% had VEA and 7.7% during leisure and ergometry.
f) VEA was connected with sleeping in 33.3% and 9.5% had VEA during both sleeping and ergometry.

B. *51 patients were symptomatic with a mean age 55.8 + 10.1 years*

1. Symptom Limited Ergometric Testing.
The target HR obtained was 128.6 + 25.3 b/min. The mean PWC for the group was 85 Watt + 25.2, 75% of the norm of healthy male individuals. The mean target double product was 21 000.

   VEA was present during the exercise test in 10.2% and 10.2% of the patients had VEA also during one of the daily activity events.

2. Heart Rate Holter Recordings.
a) During driving under heavy traffic conditions the mean HR was 88.3 + 9.5 b/min.
b) During physical exertion such as calisthenics, walking, climbing stairs, etc. the mean HR was 116.2 + 18.6 b/min.
c) 42 out of the 51 patients were recorded during desk work. The mean HR reached was 84.6% + 24.0 b/min.
d) 26 out of 51 patients were recorded during leisure time activity, mostly watching TV. The mean HR was 78.5 + 11.3 b/min.
e) During sleeping the mean HR was 48.3 + 8.0 b/min.

3. Ventricular Ectopic Activity.

(i)   46.4% of the group experienced VEA at rest and in 3.6% VEA was also present at ergometry.
(ii) During driving 32.6% had VEA and 9.3% had VEA during driving and ergometry.
(iii) 17.3% had VEA during physical exertion and 2.2% had VEA during both physical exertion and ergometry.
(iv) 38.1% experienced VEA while working at their office and 4.8% during both desk work and ergometry.
(v)   At leisure 34.6% had VEA and 11.5% during leisure and ergometry.
(vi) VEA was connected with sleeping in 28.6% and 8.2% had VEA during both sleeping and ergometry (see Table 10).

In conclusion the most important findings of our study indicates that the appearance of VEA was more pronounced during daily life activities when compared to exercise stress testing. Despite a higher target HR during the exercise test, VEA proved to be more frequent at mean heart rates, which were lower than the exercise induced acceleration of heart rate. Another finding was the relatively high appearance of VEA during sleep. In some cases ventricular tachycardia appeared and was probably connected with dreaming. This again would point to the fact that, contrary to former concepts, sleep is a dynamic process connected with arrhythmogenic properties. Finally, we should like to point out that the present study showed a

Table 10. Detection of VEA during stress testing and Holter recording, in symptomatic and asymptomatic coronary patients (percents)

	Asymptomatic				Symptomatic			
Age	52.9 ± 5.3				55.8 + 10.1			
N	42				51			
Watt	88.2 ± 23.0				85.0 ± 25.2			
Variable activity	N	VEA	VEA during event and ergometry	×HR + SD	N	VEA	VEA during event and ergometry	×HR + SD
Rest	25	54.0	10.2	66.7 ± 14.6	28	46.4	3.6	73.7 ± 11.7
Driving	34	52.9	11.7	90.8 ± 10.2	43	32.6	9.3	88.3 ± 9.5
Physical exertion	33	21.2	6.7	105.3 ± 22.8	46	17.3	2.2	116.2 ± 18.6
Sleep	42	33.3	9.5	56.0 ± 8.7	49	28.6	8.2	48.3 ± 8.0
Desk work	34	52.9	8.8	85.6 ± 24.6	42	38.1	4.8	84.6 ± 24.0
Leisure (TV etc)	26	46.2	7.7	82.0 ± 14.7	26	34.6	11.5	78.5 ± 11.3
Ergometry	41	14.6	9.7	135.4 ± 26.5	49	10.2	10.2	128.6 ± 25.3

higher incidence of VEA in the asymptomatic group when compared to symptomatic patients, especially during driving, desk work and leisure time activities.

Further follow up may disclose whether or not our findings are of any prognostic importance especially in regard to the effectiveness of an antiarrhythmic therapy.

The fact that only a small percentage of our examinees had VEA both during ergometry and daily life events may be interpreted as a poor correlation between exercise induced VEA on the one hand, and VEA induced daily routine on the other. Naturally it must be taken into consideration that all of our patients (168) were trained individuals and, therefore, the incidence of VEA during stress testing may have been decreased.

Summary

Exercise stress testing had its limitations and this should be recognised by every investigator who is directly involved with this procedure. It must also be stated that E.T. especially in the framework of C.C.C. should be used for the benefit of the patient and it should not be misused because of dogmatic approaches to certain protocols which are believed to improve specificity and sensitivity.

We have tried to discuss the broad concept of the use of exercise testing in Comprehensive Coronary Care. The most important conclusions are as follows:

1. Exercise testing can be used for vocational counselling and exercise prescription. In our experience, a 50% safety margin is recommended when the outcome of the test is translated into caloric requirements of a full day's occupation.

2. Spiroergometry can also be safely used in patients with heart failure. In our opinion, one of the most important objectives of these tests in patients with impaired ventricular function (NYHA, class III (late) or IV) is to improve quality of survival and to find proper occupational (either professional or therapeutical activities) at a level to avoid severe emotional and physical disability.

3. Our study has demonstrated that ATHR represents a useful and clinically important prognostic sign in patients with symptomatic coronary artery disease. However, repeated exercise testing is often needed to establish the severity and the dynamics of the disease. Naturally this does not exclude the use of exercise echocardiography and radionuclide methods in these patients, especially since left ventricular function has a significant influence on prognosis.

4. Various methods of E.T. and the use of Holter monitoring and telemetry prove to be necessary in order to obtain a broad and as exact as possible clinical follow-up, which in our opinion, represents an imperative part of C.C.C.

5. Exercise testing remains a valuable diagnostic technique despite the introduction of more sophisticated diagnostic procedures. Nonetheless, it is important to understand that exercise test procedures should be applied to properly selected examinees, in whom the test results may eventually contribute to diagnostic management and the assessment of the prognosis.

References

1. Kellermann JJ (1982) Cardiac rehabilitation as a secondary preventive measure—endpoints. In: Kellermann JJ (ed.): Comprehensive Cardiac Rehabilitation. Advances in Cardiology 31:134–137, S. Karger, Basel
2. Kellermann JJ (1985) Cardiac rehabilitation: An integral part of comprehensive coronary care. In: Hofman H (ed.) Primary and Secondary Prevention of Coronary Heart Disease, pp 132–138, Springer Verlag, Berlin, Heidelberg
3. Kellermann JJ, Hayet M, Fisman E (1986) Exercise testing: Intercenter variabilities, prognostic value, work and training prescription. In: Wenger NK, Almeida-Feo D, & Rosenthal J (eds) Rehabilitation of the Cardiac Patient. Advances in Cardiology 33:64–73, S. Karger, Basel
4. Ellestad MH (1986) Stress testing. 3rd edition, F.A. Davis Company, Philadelphia

5. Wenger, NK (1985) (ed.) Exercise and the heart, 2nd edition. Cardiovascular Clinics, F.A. Davis, Philadelphia

6. Wasserman K, Hansen JE, Sue DY, Whipp BJ (1987) Principles of exercise testing and interpretation, Lea and Febiger, Philadelphia

7. Kellermann JJ (1975) Rehabilitation of patients with coronary heart disease. Prog in Cardiovascular Diseases XVII:4: 303–328

8. Myocardial infarction—How to prevent, how to rehabilitate. 2nd edition, Scientific Council on Cardiac Rehabilitation of Cardiac Patients. International Society and Federation of Cardiology, 1983

9. Brody S (1945) Bioenergetics and growth. Reinhold, New York

10. Kellermann JJ, Feldman S, Levy M, Kariv I (1967) Rehabilitation of coronary patients. Journal of Chronic Diseases 20: 815–821

11. Kellermann JJ, Ben-Ari E, Chayet M, Lapidot C, Drory Y, Fisman E (1977) Cardiocirculatory response to different types of training in patients with angina pectoris. Cardiology 62:218–231

12. Ben-Ari E, Kellermann JJ (1983) Comparison of cardiocirculatory responses to intensive arm and leg training in patients with angina pectoris. Heart and Lung 12:4:337–341

13. Kellermann JJ, Ben-Ari E, Shemesh J (1988) Contraindications to physical training in patients with left ventricular impairment. European Heart Journal, Suppl (in press)

14. Kellermann JJ, Ben-Ari E, Fisman E, Hayet M, Drory Y, Haimovitz D (1986) Physical training in patients with ventricular impairment. In: Kellermann JJ and Spodick D (eds) Left Ventricular Dysfunction. Advances in Cardiology 34:131–147. S. Karger, Basel

15. Ben-Ari E, Kellermann JJ, Rothbaum DA, Fisman E, Pines A (1987) Effects of prolonged intensive versus moderate leg training on the untrained arm exercise response in angina pectoris. American Journal of Cardiology 59:231–234

16. Hayet M, Kellermann JJ (1981) The angina pectoris threshold heart rate as a prognostic sign. Cardiology 68, Suppl 2:78–83

17. Hayet M, Kellermann JJ (November 1984) Angina pectoris threshold heart rate in patients with and without rehabilitation. Proceedings II World Congress on Cardiac Rehabilitation, p. 77

18. Fisman EZ, Pines A, Rosenblum Y, Ben-Ari E, Kessler G, Drory Y, Kellermann JJ (1986) Pressure/volume ratio and pressure/volume ratio exercise quotient: an echocardiographic comparative study of left ventricular function indicators. Cardiology 73:354–367

19. Kellermann JJ, Ben-Ari E, Lederman N (1980) Frequency of ventricular ectopic activity recorded during exercise stress test and continuous Holter monitoring. In: Raineri A, Kellermann JJ, Rulli V (eds) Selected Topics in Exercise Cardiology and Rehabilitation. Plenum Publishing Corporation, pp 195–207

PART II: Ambulatory Monitoring

5. Holter ECG and the evaluation of patient's symptoms

H. WEBER, H. SCHMIDINGER, CH. AUINGER, J. WOLFRAM,
T. RIMPFL, G. NORMAN & R. SCHMID
Kardiologische Univ. Klinik, Vienna, Austria

Abstract

Various symptoms can be correlated with ECG alterations (arrhythmias as well as ischemia). A simultaneous ECG registration during a symptomatic period excludes or confirms ECG alterations as cause of the symptoms. Otherwise symptoms can be probably related to arrhythmias or ischemia, if asymptomatic precursors of a specific symptom, e.g. syncope can be found in the ECG record.

The continuous recording of an ECG over a long period (24 hr and more) enhances the chance to correlate symptoms with the ECG.

Prior to Holter monitoring (HM) 63% of the patients (total 2420 HM) had a history of one (59%) or more (41%) symptoms. During one 24 hr HM only 20% developed a typical symptomatic period, 85% patients with a symptomatic history. In 60% (290/480 HM) arrhythmias could be excluded as underlying cause of the symptoms.

Palpitations prior to HM were reported in 17–31% of the patients. During HM about 56% of the symptomatic patients complained of palpitations, whereas in 37–47% arrhythmias could be related to the symptom.

Dizzy spells, presyncopes and syncopes were reported prior to HM in 25–53%, during HM in 56–65% of the symptomatic patients, whereas in 37–47% a morphologic substrate could be found in the Holter-ECG. Therefore in patients with SY precursing arrhythmias should be taken into account, which could be detected in 36–46%. Otherwise 40–54% of patients with SY had completely uneventful HM.

Angina prior to HM occurred in 13% among our patients. During HM 20% developed typical symptoms and ST-depression, whereas 67–80% of ST-alterations were 'silent'.

V. Hombach, H. H. Hilger and H. L. Kennedy (eds), Electrocardiography and Cardiac Drug Therapy. ISBN 978-94-010-6976-2
© 1989. Kluwer Academic Publishers, Dordrecht –

48

Conclusions

In patients with symptoms possibly related to arrhythmias or ischemia HM is the method of choice to go one important step ahead on our way to register an ECG during a symptomatic period—but not more.

Introduction

Symptoms urge a patient to visit his doctor. Various symptoms can be correlated with ECG alterations (arrhythmias as well as ischemia). This simultaneous ECG registration during a symptomatic period excludes or confirms ECG alterations as cause of the symptoms. Otherwise symptoms can be probably related to arrhythmias or ischemia, if asymptomatic precursors of a specific symptom, e.g. syncope, can be found in the ECG record.

The continuous recording of an ECG over a long period (24 hr and more) enhances the chance to correlate symptoms with the ECG. The attempt will be made to review the literature and present own experiences using the Holter method (HM) in symptomatic patients.

Following questions should be answered (Figure 1):

- How many patients undergoing HM are complaining of symptoms prior to and/or only during HM?
- How frequently do symptoms occur during HM and how often do they correlate to a specific substrate?
- How often can arrhythmias or ischemia be detected during HM without symptoms?

HOLTER–TECHNIQUE IN SYMPTOMATIC PATIENTS

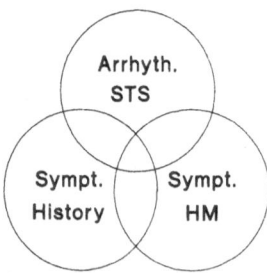

Figure 1. Holter technique in symptomatic patients. Symptoms occur prior to (symptomatic history) and/or during (sympt. HM) Holter Monitoring (HM) without and/or with arrhythmias or ST-segment changes (Arrhyth. STS).

$$\frac{F \times L}{V} = \text{const.}$$

Figure 2. Relation between frequency (F) of a phenomenon (i.e. symptom, arrhythmia, ischemia), it's variability (V) and the ECG recording length (L).

Shortcomings of the Holter technique and the symptoms

Prior to a detailed analysis we have to take into account the limitations of the Holter method. Similar to arrhythmias frequent symptomatic periods (F) have a low variability (V) and can appear easily during a 24-hr Holter period (L), so that symptoms can be clearly correlated with an ECG (Figure 2).

Otherwise infrequent symptoms (F) demonstrate a high spontaneous variability (V) beyond the circadian variability, which will be excluded using records over 24 hours continuously, so that the recording duration has to be enhanced dramatically until the symptom occurs during an ECG-recording (Figure 2).

Another problem is that dealing with 'symptoms' means dealing with 'subjective feeling', two soft parameters, which are felt subjectively different from each individual patient. Therefore we reduced our tasks on characteristic symptoms like palpitation, dizzy spells, presyncopes and syncopes, which can be related to arrhythmias and at last but not at least to angina related to ischemia also detectable in the Holter ECG.

Prevalence of symptoms prior to HM

Patients and methods

Since 1980 each of our patients undergoing HM introduced a database (PDP 11/73), where prospectively 56 different parameters were stored: Patient data, underlying diseases, drug therapy, symptoms prior and during HM, indication for HM, HM-results (heart rates, number of beats, PVCs, SVPB, complex ventricular arrhythmias, artefacts, patient events, etc.). These data were analysed using a UNIX-3 system [1].

The Holter records were analysed using the computer assisted (PDP-11/60) 'Multipass-Scanning' system [2]. Data were collected by analysing

Table 1. Prevalence of symptoms prior to HM.
irreg. HR = heart rate irregularities;
par. tach. = paroxysmal rapid heart beating (tachycardia)

PREVALENCE OF SYMPTOMS
PRIOR HOLTER MONITORING
(N=2420)

SYMPTOM	N	%
Palpitation	1065	44
irreg. HR	699	29
par. tach.	366	15
Dizzy spells	440	18
Syncope	366	15
Angina	193	8
one sympt.	894	59
more sympt.	631	41
total	1525	63

2420 consecutive Holter records in 1688 patients (3/12–88 years old, 1062 male, 626 female) with following diseases: 20% coronary artery disease, 8% dilated cardiomyopathy, 3% HCM, 4% aortic or mitral valve disease, 6% mitral valve prolapse, 4% sick sinus or carotid sinus syndrome, 2% WPW, 7% electrical heart disease, 11% symptoms possibly related to arrhythmias, other diseases 11%. From the remaining patients no more information was available prior to HM.

Results

Prior to Holter monitoring 63% of our patients and 72% in the study of Zeldis [3] complained of symptoms in their history, 59% among them of one and the remaining 41% of more than one symptom (Table 1). 44% reported of palpitations, 29% in the manner of irregular heart beating, and 15% of paroxysmal rapid heart beating (Table 1). 33% complained of dizzy spells and/or syncopes vs 41% in Zeldis' study [3] and 8% vs 19% complained of angina prior to Holter monitoring. In about 50% of these patients with a symptomatic history Zeldis found 'significant arrhythmias' and in 1/3 'major' arrhythmias including frequent PVBs, CPL, ventricular tachycardia etc. [3].

Prevalence of symptoms during HM

78% of the patients were asymptomatic during HM, whereas in 20% typical symptoms occurred while undergoing HM (Table 2). In 60% of the

51

Table 2. Symptoms and arrhythmias during one 24 hour HM.
no symptoms = asymptomatic during HM;
sy +, arrh − = symptoms during HM, but no rhythmogenic substrate;
sy +, arrh + = symptoms during HM could be clearly related to arrhythmias;
no diary = results of a patient's diary were not available

SYMPTOMS AND ARRHYTHMIAS
DURING 24 HR HOLTER

DIARY	N	%
no symptoms	1900	78
sy +, Arrh −	290	12
sy +, Arrh +	190	8
no diary	40	2
total	2420	100

Weber 86

symptomatic patients arrhythmias could be excluded as underlying cause for the symptoms similar to the results of Zeldis [3]. Symptoms could be correlated with arrhythmias in only 8% of the patients demonstrating the 'lack of correlation' between arrhythmias and symptoms but also vice versa [4].

Specific symptoms prior and during HM

'Palpitations'

'Palpitations' were defined by E. Braunwald as the 'unpleasant awareness of the beating of the heart' [5].

If you ask the patient carefully palpitation can be felt frequently either as regular or irregular rapid heart-beating or as 'stumbling' of the heart. So the symptom palpitation could be related to an amount of different arrhythmias! In 17 to 44% palpitation led to a longterm-ECG recording (Table 3) [3, 6]. In 10 to 29% palpitation occurred during Holter recording, whereas in about 2/3 arrhythmias could be excluded and in the remaining patients confirmed as cause for this symptom (Table 3) [3, 6]. The rhythmogenic substrate varied between the different studies (Table 4) and were predominantly related to PVCs, SVPBs and paroxysmal supraventricular tachycardias as expected due to Braunwald's definition of palpitations.

Table 3. Prevalence of palpitations in HM.
HM = Holter monitoring

SYMPTOM: PALPITATION

Study	N	HM (%)		ARRH (%)	
		prior	during	pos.	neg.
ZELDIS 80	518	31	18	37	63
BURCKHARDT 82	950	17	10	36	64
WEBER 86	2420	44	29	48	52

Table 4. Symptom palpitation and the ECG.
SV-TACH = paroxysm. supraventr. tachycardia;
VTACH   = not sustained ventricular tachycardia;
BRADY   = supraventr. brady-arrhythmia;
PVC, CPL = premature ventric. contractions, couplets;
SVPB   = supraventr. premature beats;
NO   = no rhythmogenic substrate

SYMPT. PALPITATION AND ECG

ECG	Study (%)		
	Zeldis 80	Burckhardt 82	Weber 86
SVTACH	9	11	24
VTACH	7	–	–
BRADY	–	–	–
PVC, CPL	35	35	48
SVPB	–	27	3
NO	49	27	25
N	223	165	1065

Table 5. Prevalence of dizziness and syncope in HM

SYMPTOM: DIZZINESS AND SYNCOPE

Study	N	HM (%)		ARRH (%)	
		prior	during	pos.	neg.
ZELDIS 80	518	29	21	22	78
BURCKHARDT 82	950	25	20	41	59
WEBER 86	2420	33	24	46	54

Table 6. Symptom dizziness/syncope and the ECG

SYMPT. DIZZINESS/SYNCOPE AND ECG

ECG	Study (%)		
	Zeldis 80	Burckhardt 82	Weber 86
SVTACH	12	10	15
VTACH	5	–	–
BRADY	–	15	11
PVC, CPL	14	–	20
SVPB	–	–	–
NO	71	75	64
N	158	240	806

Symptoms 'dizziness and syncopes'

25–33% of the patients undergoing a Holter recording are suffering from these symptoms, whereas during HM in 20–24% these symptoms were reported in the patients diaries (Table 5). In 54–78% no arrhythmogenic substrate could be found [3, 6]. In 22–46% of the patients dizziness and syncopes could be related to supraventricular tachycardias, to bradyarrhythmias or to ventricular arrhythmias (Table 6).

Symptom 'syncope'

This sudden unexpected loss of consciousness without a following neurologic deficit is a dangerous situation not only for the patient himself, but also for his environment. 15–21% [3] of the patients undergoing Holter monitoring complained anamnestically of syncopes. In 43–66% significant arrhythmias could be found (Table 7), which were defined as supraventricular tachycardia >130 b.p.m., SB < 50 b.p.m., AV-blocks II–III,

Table 7. HM in patients with syncopes

HM IN PTS. WITH SYNCOPES

	Zeldis 80	Müller 86
HM: 0 (%)	67	44
ARRH.+	43	66
SYMPT.	46	24
SY. + ARRH.	14	12
Addit. Inf.	–	40
total (N)	125	126

54

paroxysm, AFib. or ventricular arrhythmias as frequent PVBs, Cpl etc. [7]. In 36–60% of these patients symptoms occur during Holter recording, but no syncope (Table 7). In only 12–14% these symptomatic but non-syncopal periods can be related to arrhythmias! We concluded that in 40% of our 126 patients we got additional information using the Holter analysis taking other methods into account [7].

The ECG recording during a typical syncopal attack can be expected only by chance in the promille range using one 24 hr Holter record. Among more than 20.000 HM we could capture only one typical Gerbezius–Morgagni–Adams–Stokes attack. It is worth to mention, that our compatriot Gerbezius first observed such an attack in 1717 followed by Morgagni (1761), Adams (1826) and Stokes (1846) [8].

As mentioned above that infrequent symptoms can be captured only by chance, we should increase our chance to register an ECG during a typical syncopal attack by increasing the recording duration beyond 24 hrs (Figure 3).

Johansson was successful in about 50% of his patients with syncopes to achieve a HM during the attack while recording the ECG for mean 7 days continuously [9]. 75% of the patients complained of other symptoms like dizzy spells presyncopes or syncopes after 9 days continuous recording duration (Figure 3) [9].

This enormous prolongation of the recording period increases costs, affects patient's quality of life and prejudices other patients, obtaining a symptom-simultaneous ECG recording in only 50% after mean 7 days! Furthermore it is not surprising, that—despite an amount of different diagnostic tools—in only 50% the underlying mechanism of syncopes can be recognized clearly at present [10]!

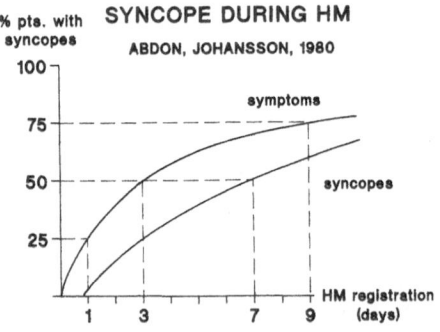

Figure 3. Syncope during Holter Monitoring.

Symptom 'angina'

It can be related to arrhythmias as well as to ischemia. Both can be analysed using the Holter method. Prior to HM only 10–13% of all patients complained of angina, whereas during HM 15–20% are reporting this symptom in their diaries [3 and own results]. In 21–30% angina can be related to arrhythmias (whereas we never know exactly what is the hen and what's the egg!) [3 and own results] and in 46–62% to ischemia [11, 12].

Nevertheless the majority of ischemic attacks are asymptomatic and silent [11–14]!

Alternatives to HM in symptomatic patients

Using the Holter technique we have to be aware of the advantages and disadvantages of this technique and of other alternative techniques to reach our aim of an ECG registration during a symptomatic period [15]. The duration of a symptomatic period can be neglected in the Holter method, if the symptom occurs minimal once during the recording period (normally 24 hrs). If the duration of the symptom exceeds about 20 seconds patient activated event recorders or if the symptoms are lasting for more than about 3 minutes the ECG-Telefone Transmission can be used successfully [15, 16]. If the duration of the symptoms is too short and they occur too infrequently only extensive prolongation of HM—as demonstrated above—or other investigations, e.g. electrophysiologic methods, can be used to increase the success rate predominantly in patients with syncopes [17].

Summary of the results

- 'Symptom' means 'subjective feeling' which includes two imprecise parameters ('subjective' and 'feeling'). To verify or exclude arrhythmias or ischemia as underlying cause of a symptomatic period an ECG record has to be achieved during the symptomatic period.
- This depends on the duration and on the frequency of the symptomatic period.
- HM is a valuable tool in symptomatic patients if:

1. the symptom occurs during HM (frequency) independent from the duration;

SYMPTOMS AND THE HOLTER TECHNIQUE

(N=2420)

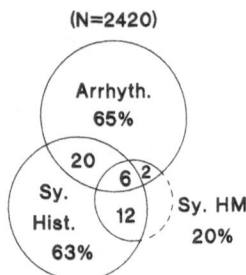

Figure 4. Symptoms and the Holter Technique—Results. sy. hist. = symptomatic history (prior HM); sy HM = symptoms during HM; arrhythm. = arrhythmias detected by HM.

2. 'precursors' of symptoms can be detected during HM (cave: imprecise definition !);
3. ST segment alterations occur in the two recorded leads.

- 2/3 of all patients are complaining of symptoms prior to HM or are symptomatic during HM, but only 20% are suffering from a typical symptomatic period during HM (Figure 4).
- In 8% the symptoms can be related clearly to arrhythmias, whereas in the remaining 12% arrhythmias can be excluded producing the symptoms (Figure 4).
- The discrepancy between those 2/3 of the patients with symptoms prior to HM and only 20% during HM demonstrates one limitation of the method.
- If an ECG can be registered during a symptomatic period no morphologic substrate could be found in about 2/3 of these patients (Figure 4).
- Palpitations, dizzy spells and angina can be more frequently related to a morphologic substrate than dyspone or syncopes.

Conclusion

In symptomatic patients HM is one important step to register an ECG *during* a symptomatic period—*but not more*!!

References

1. Dolotta TA, Olsson SB, Petrucelli AG (1980) UNIX User's Manual, Bell Laboratories
2. Joskowicz G, Balatka H, Glogar D, Weber H, Steinbach K (1979) A high speed digital Holter tape analysis with full editing capability. IEEE Proc Comp Card pp 277–279

3. Zeldis SM, Levine BJ, Michelson EL, Morganroth J (1980) Cardiovascular complaints—correlation with cardiac arrhythmias on 24-hour electrocardiographic monitoring. Chest 78:456–462

4. Clark PJ, Glasser SP, Spoto Jr E (1980) Arrhythmias detected by ambulatory monitoring—lack of correlation with symptoms of dizziness and syncope. Chest 77:722–725

5. Braunwald E (1980) Heart Disease; WB Saunders Comp, p 9

6. Burckhardt D, Luetold BE, Jost MV, Hoffmann A (1982) Holter monitoring in the evaluation of palpitation, dizziness and syncopes, In: Roelandt J, Hugenholtz PG (eds) Long-term ambulatory electrocardiography. Dordrecht: Martinus Nijhoff Publishers, pp 29–39

7. Mueller C, Kiss H, Weber H, Kaindl F (1986) Longterm ECG in patients with syncopes. Z Kardiol 75:730–736

8. Snellen HA (1984) History of cardiology. Rotterdam: Dorher Academic Publications, p 137

9 Johansson BW (1980) Evaluation of alterations of consciousness and palpitations. In: Wenger NK, Mock MB, Rinquist I (eds) Ambulatory electrocardiographic recording. Year Book Med Publ pp 321–330

10. Kapoor WN, Karpf M, Wieand S, Peterson JR, Levey GS (1983) A prospective evaluation and follow-up of patients with syncope. N Eng J Med 109:197–204

11. Stern S, Tzivoni D, Stern Z (1975) Diagnostic accuracy of ambulatory monitoring in ischemic heart disease. Circulation 52:1045–1049

12. Cohn PF (1980) Silent myocardial ischemia in patients with a defective anginal warning system. Am J Cardiol 10:59–69

13. Pepine CJ (1978) Asymptomatic myocardial ischemia during daily activities. Observations in persons with and without coronary heart disease. In: Stern S (ed.) Ambulatory ECG monitoring. Year Book Med Publ, Chicago: p 107

14. Selwyn AP, Fox K, Eves M, Oakley D, Dargie H, Shillingford J (1978) Myocardial ischemia in patients with frequent angina pectoris. Brit Med J 2:1594

15. Weber H, Joskowicz G, Kiss H, Glogar D, Steinbach K, Probst P, Kaindl F (1985) Transtelephonic telemetry of cardiac arrhythmias and pacemaker surveillance. In: Hombach V, Hilger HH (eds) Holter monitoring technique. Stuttgart – New York: Schattauer Verlag, pp 75–84

16. Grodman RS, Capone RS, Most AS (1979) Arrhythmias surveillance by transtelephonic monitoring. Comparison with Holter monitoring in symptomatic ambulatory patients. Am Heart J 98:459

17. Doherty JU, Pembroo-Rogers D, Grogan EW, Falcone RA, Buxton AE, Marchlinski FE, Cassidy DM, Kienzle MG, Almendral JM, Josephson ME (1985) Electrophysiologic evaluation and follow-up characteristics of patients with recurrent unexplained syncope and presyncope. Am J Cardiol 55:703–708

6. Holter ECG and the diagnosis of cardiac arrhythmias

HAROLD L. KENNEDY & ROBERT D. WIENS

The Division of Cardiology, Department of Internal Medicine, St. Louis University School of Medicine, St. Louis, Missouri, U.S.A.

Introduction

Ambulatory (Holter) electrocardiography is a continuously evolving science with regards to both its technology and clinical applications. Ambulatory electrocardiography is most useful when the information obtained is interpreted for the specific population examined, the type of technical examination employed, and the duration of the examination. Thus, to obtain the full clinical value of ambulatory electrocardiography demands that clinicians be aware of these various aspects which affect interpretation of the data. This chapter reviews ambulatory electrocardiography Holter technology, and its clinical application in the diagnostic value of evaluating patient symptoms, the prognostic value of assessing risk, and the evaluation of the efficacy of therapeutic interventions.

Holter technology

Continuous 24 and 48 hour ambulatory electrocardiogram
The continuous 24 or 48 hour ambulatory electrocardiogram is obtained either by a) conventional tape Holter recorder and playback instrumentation systems, or b) real-time analysis microcomputer and report generator technology [1].

Conventional ECG systems. The conventional ambulatory ECG or Holter system is defined as a continuous tape recording of all ambulatory electrocardiographic data for a minimum of 24 or 48 hours and its playback analysis. This technology employs a small, light weight, battery operated electromagnetic tape recorder that records from two bipolar leads either two or three channels of electrocardiographic data on magnetic tape cassette or reel-to-reel. State-of-the-art recorders have patient activated

V. Hombach, H. H. Hilger and H. L. Kennedy (eds), Electrocardiography and Cardiac Drug Therapy. ISBN 978-94-010-6976-2
© 1989, Kluwer Academic Publishers, Dordrecht –

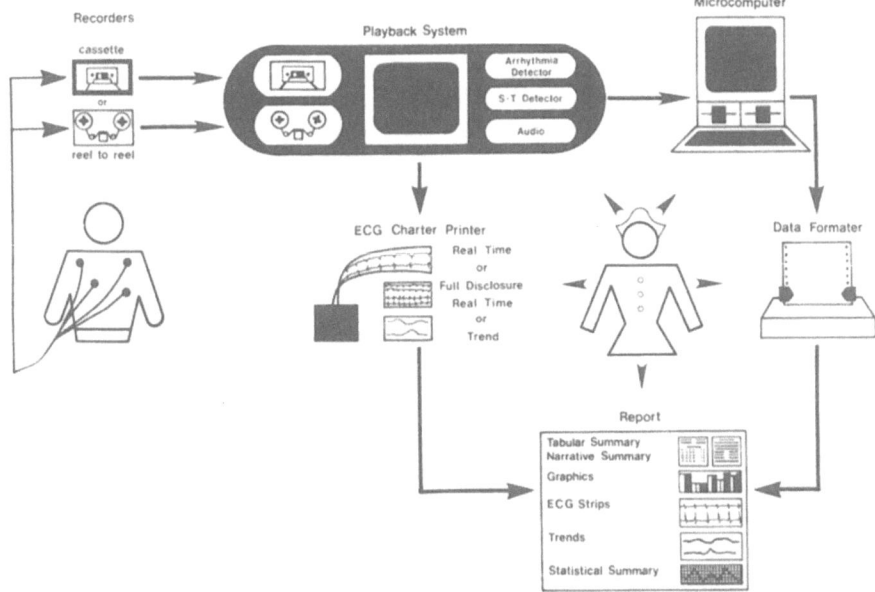

Figure 1. Components of a conventional tape based Holter instrument system.

event markers, encoded time or time markers, and are the size of a small book. The cassettes or reels of magnetic tape are analyzed following patient examination with a playback instrument system that demands operator interaction with regards to an arrhythmia analyzer, ST computer, and audiovisual detection devices. Varying degrees of operator interaction are required to accurately identify and quantitate electrocardiographic data, and to present tabular, trend, and real-time printouts of electrocardiographic phenomena (Figure 1).

Real-time analysis. Real-time analysis instruments consist of a small light weight battery operated microcomputer that analyzes and records the ambulatory electrocardiogram, and a report generator that receives the data from the real-time analysis recorder and permits editing, generation of analog and graphic hard copy results, and data storage and retrieval (Figure 2). This instrumentation typically also evaluates continuous two or three channels of electrocardiographic data from bipolar leads for 24 hours. Some instruments purport to examine continuous ambulatory electrocardiographic data (with battery changes) for extended periods up to five days [1]. This continuous technology examines ambulatory ECG data as it occurs beat-by-beat (i.e. during real-time) to determine a variety of decision analysis diagnoses within the capability of the algorithm of the

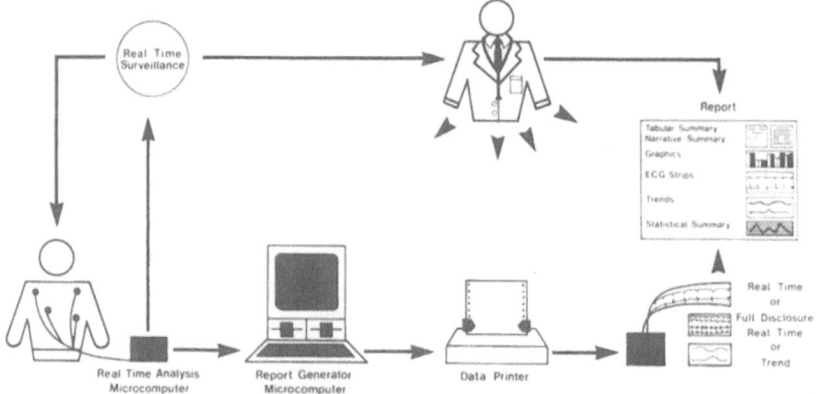

Figure 2. Components of a real-time analysis microcomputer instrument system.

specific microcomputer. Although this technique examines electrocardiographic data in a continuous manner, because of the constraints of data storage techniques in these microcomputers, they can usually only record and document selected electrocardiographic examples. Thus, most real-time analysis instruments store their decision analysis in a computational or summary data format in either solid-state memory or on tape storage, and are forced to present the evidence of that decision analysis with noncontinuous excerpted electrocardiographic examples. More recently, however, innovative data compression techniques have resulted in some systems being capable of storing all 'abbreviated' electrocardiographic complexes which occur during a continuous 24 hour examination [1]. Playback computer techniques fill in these abbreviated waveforms, giving the appearance of stored 'full disclosure' continuous electrocardiographic recording. Whether important electrocardiographic data are lost with these techniques has not been determined yet. Whereas the major advantage of real-time analysis technology is cited to be the preprocessing of electrocardiographic data making it immediately available upon completion of the examination, the major disadvantage of most systems is the absence of continuous storage of all ECG data for subsequent analysis and verification [1].

Intermittent and noncontinuous ambulatory ECG

Noncontinuous ambulatory electrocardiography data of an intermittent nature is recorded by a) pre-programmed sampling devices or b) trans-telephonic devices which are with or without memory capability.

Pre-programmed sampling devices employ intermittent recorders which often can be worn for prolonged periods of time, and are programmed to record ECG samples intermittently at pre-selected times, when heart rates exceed certain limits, or when activated by the patient with an event button. These recordings occur without any ECG analysis and the stored data are commonly retrieved on a standard electrocardiographic instrument for direct physician evaluation. These devices are not widely used because of the known limitations of the detection of cardiac arrhythmias by sampling techniques due to inherent cardiac arrhythmia variability and the inability to correctly characterize patient populations [2, 3]. Moreover, the development of transtelephonic devices seems to be supplanting a necessity for such instrumentation.

Transtelephonic electrocardiographic devices exist as several forms of transtelephonic recorders and transmitters capable of direct transmission of an ECG as an audio signal by telephone (Figure 3). These ECG signals are received at a base station equipped with a demodulator and an electrocardiographic strip chart recorder. The base station may be staffed by a cardiovascular technician or nurse on a 24-hour availability basis, or may at

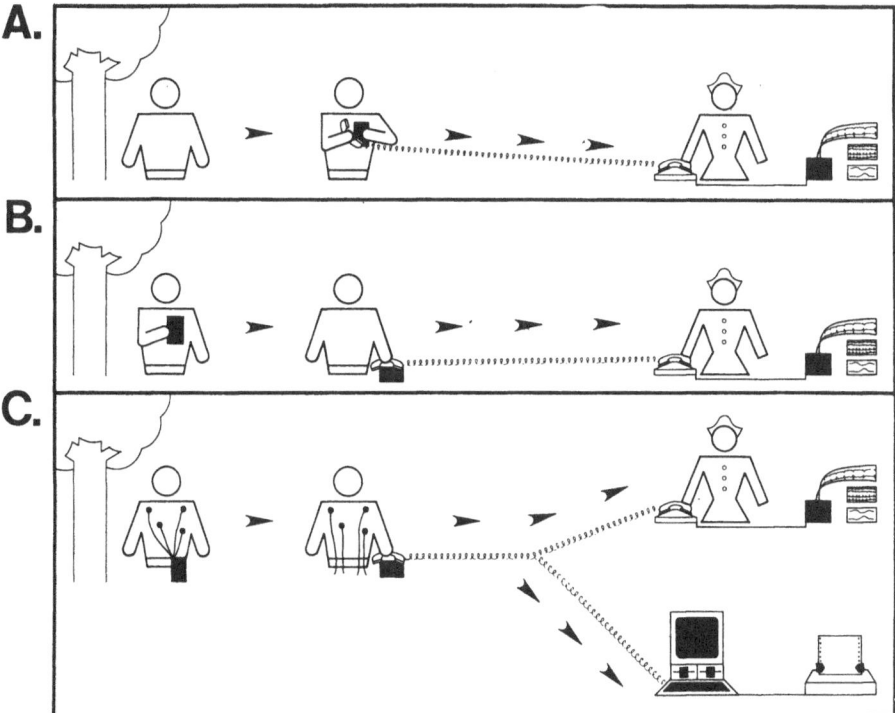

Figure 3. Components of transtelephonic electrocardiographic devices (A). Noncontinuous device without memory (B). Noncontinuous device with memory (C). Continuously applied device with memory transmitting to the base station or automatic microcomputer storage.

times be interfaced to a microcomputer capable of receiving and storing the data for interpretation at a later time (Figure 3). These devices are growing in popularity in the United States and with the recent availability of fiberoptic digital telephone communication lines, now widespread in North America, are technically very acceptable. Although such devices most commonly provide limited noncontinuous sample electrocardiographic data, the type of examination required may necessitate noncontinuous or continuous application of the recording device.

Noncontinuously applied transtelephonic devices without and with memory are small, (cigarette case size) light weight devices that are generally inexpensive. These devices are carried by the patient, and can be applied with temporary contact either directly to the precordial area or with the use of non-gel electrodes be placed in the axilla or on the wrist. One version of the device (without memory) requires immediate access to a telephone to perform transmission of the electrocardiographic data on-line to the base station (Figure 3A). This technology is most widely employed for routine pacemaker follow-up of a limited electrocardiographic sample [4], but may also be used to provide a prolonged (5 or 7 minutes) electrocardiographic sample in specific patient populations under surveillance [5, 6, 7]. Noncontinuously applied transtelephonic devices with memory on the other hand are the same recorders with limited solid state memory (usually 3 minutes), whose major advantage resides in the capability of recording a sample of data without the necessity for immediate access to telephone transmission (Figure 3B). Patients in the latter instance may apply the device to the precordial area and obtain a recording of electrocardiographic data into solid state memory, and at a later time (when telephonic transmission is available) transmit the electrocardiographic data for interpretation. These circumstances facilitate the examination of patients with intermittent or rare symptoms to record electrocardiographic data during such symptoms, although it requires that the patient is not incapacitated during the symptom and has a reasonable amount of physical dexterity to apply the device.

Continuously applied transtelephonic devices are employed to take advantage of a memory loop circuitry through constant examination by continuously applied conventional bipolar electrodes (Figure 3C). More recently, hybrid devices of real-time analysis technology are also used for shorter periods of time (6 or 8 hours) for electrocardiographic surveillance (see below). Patients wearing such a continuously applied transtelephonic device with memory, therefore, can activate the device permitting recording of stored data prior to the event (typically 30 to 60 seconds) as well as observations (30 to 60 seconds) after the event. At a later time, the patient can send the electrocardiographic recording via telephone transmission to the base station for interpretation or it may be automatically stored on microcomputer for later review (Figure 3C). Since such devices continuously have the electrocardiogram in memory prior to activation, they are excellent for documenting transient symptomatic or incapacitating events and the antecedant onset and offset electrocardiographic data. This technology obviates the necessity for rapid manual dexterity such as with applied precordial devices and are more suitable for persons who are physically distraught or incapacitated by their symptoms or have limited manual dexterity.

Surveillance electrocardiography

Surveillance ambulatory ECG employs a) telemetry in a *hospital* or *home* setting, or b) real-time analysis preprocessed data to provide limited or extended examination with transtelephonic accessibility.

Hospital telemetry provides continuous electrocardiographic monitoring within the setting of the coronary care unit or the intermediate care unit and continues to be the mainstay of surveillance monitoring of patients who are seriously ill or have life-threatening cardiac arrhythmic disturbances. More recently, improvement of telemetry systems to accommodate two channels of electrocardiographic data permit analysis of both cardiac arrhythmias and ST segment changes [8]. Abnormal electrocardiographic events can then receive continuous attention from medical staff, and permit immediate intervention if required. Even outside of the setting of the coronary care unit, the technology appears to be cost-effective in patients at moderate risk of life-threatening arrhythmias, and has been found to be valuable in patients with definite or suspected coronary artery disease or previously documented arrhythmias [9, 10, 11].

Home telemetry, a recent introduction, represents an emerging field of ambulatory electrocardiography which seeks to utilize the availability of the resources of the trained hospital medical staff of coronary care and intermediate care settings that are constantly surveying patients. Home telemetry systems employ transtelephonic devices to transmit their data periodically from a transmitter in the home to the receiving base station in the coronary care or intermediate care unit [12, 13]. Such devices permit immediate response (via paramedics or physician interaction) should a life-threatening arrhythmic event occur. Employment of these strategies are currently being directed at specific high-risk stratified patient groups identified early after post myocardial infarction or after recovery from sudden death [6, 7]. These devices would appear also to be of use in intermediate risk patients, in whom therapeutic interventions can be directed if their electrocardiographic status changes during prolonged follow-up.

It requires close cooperation between monitoring cardiovascular technicians or nurses, coronary and intermediate care units, physicans and paramedics. Home monitoring is purported to allow more cost-effective management of many patients, and provide benefits to specific high risk groups [12, 13].

Real-time analysis surveillance is a new emerging application of extended capacity real-time analysis ambulatory ECG and transtelephonic transmission. This technology employs a real-time analysis microcomputer equipped for transtelephonic transmission and allows the preprocessed real-time ambulatory ECG analysis collected for extended periods (several hours up to 24 hours) to be sent to a physician or technician/nurse monitored base station. Obviously, this technology provides a more comprehensive surveillance of all patients in the home setting because of the availability of having continuous electrocardiographic data assessed for either cardiac arrhythmia or ST segment changes over an extended period of time. In addition, such systems are being developed to contain either warning lights or non-alarming audio signals to advise the patient to make transmission of data because of a specific detected cardiac abnormality. Although studies using such technology are not yet reported, the implementation of this technology may allow identification of the increase in density in ventricular arrhythmias said to precede sudden cardiac death [14], or possibly may detect an increasing ischemic burden which may precede an acute ischemic myocardial event.

Special applications

Special applications of ambulatory Holter electrocardiography technology include its use for evaluation of pacemakers, esophogeal, intracavitary, and late-potential electrocardiography.

Pacemaker Holter ECG recorders have been adapted to display one channel of electrocardiographic data, and another dedicated channel of data to augment and display pacemaker signals permitting easier interpretation [15, 16]. The current instrumentation facilitates the interpretation of both single- and dual-chamber pacing devices and permits automatic analysis, although automatic analysis of such recordings with conventional playback instrumentation is confined to only single-chamber pacing devices (VVI, AAI, V00, A00). Although several real-time analysis manufacturers purport to perform pacemaker analysis, these claims to the author's knowledge are unsubstantiated [1].

Esophageal electrocardiography employing either telemetry or ambulatory electrocardiography [17, 18] is feasible with little discomfort using a small bipolar recording pill electrode. Such recordings permit identification of large amplitude atrial electrograms, and are of most value in establishing the supraventricular nature of a specific cardiac arrhythmia. Typically, these esophageal electrocardiograms are combined with either one or two surface leads of long-term electrocardiographic data and provide insight into the mechanisms of a specific cardiac arrhythmia. These methods are said to result in good quality tracings in approximately 70% of patients, and have contributed to the diagnosis of arrhythmia in approximately 40% of patients [18].

Intracavitary ECG recordings have not been widely adapted in America but again have been reported to have adjunctive value in the coronary care setting as obtained by either a floating pacing electrode or balloon monitoring catheter [8]. The electrocardiographic data recorded in such instances is analogous to esophageal recordings in permitting enhancement of the atrial electrogram.

Late potential ambulatory electrocardiography employs conventional continuous ambulatory electrocardiography instrumentation to record and play back into special adapted playback instrumentation on a beat-by-beat basis a high resolution electrocardiogram [19]. Such methods are entirely investigational at this time, and are being examined to see if such electrocardiographic information will permit identification of high risk groups [19].

Holter ECG clinical applications

Clinical applications of ambulatory (Holter) electrocardiography pertain to three general areas: a) its diagnostic value in evaluating patient symptoms, b) its prognostic value in assessing risk in specific patient populations, and c) the evaluation of therapeutic interventions including pharmacologic, pacing and cardioversion, and rehabilitation.

Diagnostic value in evaluating symptoms

Ambulatory electrocardiography is the most widely employed technology to evaluate patient symptoms. Complaints of a) perception of abnormal heart beat that is either brief or sustained, b) suggestive of cerebral ischemia e.g., dizziness, light headedness, 'passing out', or syncope, and c) unpredictable or nonprovokable chest pain and discomfort are frequently investigated by long-term electrocardiography. Whereas clinical experience has shown that cardiac electrocardiographic abnormalities are often associated with such complaints, it is imperative to correlate the simultaneous electrocardiographic rhythm with the occurrence of such symptoms. Ambulatory (Holter) electrocardiography is the most commonly used technology to evaluate such patient symptoms, often for extended periods of monitoring. The type of Holter ECG technology employed depends on the nature of the symptoms (disturbing vs. incapacitating) the frequency and duration of the symptom, and the necessity to observe electrocardiographic data before and after the complaint (onset and offset). Moreover, the electrocardiographic importance of establishing the inherent baseline cardiac arrhythmias present in an individual patient, and the practical medical aspects of patient safety and participation during such monitoring (elderly patients may have difficulty in activating some devices) all determine the ambulatory ECG technology to be used. In most instances, all patients benefit from being examined initially either for 24 or 48 hours with conventional continuous ambulatory electrocardiography to examine their underlying cardiac rhythm and assess background arrhythmias or conduction disturbances that may be present. The symptoms that occur daily can then be readily correlated with the onset and offset of complaints and evaluated for their causal nature. More often than not, such examinations serve to exclude cardiac arrhythmias as a specific cause of a patient's complaint. For less frequently occurring symptoms, transtelephonic monitoring or real-time analysis surveillance systems may be better suited and more cost effective in the examination of an intermittent or sporadic complaint. On the other hand, if symptoms are severe and potentially life-threatening (syncope, presyncope, sustained lightheadedness, etc.), it is probably more appropriate to admit the patient to the hospital for coronary care or intermediate care telemetry monitoring, or to utilize continuous 24 or 48 hour ambulatory Holter ECG examination within the safety of the hospital environment.

Notwithstanding, the available spectrum of Holter technology which is now becoming generally available, it may be appropriate in instances of severe incapacitating symptoms (e.g. syncope) which occur infrequently or unpredictably that intracardiac electrophysiologic studies and exercise testing are used adjunctively with ambulatory electrocardiography techniques [20, 21], particularly when such patients are disclosed by ambulatory electrocardiography to have frequent or repetitive ventricular ectopy, which has been shown to be a predictor of sudden death and mortality in such patients [22].

Many studies have documented the clinical efficacy of ambulatory electrocardiography in the examination of such symptoms [23, 24, 25]. While early studies were comprised of patients with symptoms of palpitation as well as disturbances of consciousness [23, 26], more recent studies have focused on patient symptoms associated with hemodynamic instability, such as dizziness, presyncope and syncope [22, 27]. Approximately 25% to 50% of patients will experience a complaint during a 24-hour ambulatory ECG, and approximately 2% to 15% will have a causal cardiac arrhythmia and 35% will have a complaint without ECG abnormality [22, 26, 27, 28]. In the case of syncope or presyncope, when the recording is extended to three days, half of the patients have symptoms, and if it is extended to 5 to 21 days (mean 9) 75% have symptoms [28].

These data are difficult to interpret precisely because they are comprised of various population groups, examined for various durations of electrocardiographic monitoring, with varying definitions of electrocardiographic abnormalities, which may or may not have sought temporal correlation of the symptom to the electrocardiographic abnormality. Moreover, detected electrocardiographic abnormalities of sinus bradycardias, sinus pauses, supraventricular arrhythmias, and ventricular arrhythmias are known to occur in normal asymptomatic populations. Therefore, the occurrence of such arrhythmias does not necessarily establish a causal mechanism for the disturbance in consciousness.

Recent data of Kapoor [22] focuses on these diagnostic dilemmas and reported the ultimated clinical outcome in such patients. First, demanding temporal correlation between symptoms and electrocardiographic findings will underestimate the prevalence of important arrhythmias and will be demonstrated in only 2% to 3% of patients [22, 27, 29]. Although important benefit of excluding arrhythmias as a causal phenomena during such complaints will be found in 20% to 35% of patients. Second, the criteria for what should be considered a casual arrhythmia are quite arbitrary, and are constantly changing. Whereas many authors have indicated that sinus pauses of 2.0 seconds are usually abnormal, recent data demonstrates that sinus pauses of 3 seconds or longer may not cause symptoms and do not predict adverse prognosis [30, 31]. In the latter instance, only the presence of correlating symptoms with the sinus pause was an indication for intervention. Finally, Kapoor et al. [22] related detected arrythmias to ultimate outcome. This prognostic data showed that patients with frequent and complex ventricular arrhythmias who sustained syncope had a higher incidence of sudden death. Recurrent syncope was not a reliable end-point in defining prognosis. Thus, specific therapeutic intervention perhaps should be directed at patients, who sustain syncope with frequent and repetitive ventricular ectopy regardless of whether or not the ectopy produces symptoms.

Prognostic value in assessing risk

Ambulatory electrocardiography is useful to assess risk associated with cardiac arrhythmias in specific asymptomatic and symptomatic populations. This most commonly is performed with the conventional 24 hour ambulatory ECG recording. Asymptomatic populations include patients with coronary heart disease, especially those post-myocardial infarction; patients with cardiomyopathy, both hypertrophic and dilated, and apparently healthy persons without evidence of cardiac disease. Symptomatic patients presenting with hemodynamically unstable ventricular tachycardia or ventricular fibrillation resulting in sudden death most commonly present with severe cardiac disease and can also be assessed for prognosis with ambulatory electrocardiography.

Coronary heart disease. In post-myocardial infarction patients, the Coronary Drug Project called attention to the prognostic value of frequent and complex ventricular arrhythmias in identifying patients at excess risk of death, including sudden death [32, 33]. This finding was confirmed by others [34, 35] and found to have an excess two-fold risk of death from all causes and three-fold increased risk of sudden death in men with complex forms [35]. On longer 5 year follow-up, age-adjusted risk for sudden coronary death in men with ventricular tachycardiac or early-cycle beats was found to be four to five times greater than men without ventricular arrhythmias (Figure 4) [36]. Although some debate ensued with regards to whether or not ventricular arrhythmias were an independent variable [37], further studies unequivocally demonstrated that ambulatory electrocardiography detected ventricular arrhythmias had independent prognostic risk for frequency and complexity which was additive to increased risk of an adverse outcome associated with decreased left ventricular function [38]. More recently, ambulatory ECG studies of postmyocardial infarction patients have shown that heart rate variability as measured by the standard deviation of the RR intervals in sinus rhythm was a powerful predictor of prognosis, independent of ventricular arrhythmias or left ventricular function [39]. The study suggests that patients with decreased heart rate variability have decreased vagal tone or increased sympathetic tone and may have higher risk of ventricular fibrillation. Decreased heart rate variability has been identified in patients, who sustained sudden death during ambulatory electrocardiography [40].

Cardiomyopathy. Sudden death is not an uncommon event in the natural history of patients with hypertrophic or dilated cardiomyopathy. Ambulatory electrocardiography in patients with hypertrophic cardiomyopathy

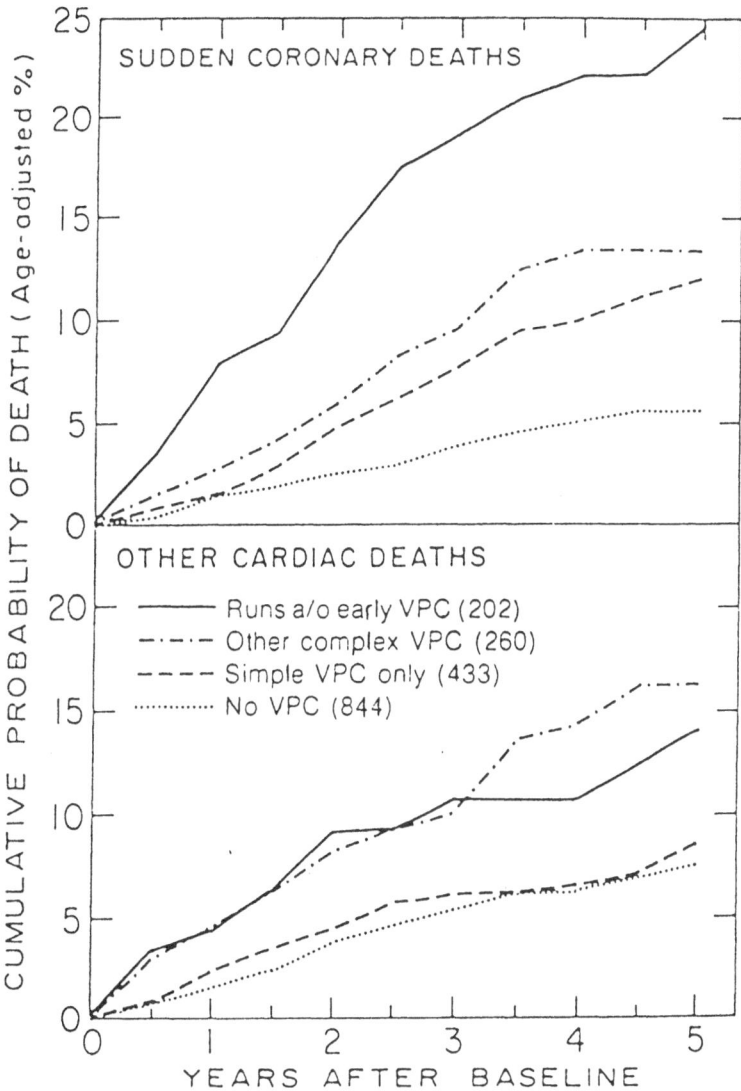

Figure 4. Sudden and nonsudden cardiac death over 5 years in male survivors of myocardial infarction in relation to type of ventricular premature complexes (VPC) during 1 hour of baseline monitoring. Reproduced with permission: Ruberman W et al., Circ 1981; 64:297

discloses that approximately 2/3's of patients have frequent and complex ventricular arrhythmias, and the presence of ventricular tachycardia (found in approximately 25%) predicts those patients with the subsequent occurrence of sudden death [41, 42]. Recent evidence suggests that amiodarone prevents sudden death in this subset of patients by ablating ventricular tachycardias assessed by 48-hour ambulatory electrocardiography [43]. Similarly, in ischemic or non-ischemic dilated cardiomyopathy complex and frequent ventricular arrhythmias are detected by ambulatory ECG in 80% to 90% of patients, and although some investigators have cited they do not predict prognosis [44], prospective follow-up studies have shown that complex repetitive ventricular arrhythmias are an independent predictor of sudden death in representative dilated cardiomyopathy populations [45, 46]. This association appears to be independent of hemodynamic or neuroendocrine variables [46], and sudden death may occur despite a seemingly favorable clinical response to medical therapy [47].

Apparently healthy persons. Ventricular arrhythmias are found in 40 to 75 percent of normal persons as assessed by 24 to 48 hours of continuous ambulatory electrocardiography [48–53]. The incidence and frequency of ventricular ectopy increase with age, and even frequent and complex forms have been found in 1 to 4 percent of the general population [51, 53, 54]. When apparently healthy persons with frequent and complex ventricular ectopy are examined by non-invasive cardiologic evaluation and found to have no overt evidence of myocardial dysfunction or fibrosis, such persons have a favorable long-term prognosis [55]. This good prognosis was even true in the presence of asymptomatic coronary artery disease [55]. Thus, ventricular arrhythmias in apparently healthy persons are not associated with an increased adverse prognosis.

Symptomatic ventricular tachycardia or ventricular fibrillation. An increasing number of patients have been resuscitated from sudden cardiac death or have severe coronary artery disease, which predisposes to recurrent symptomatic ventricular tachycardia. These patients have a high recurrence rate of malignant ventricular arrhythmias when they are untreated or are treated empirically, and a decreased long-term survival [56, 57]. Grayboys et al. [58] has shown that ambulatory electrocardiography assessment of antiarrhythmic therapy, that abolishes repetitive ventricular activity in conjunction with exercise testing, correctly predicted long-term survival in 98 patients, in which this was accomplished for a 2.3% annual mortality rate. In contrast, in 25 patients in whom advanced ventricular arrhythmias could not be controlled, 17 died suddenly and the annual mortality rate was 52.5% [58]. Similar observations have been suggested by Hoffman et al., in patients with chronic coronary artery disease and frequent and complex ventricular ectopy without malignant ventricular arrhythmias [59]. Importantly, continued follow-up of this high risk group of patients by Grayboys showed that when antiarrhythmic drug therapy was discontinued because of adverse drug effect or the necessity to reassess the need for continued drug therapy, 12 of 24 patients (50%) had recurrence of malignant ventricular tachycardia or fibrillation or died suddenly [60]. Continuing follow-up of these patients by the Boston group attests to the consistency of this observation [61]. Thus, ambulatory electrocardiography evaluation of antiarrhythmic therapy in this patient group has predictive value.

Evaluation of therapeutic interventions

Ambulatory electrocardiography has proven valuable for evaluating a variety of therapies used to treat cardiac arrhythmias. Most commonly, evaluation of antiarrhythmic drug therapy, pacemaker function, and patient cardiac status during rehabilitation are the major indications for evaluation.

Antiarrhythmic drug therapy. Conventional 24 or 48 hour continuous ambulatory electrocardiography is most commonly used to assess a patient's baseline cardiac arrhythmias. When serious ventricular arrhythmias are discovered in a patient with underlying organic heart disease, physicians often treat such arrhythmias with antiarrhythmic drugs in the hope of altering an adverse prognosis. This rationale seems logical in view of studies previously discussed (see above), but as of yet, the hypothesis is unsubstantiated. Currently a large scale multicenter, multinational clinical trial (the Cardiac Arrhythmia Suppression Trial) is in progress to establish the merit of this hypothesis. Nevertheless, most physicians ascribe to this medical practice and must be aware of the spontaneous variability of ventricular arrhythmias in populations being treated [62, 63], cognizant of baseline arrhythmia changes over time [64], and careful to guard against the occurrence of proarrhythmic effects [65]. The continuous conventional 24 or 48 hour ambulatory ECG examination is the 'mainstay' of such evaluations and are used in or out-of-hospital to document suppression of asymptomatic arrhythmias. Commonly, suppression of mean freqency of total ventricular ectopy (70 to 90%) and all repetitive forms (runs and couplets) are sought to demonstrate antiarrhythmic efficacy [63]. In addition, transtelephonic monitoring has also been used to evaluate antiarrhythmic therapy [66, 67, 68, 69] and has been extended to provide 'surveillance' of specific high-risk subgroups [7, 70]. It would seem that transtelephonic monitoring combined with real-time analysis surveillance would be especially beneficial in this latter high-risk subgroup. Although studies exist that substantiate the value of transtelephonic monitoring in antiarrhythmic drug assessment programs [66, 67], these trials were not directed at specific high-risk subgroups. Somewhat along these lines Capone [71] showed that 161 post myocardial infarction patients who received patient education and were followed by transtelephonic monitoring in cardiac care unit control intervention (the use of lidocaine IM and prompt dispatchment of an ambulance) sustained a 5.8% cardiac annual mortality vs. 12.9% in 124 control patients receiving the usual medical care. This suggested that the program did not effect the acute incident, but rather the mortality subsequent to it. On the other hand, David et al. [72] could not demonstrate significant differences in a similar program, of 216 treated patients compared to 230 controls. These findings indicate that the discipline of transtelephonic monitoring and perhaps transtelephonic surveillance can be expected in the next few years to be applied to specifically identified high risk subgroups, in which such monitoring will assure that an efficacious antiarrhythmic program has been obtained in the home out-patient setting, and should provide benefits in terms of decreased long-term mortality.

Pacemaker function. It is estimated that about 90% of pacemaker patients are followed by their private physician or pacemaker surveillance service [73]. With the emergence of pacemaker technology in recent years, the need for a dedicated cardiac pacemaker follow-up clinic has become apparent [74]. These pacemaker clinics provide education, major record keeping, safe maximal use of the power source, detection of abnormal pacemaker function, and non-invasive correction of pacing problems (with multiple programmability) [74]. Pacemaker clinics in the past have traditionally utilized history and physical examination, chest x-ray and fluoroscopy, standard electrocardiograms, and oscilloscopic analysis of the pacing artifact stimulus to determine normal function [75]. More recently, digital counters, exercise testing (for rate responsive pacing), transtelephonic surveillance [76], and ambulatory electrocardiography [16, 77, 78, 79] have all proven to be valuable adjunctive assessors of pacemaker function. Because of the limited time of examination provided by the traditional clinic visit, the use of ambulatory electrocardiography has increased the diagnosis of pacemaker malfunction by examining the patient over 24 hours or more during daily activities [16]. Enhanced detection of pacemaker dysfunction by ambulatory electrocardiography has also proven valuable in the early post implant period as compared to in-hospital telemetry monitoring, and has allowed therapeutic intervention prior to discharge [79]. The increased diagnostic yield associated with ambulatory electrocardiography is not simply related to the more prolonged time of examination, but has been facilitated by Holter technology, that permits detection and recognition of the pacing stimulus artifact with amplification, and recording of it on a separate dedicated channel [15]. Thus information concerning failure to capture, failure to sense, failure to output, the number of pacing stimuli, and the percent of beats paced are all provided by the current ambulatory ECG assessment of pacemaker function.

While these methods are currently reliable for single-chamber pace-makers, the technology needs additional refinement for the automatic evaluation of dual-chamber pacemakers. Nevertheless, this latter tech-nology has proven to be a valuable aid in the visual interpretation of electrocardiograms from dual chamber pacemakers [16]. To date, only the conventional continuous Holter recordings have enjoyed success in such applications. Real-time analysis systems have not been substantiated or validated in studies of pacemaker patients to our knowledge [1]. On the other hand, the use of routine transtelephonic transmissions is now a part of the official recommendations of pacemaker follow-up as indicated by the policy conference of the North American Society for Pacing and Elec-trophysiology [80]. Such transtelephonic devices most commonly assess pacemaker rate, but on modern programmable models may allow varying forms of interrogation. It might be anticipated that such studies in the future will address not only pacemaker function, but antiarrhythmic con-trol. The latter is particularly true with the recent application of antitachy-arrhythmia devices which currently constitute only a small fraction of the overall volume of pacemaker implants.

Cardiac status during rehabilitation. The importance of rehabilitation in the ischemic heart disease patient following myocardial infarction or inter-ventional therapy (coronary artery bypass surgery or PTCA) is increasingly recognized and receiving clinical attention. Such rehabilitative measures commonly employ medically supervised exercise sessions, which use in-creasing total body work to increase the efficiency of the heart and peripheral muscle metabolism or improve oxygen delivery to the myocar-dium. Exercise stress testing is most commonly used to determine the patient's initial physical fitness and the progress in such programs. Thereafter, a 'standard prescription' of exercise during supervised group sessions and home exercise is targeted and guided by achieving an exercise intensity indicated by a particular percentage of the individual's maximal attainable heart rate (commonly 70 to 85%) for a particular duration, frequently 20 to 30 minutes [81]. Ambulatory electrocardiography has proven useful in the evaluation and management of such patients, and has employed the form of both telemetry monitoring as well as standard conventional 24 hour Holter recordings [82]. Monitoring during a super-vised exercised session facilitated detection of complex and frequent arr-hythmias, which perhaps require alteration of exercise activities or in-stitution of antiarrhythmic therapy. Moreover, adherence to a target heart rate during such sessions could be more specifically examined, and the patient educated to the necessity of program adherence or the exercise

74

program modified [82]. Certainly, one revealing aspect of such examinations are the insight they provide in evaluating the patient in his home or work environment and for prescribed home exercise. Heart rate, which is highly correlated with exercise intensity, has more recently been assessed in a home-based exercise training program using a real-time analysis microprocessor instrument [83]. These devices are thought to contribute to the high level of adherence to a home-based moderate intensity exercise training program by allowing self-monitoring of exercise intensity and providing immediate feedback regarding the appropriate level of exertion [84].

Conventional ambulatory electrocardiography has proven particularly useful in evaluating the cardiovascular response of patients during sexual activity. Early studies of sexual activity in post myocardial infarction patients have shown that the average duration of coitus ranges from 16 to 19 minutes and is accompanied by an average peak heart rate of 107 to 118 beats per minute with approximately 20% of patients showing serious arrhythmic abnormalities during sexual activity [85, 86]. Although it is commonly held that the cardiac work of coitus is comparable to climbing one flight of stairs (mean heart rate 118 beats per minute) [85], clinical observations of excessive ST segment changes or complex ventricular arrhythmias occurring at modest heart rates during sexual intercourse strongly suggest that other factors (neuroendocrine) are also operative in affecting myocardial oxygen and electrical stability. There have been no reported transtelephonic or surveillence studies in such patients.

References

1. Kennedy HL, Wiens RD (1987) Ambulatory Holter Electrocardiography using real-time analysis. Am J Cardiol 59:1190–1195
2. Ryden L, Waldenstrom A, Holmberg S (1975) The reliability of intermittent ECG sampling in arrhythmia detection. Circulation 52:540–545
3. Winkle RA (1978) Antiarrhythmic drug effect mimicked by spontaneous variability of ventricular ectopy. Circulation 57:1116–1121
4. Furman S, Escher DJW (1975) Telephone pacemaker monitoring. Ann Thorac Surg 20:326–328
5. Antman EM, Ludmer PL, McGowan N, Bosak M, Friedman PL (1986) Transtelephonic electrocardiographic transmission for management of cardiac arrhythmias. Am J Cardiol 58:1021–1024
6. Pratt CM, Slymen DJ, Wierman AM, Francis M, Thornton B, Young JB, English LD, Stone CL, Sarnoff SJ, Roberts R (1987) Asymptomatic telephone ECG transmissions as an outpatient surveillance system of ventricular arrhythmias: Relationship to quantitative ambulatory ECG recordings. Am Heart J 113:1–7
7. Chadda KD, Harrington D, Kushnik H, Bodenheimer MM (1986) The impact of

transtelephonic documentation of arrhythmia on morbidity and mortality rate in sudden death survivors. Am Heart J 112:1159–1165

8. Hasin Y, Freiman I, Gotsman MS (1984) Two-channel ECG monitoring in the coronary care unit. Clin Cardiol 7:102–108

9. Hubner PJB, Goldberg MJ, Lawson CW (1969) Value of routine cardiac monitoring in the management of acute myocardial infarction outside a coronary care unit. Br Med J 1:817–817

10. Rawles JM, Crockett GS (1979) Automation on a general medical ward: monitron system of patient monitoring. Brit Med J 3:707–711

11. Lipskis DJ, Dannehl KN, Silverman ME (1984) Value of radiotelemetry in a community hospital. Am J Cardiol 53:1284–1287

12. Karz AE, Eckel K, Tilkian A, Guzy P, Cocco J, Haber L, Lyons H (1983) Home ECG monitoring of high risk cardiac outpatients. J Am Coll Cardiol 1:598 (abstract)

13. Karz AE, Eckel KJ, Tilkian AG, Guzy PM, Wiener I, Haber LP, Agonafir B, Lyons H (1984) Home ECG monitoring for the recognition and treatment of ventricular tachycardia. Circulation 70 (Supp II):368 (abstract)

14. Lewis BH, Antman EM, Grayboys TB (1983) Detailed analysis of 24 hour ambulatory electrocardiographic recordings during ventricular fibrillation or Torsade de pointes. J Am Coll Cardiol 2:426–436

15. Kelen GJ, Bloomfield DA, Hardage M, Gomes JA, Khan R, Gopalaswamy C, El Sherif N (1980) A clinical evaluation of an improved Holter monitoring technique for artificial pacemaker function. PACE 3:192–197

16. Famularo MA, Kennedy HL (1982) Ambulatory electrocardiography in the assessment of pacemaker function. Am Heart J 104:1086–1094

17. Schuchard GH, Tristani FE (1986) A new use for the esophageal lead: Continuous telemetry monitoring. Am Heart J 111:1007–1009

18. Schnittger I, Rodriques IM, Winkle RA (1986) Esophageal electrocardiography: A new technology revives an old technique. Am J Cardiol 57:604–607

19. Kelen GJ, Henkin R, Restivo M, Zeiler RH, Caref EB, El Sherif N (1986) Signal averaging of high gain Holter EKG recordings—validation of a new technique for detection of after potentials. J Am Coll Cardiol 7:104 (abstract)

20. Boudoulas H, Geleris P, Schaal SF, Leier CV, Lewis RP (1983) Comparison between electrophysiologic studies and ambulatory monitoring in patients with syncope. J Electrocardiol 16:91–96

21. Boudalas H, Schaal SF, Lewis RP, Robinson JL (1979) Superiority of 24-hour outpatient monitoring over multi-stage exercise testing for the evaluation of syncope. J Electrocard 12:103–109

22. Kapoor WN, Cha R, Peterson JR, Wieand HS, Karpf M (1987) Prolonged electrocardiographic monitoring in patients with syncope. Am J Med 82:20–28

23. Lipski J, Cohen L, Espinoza J, Motro M, Dacks, Domoso E (1976) Value of Holter monitoring in assessing cardiac arrhythmias in symptomatic patients. Am J Cardiol 37:102–107

24. Hertzenau H, Yahini JH, Neufeld NH (1979) Holter monitoring in dizziness and syncope. Acta Cardiol (Brux) 34:375–383

25. Goldberg AD, Raftery EB, Cashman PMM (1975) Ambulatory electrocardiographic records in patients with transient cerebral attacks or palpitation. Br Med J 6:569–571

26. Zeldis SM, Levine BJ, Michelson EL, Morganroth J (1980) Cardiovascular complaints. Correlation with cardiac arrhythmias on 24-hour electrocardiographic monitoring. Chest 78:456–462

27. Gibson TC, Heitzman MR (1984) Diagnostic efficacy of 24-hour electrocardiographic monitoring for syncope. Am J Cardiol 53: 1013–1017

76

28. Johansson BW (1981) Evaluation of alteration of consciousness and palpitations. In: Wenger NK, Mock MB, Ringquist I (eds) Ambulatory electrocardiographic recording. Chicago: Year Book Medical Publishers, pp 321–330
29. Clarke JM, Hamer J, Shelton JR, Taylor S, Venning GR (1976) The rhythm of the normal human heart. Lancet 11:508–512
30. Hilgard J, Ezri MD, Denes P (1985) Significance of ventricular pauses of three seconds or more detected on twenty-four hour Holter recordings. Am J Cardiol 55:1005–1008
31. Mazuz M, Friedman HS (1983) Significance of prolonged electrocardiographic pauses in sinoatrial disease: Sick sinus syndrome. Am J Cardiol 52:485–489
32. The Coronary Drug Project Research Group (1973) Prognostic importance of premature beats following myocardial infarction. JAMA 223:1116–1124
33. Kotler MN, Tabatznik B, Mower MM, Tominaga S (1973) Prognostic significance of ventricular ectopic beats with respect to sudden death in the late post-infarction period. Circulation 47:959–966
34. Moss AJ, Davis HT, DeCamilla J, Bayer LW (1979) Ventricular ectopic beats and their relation to sudden and nonsudden cardiac death after myocardial infarction. Circulation 60:998–1003
35. Ruberman W, Weinblatt E, Goldberg JD, Frank CW, Shapiro S (1977) Ventricular premature beats and mortality after myocardial infarction. N Engl J Med 297:750–757
36. Ruberman W, Weinblatt E, Goldberg JD, Frank CW, Chaudhary BS, Shapiro S (1981) Ventricular premature complexes and sudden death after myocardial infarction. Circulation 64:297–305
37. Schultze RA Jr, Straus HW, Pitt B (1977) Sudden death in the year following myocardial infarction. Relation to ventricular premature contractions in the late hospital phase and left ventricular ejection fraction. Am J Med 62:192–199
38. Bigger JT, Fleiss JL, Kleiger R, Miller JP, Rolnitzky LM (1984) The relationships among ventricular arrhythmias, left ventricular dysfunction, and mortality in the 2 years after myocardial infarction. Circulation 69:250–258
39. Kleiger RE, Miller JP, Bigger JT, Moss AJ, and the Multicenter Post-Infarction Research Group (1987) Decreased heart rate variability and its association with increased mortality after acute myocardial infarction. Am J Cardiol 59:256–262
40. Martin GJ, Magid NM, Myers G, Barnett PS, Schaad JW, Weiss JS, Lesch M, Singer DW (1987) Heart rate variability and sudden death secondary to ambulatory electrocardiographic monitoring. Am J Cardiol 60:86–89
41. Maron BJ, Savage DD, Wolfson JK, Epstein SE (1981) Prognostic significance of 24 hour ambulatory electrocardiographic monitoring in patients with hypertrophic cardiomyopathy: a prospective study. Am J Cardiol 48:252–257
42. McKenna WJ, England D, Dio YL, Deanfield JE, Oakley CM, Goodwin JF (1981) Arrhythmia in hypertrophic cardiomyopathy: Influence on prognosis. Br Heart J 46:168–72
43. McKenna WJ, Oakley CM, Krikler DM, Goodwin JR (1985) Improved survival with amiodarone in patients with hypertrophic cardiomyopathy and ventricular tachycardia. Br Heart Jr 53:412–416
44. Huang SK, Messer JV, Denes P (1983) Significance of ventricular tachycardia in idiopathic dilated cardiomyopathy: observations in 35 patients. Am J Cardiol 51:507–512
45. Meinertz T, Hofmann T, Kasper W, Terese N, Bechtold H, Stienen U, Pop T, Leitner ER, Anresen D, Meyer J (1984) Significance of ventricular arrhythmias in idiopathic dilated cardiomyopathy. Am J Cardiol 53:902–907
46. Holmes J, Kubo SH, Cody RJ, Kligfield P (1985) Arrhythmias in ischemic and nonischemic dilated cardiomyopathy: Prediction of mortality by ambulatory electrocardiography. Am J Cardiol 55:146–151

47. Chakkao CS, Gheorghiade M (1985) Ventricular arrhythmias in severe heart failure: Incidence, significance, and effectiveness of antiarrhythmic therapy. Am Heart J 109:497–504

48. Brodsky M, Wu D, Denes P, Kanakis C, Rosen KM (1977) Arrhythmias documented by 24 hour continuous electrocardiographic monitoring in 50 male medical students without apparent heart disease. Am J Cardiol 39:390–395

49. Sobotka PA, Mayer JH, Bauernfeind RA, Kanakis C Jr, Rosen KM (1981) Arrhythmias documented by 24-hour continuous ambulatory electrocardiographic monitoring in young women without apparent heart disease. Am Heart J 101:753–759

50. Raftery EB, Cashman PMM (1976) Long-term recording of the electrocardiogram in a normal population. Postgrad Med J 52:Suppl 7:32–37

51. Bjerregaard P (1982) Premature beats in healthy subjects 40–79 years of age. Eur Heart J 3:493–503

52. Fleg JL, Kennedy HL (1982) Cardiac arrhythmias in a healthy elderly population: detection by 24-hour ambulatory electrocardiography. Chest 81:302–307

53. Kostis JB, McCrone K, Moreyra AE, et al (1981) Premature ventricular complexes in the absence of identifiable heart disease. Circulation 63:1351–1356

54. Kennedy HL, Underhill SJ (1976) Frequent and complex ventricular ectopy in apparently healthy subjects: a clinical study of 25 cases. Am J Cardiol 38:141–148

55. Kennedy HL, Whitlock JA, Sprague MK, Kennedy LJ, Buckingham TA, Goldbert RJ (1985) Long-term follow-up of asymptomatic healthy subjects with frequent and complex ventricular ectopy. N Engl J Med 312:193–197

56. Schaffer WA, Cobb LA (1975) Recurrent ventricular fibrillation and modes of death in survivors of out-of-hospital ventricular fibrillation. N Engl J Med 293:259–262

57. Eisenberg MS, Hallstrom A, Bergner L (1982) Long-term survival after out-of-hospital cardiac arrest. N Engl J Med 306:1340–1343

58. Grayboys TB, Lown B, Podrid PRJ, DeSilva R (1982) Long-term survival of patients with malignant ventricular arrhythmia treated with antiarrhythmic drugs. Am J Cardiol 50:437–443

59. Hoffmann A, Schutz E, White R, Follath F, Burckhardt D (1984) Suppression of high-grade ventricular ectopic activity by antiarrhythmic drug treatment as a market for survival in patients with chronic coronary artery disease. Am Heart J 107:1103–1108

60. Grayboys TB, Almeida EC, Lown B (1986) Recurrence of malignant ventricular arrhythmia after antiarrhythmic drug withdrawal. Am J Cardiol 58:59–62

61. Hohnloser SH, Raeder EA, Podrid PJ, Grayboys TB, Lown B (1987) Predictors of antiarrhythmic drug efficacy in patients with malignant ventricular tachyarrhythmias. Am Heart J 114:1–7

62. Winkle RA (1978) Antiarrhythmic drug effect mimicked by spontaneous variability of ventricular ectopy. Circulation 57:1116–1121

63. Morganroth J, Michelson EL, Horowitz LN, Josephson ME, Pearlman AS, Dunkman WB (1980) Limitations of routine long-term electrocardiographic monitoring to assess ventricular ectopy frequency. Circulation 61:690–695

64. Pratt CM, Delclos G, Wierman Am, Maher SA, Seals AA, Leon CA, Young JB, Quinones MA, Roberts R (1985) The changing baseline of complex ventricular arrhythmias. N Engl J Med 313:1444–1449

65. Velebit V, Podrid P, Lown B, Cohen BH, Grayboys TB (1982) Aggravation and provocation of ventricular arrhythmias by antiarrhythmic drugs. Circulation 65:886–894

66. Hasin Y, David D, Rogel S (1976) Diagnostic and therapeutic assessment by telephone electrocardiographic monitoring of ambulatory patients. Br Med J 2:609–612

67. Pritchett ELC, Zimmerman JM, Hammill K, Reiter MJ, Hammill SC (1982) Electrocardiogram recording by telephone in antiarrhythmic drug trials. Chest 81:473–476

68. Antman EM, Ludmer PL, McGowan N, Bosak M, Friedman PL (1986) Transtelephonic electrocardiographic transmission for management of cardiac arrhythmias. Am J Cardiol 58:1021–1024

69. Shen WK, Holmes DR, Hammill SC (1987) Transtelephonic monitoring: Documentation of transient cardiac rhythm disturbances. Mayo Clin Proc 62:109–112

70. Pratt CM, Slymen DJ, Wierman AM, Francis M, Thornton B, Young JB, English LD, Stone CL, Sarnoff SJ, Roberts R (1987) Asymptomatic telephone ECG transmissions as an outpatient surveillance system of ventricular arrhythmias: Relationship to quantitative ambulatory ECG recordings. Am Heart J 113:1–7

71. Capone RJ, Visco J, Curwen E, Van Every S (1984) The effect of early prehospital transtelephonic coronary intervention on morbidity and mortality: Experience with 284 post-myocardial infarction patients in a pilot program. Am Heart J 107:1153–1160

72. David D, Kaplinsky E (1985) The role of outpatient transtelephonic monitoring and self-medication following acute myocardial infarction. In: Califf GM, Wagner GS, (eds): Acute coronary care: principles and practice. Boston, Martinus Nijhoff Publishing, Ch 56, pp 531–536

73. Parsonnet V, Bernstein AD (1986) Pacing in perspective: concepts and controversies. Circulation 73:1087–1093

74. Griffin JC, Schuenemeyer TD (1984) Current concepts in pacemaker follow-up. Intell Report in Cardiac Pacing and Electrophysiologic 2:1–5

75. Griffin JC, Schuenemeyer TD (1983) Pacemaker follow-up: An introduction and overview. Clin Progr Pacing Electrophysiol 1:30

76. Dreifus LS, Zinberg A, Hurzeler P, Puziak AD, Pennock R, Feldman M, Morse DP (1986) Transtelephonic monitoring of 25,919 implanted pacemakers. PACE 9:371–378,

77. Breivik K, Ohm OJ (1980) Myopotential inhibition of unipolar QRS inhibited (VVI) pacemakers, assessed by ambulatory Holter monitoring of the electrocardiogram. PACE 3:470–478

78. Jacobs LJ, Kerzner JS, Diamond MA, Berlin HF, Sprung CL (1982) Pacemaker inhibition by myopotentials detected by Holter monitoring. PACE 5:30–33

79. Janosik DL, Redd RM, Buckingham TA, Blum RI, Wiens RD, Kennedy HL. The utility of ambulatory electrocardiography in detecting pacemaker dysfunction in the early post-implant period. Am J Cardiol (in press)

80. Levine PA, Belott PH, Bilitch M, Boal B, Escher DJW, Furman S, Griffin JC, Hauser RG, Maloney JD, Morse D, Semler HJ (1983) Recommendations of the NASPE Policy Conference on Pacemaker Programmability and Follow-up. PACE 6:1222–1223

81. Sheuer J, Greenberg MA, Zohman LR (1978) Exercise training in patients with coronary artery disease. Mod Concepts Cardiovasc Dis 47:85–90

82. Fletcher GF, Cantwell JD (1977) Continuous ambulatory electrocardiographic monitoring. Use in cardiac exercise programs. Chest 71:27–32

83. Mueller JK, Gossard D, Adams FR, Taylor CB, Haskell WL, Kraemer HC, Ahn DK, Burnett K, DeBusk RF (1986) Assessment of prescribed increases in physical activity: Application of a new method for microprocessor analysis of heart rate. Am J Cardiol 57:441–445

84. Rogers F, Juneau M, Taylor CB, Haskell WL, Kraemer HC, Ahn DK, Debusk RF (1987) Assessment by a microprocessor of adherence to home-based moderate-intensity exercise training in healthy, sedentary middle-aged men and women. Am J Cardiol 60:71–75

85. Hellerstein HK, Friedman EH (1970) Sexual activity and the post-coronary patient. Arch Intern Med 125:987–999

86. Johnston BL, Fletcher GF (1979) Dynamic electrocardiographic recording during sexual activity in recent post-myocardial infarction and revascularization patients. Am Heart J 98:736–741

7. Silent myocardial ischemia on ambulatory Holter monitoring and exercise testing: detection, characteristics and significance

SHLOMO STERN & DAN TZIVONI

The Heiden Department of Cardiology, Bikur Cholim Hospital and The Hebrew University-Hadassah Medical School, Jerusalem, Israel

Introduction

The pioneer of ambulatory long-term monitoring of the electrocardiogram Norman J. Holter [1] described already in his first publication in 1961 ischemic changes during daily activities. A few years later, Norland and Semler [2] and Corday and coworkers [3] stressed that not only arrhythmias but also angina pectoris can be documented by telemetry. In spite of this, for almost 10 years no further advance was made in this field, mainly due to the caution advocated in 1967 by Hinkle [4] concerning the poor low-frequency response of the recorders available at that time. However, improvements and modifications made by manufacturers led to an adequate low-frequency response in the newer tape recorders [5]. Since then many investigators started to use the Holter tapes to study the frequency of ischemic episodes under dynamic conditions.

In 1974 [6] we described the presence of frequent transient ST depressions during daily activities in 50 patients; many of these episodes were not accompanied by pain. This investigation seems to be the first published description of silent ischemic episodes. In 1975 we proved that patients who had ST depression on ambulatory ECG monitoring had arteriographic evidence of coronary disease [7]. In 1975 Allen and Gettes [8] called attention to the frequent lack of pain during myocardial ischemia and in 1977 Schang and Pepine [9] confirmed the presence of silent ST depression on Holter monitoring during daily activities. These authors pointed out that the ischemic episodes during everyday activities may appear without any physical stress and very frequently at heart rates lower than those observed during anginal attacks during treadmill testing.

V. Hombach, H. H. Hilger and H. L. Kennedy (eds), Electrocardiography and Cardiac Drug Therapy. ISBN 978-94-010-6976-2
© 1989, Kluwer Academic Publishers, Dordrecht –

Hemodynamic and metabolic proof of the ischemic nature of the silent episodes

Significant hemodynamic alterations during transient ST depressions, silent or symptomatic, such as an increase in left ventricular end-diastolic pressure were described during atrial pacing [10], or during spontaneous angina [11]. In the coronary care unit Maseri et al. [12, 13] showed that silent ST deviations were accompanied by an increase in left ventricular end-diastolic or pulmonary artery pressures or a decrease in dp/dt or both, changes similar to those observed during painful episodes. A concurrent reduction of coronary sinus oxygen saturation during episodes of silent ST-T changes compatible with acute transient myocardial ischemia was also demonstrated by the same investigators [14]. Deanfield and co-workers [15] used rubidium-82 positron tomography to document that the same regional myocardial perfusion defects were present during positive exercise and cold pressor tests, as well as during unprovoked silent ST depressions. Cohn and coworkers [16] examined purely asymptomatic patients by exercise radionuclide ventriculography, and found a decrease in regional wall-motion during silent ST depression. Thus, there is ample and convincing evidence now that the ST segment alterations during daily activities, even without symptoms, indicate myocardial ischemia.

Deanfield and coworkers [17] showed that not only physical but also mental stress can induce myocardial ischemia. These authors studied 16 patients with angina pectoris by Holter monitoring and by Rubidium 82 tomography. Twelve (75%) of them developed ischemic changes during mental stress (arithemetic testing). In 8, this was not accompanied by chest pain. During exercise testing the patients developed ischemic changes that were of similar severity to those observed during mental stress, however, during physical stress, 15 patients developed chest pain as compared to only 4 during mental stress.

Silent ischemia on Holter monitoring and on treadmill testing

In 1985 we reported 144 patients [18] who underwent a Bruce protocol treadmill exercise test during which electrocardiograms were recorded simultaneously both with a 2-channel Holter recorder with bipolar V_3 and V_5-like leads and with a conventional 12-lead system. Sixty-eight patients had no ST depression on either the Holter or on the 12-lead ECG during the exercise test, whereas in 70 patients ischemic changes were recorded by both methods; thus, in 138 of the 144 patients (96%), the results of the 2 tests were concordant. The heart rate at which ischemic changes were first noted and the maximal ST depression observed, were similar on both recording systems. The Holter system identified 6 of the 7 patients whose ischemic changes were confined to the inferior wall on the 12-lead ECG. The addition of the V_3 lead as a second ischemic lead increased the ischemia detection by 10%. Thus, the 2-channel Holter recording system with bipolar V_3 and V_5-like leads was as accurate as the 12-lead system in detecting ischemic changes during exercise and proved that ambulatory monitoring system can reliably reproduce ST segment. Both Selwyn et al. [19], and Pepine and coworkers [20] performed similar studies on smaller groups of patients and found that both AM and FM systems reproduced the ST segment accurately, and also that there is no need for extended low frequency range (such as found in FM system) for accurate reproduction of ST segment shifts.

The myocardial ischemia precipitated during exercise testing in patients with known ischemic heart disease, was found to be silent in 29% of 302 patients in the study of Weiner and coworkers [21]. The prevelance of multivessel disease was similar in the subgroup with silent myocardial ischemia compared with the patients who developed angina during the exercise testing. The prognostic implication of silent ischemia during exercise testing in patients with ischemic heart disease was studied by Bonow et al. [22] who evaluated the exercise test data of 117 patients who were either asymptomatic or mildly symptomatic and found that the 4-year survival of patients with ischemic ST segment depression during exercise testing was 92%. In a similar group of patients from the CASS Registry [23] the 5 year survival rate of patients with ischemic ST depression was 85%. In both studies the presence of "asymptomatic" ST segment depression during exercise testing placed the patient with established coronary artery disease at a higher risk.

Cecchi and coworkers [24] found that patients who had silent ischemia on treadmill, had higher frequency of silent ischemia also on Holter monitoring during daily activities. Campbell and coworkers [25] assessed the exercise test parameter, which can predict the presence of ischemic changes during daily activities. They studied 32 patients with documented coronary artery disease, who had a positive treadmill stress test; two-thirds of them had ischemic episodes also during daily activities. In patients who, during exercise testing developed ischemic changes before six minutes or at heart rate below 150 beats/min, and in those whose ST depression persisted for more than 5 minutes after the exercise, the spontaneous ischemic episodes were more numerous and the total duration of transient ischemia per 24 hour was longer. They found no relationship between out-of-hospital transient ischemia and other treadmill variables such as the presence of chest pain, total exercise duration, maximal heart rate, maximal blood pressure or double product.

We [26] performed Holter monitoring during daily activities and a treadmill testing in 210 patients. The results indicated that Holter monitoring during daily activity disclosed pathologic ST-segment depression less frequently than treadmill testing, as only 77% of those who had ST depression during the provocation of the treadmill exercise had similar changes on the same day during their usual activities. It could be confirmed in these patients that the mechanism responsible for ischemic changes during daily activities is different from the mechanism of ischemia during stress, as the heart rate at which these changes were noted during daily activity was significantly lower (94 beats/min) than the heart rate at which such changes were observed during stress test (109 beats/min).

On the basis of these results, we suggested that if the primary goal of the clinician is to diagnose the presence or absence or ischemic heart disease, ambulatory Holter monitoring is not an alternative to stress testing. However, in patients with strongly suspected or proven coronary disease judging the severity and activity of the disease only by the presence of chest pain may underestimate the true extent and activity of the disease and important additional information can be gained from this ambulatory Holter monitoring.

The characteristics of silent ischemic episodes

The characteristics of silent vs. symptomatic ischemic episodes during daily activities was studied in 191 patients [27]. All patients had transient ST depression on 24-hour ambulatory Holter monitoring and positive treadmill tests; 116 of the patients had coronary arteriograms. Monitoring detected 424 silent (72.3%) and 163 symptomatic (27.7%) episodes. There were no statistically significant differences between the silent and the symptomatic episodes as to the mean duration of an episode (15.1 vs 14.3 min, respectively), heart rate at onset of ST depression (93 vs. 96 beat/min, respectively), heart rate at the time of maximal ST depression (114 beat/min for both) and mean maximal ST depression (1.9 vs. 2.0 mm, respectively).

One hundred and four patients had only silent, 33 only symptomatic and 54 had both types of episodes ("mixed"). Patients with silent, symptomatic and mixed episodes, had similar extent of angiographically documented coronary disease. However, mixed patients had significantly more ischemic episodes/day (4.8) than silents (2.6) or symptomatics (1.9); $p < 0.001$ for both, and a longer total period of ischemia/day (60 min), than silents (36 min) or symptomatics (28 min); $p < 0.001$ for both. Ninety-seven patients had a previous myocardial infarction and the characteristics of their silent and symptomatic episodes were similar to those of the 94 non-infarction patients, except for a longer duration of the silent episodes. Post-infarction patients had a higher frequency of silent episodes (75%) than non-infarction patients (65%; $p < 0.02$).

Prognostic significance of silent coronary artery disease

The prognostic significance of spontaneous ischemic changes has not been evaluated yet in a large patient propulation. Nademanee et al. [28] suggested that silent myocardial ischemia documented on Holter recordings in patients with unstable angina is of prognostic significance. This conclusion was reached after studying 30 patients with unstable, 24 with stable angina and six with normal coronaries but with spasm, who had a total of 407 ischemic episodes. It was found that only 28% were symptomatic and in 18% the episodes were associated with ventricular arrhytmias. In 310 episodes it was seen that in only 32 (10%) was there a heart rate increase of 6 beats/min or greater preceding the onset of the ischemia, while in the remaining 278 episodes there was either no change or a decrease. During the peak of ischemia, heart rate increased in all 310 episodes. In a recent report Gottlieb et al. [29] found that 60 minutes of ischemia per 24 hour in patient with unstable angina was associated with unfavourable outcome.

Recently we presented [30] a 2 years follow-up of 356 stable ischemic heart disease patients with ischemic episodes on Holter monitoring during everyday activities. Cardiac events (death, recurrent infarction, balloon angioplasty or by-pass surgery) were significantly more common in the 211 post-infarction patients who had episodes of ST depression (30%), as compared to those without ST depression (9%); $p < 0.01$. In the 145 patients without a previous infarction a 30% event rate was observed in those with ST depression during the 2 years follow-up period, significantly higher than those without ST depression (13%); $p < 0.025$. It seems therefore that the presence of episodes of ST depression on Holter monitoring is a powerful predictor for cardiac events in post-infarction and no-infarction patients.

The incidence of silent myocardial infarctions is about 25%, as reported by Kannel and Abbott in the Framingham study [31]. The mortality in patients with unrecognized infarction was similar to that of patients with recognized (symptomatic) infarctions. Whether the patients in the study by Kannel and Abbott who developed silent myocardial infarctions might have exhibited silent ischemia before the development of infarction remains uncertain.

More prospective and prognostic studies of symptomatic and silent individuals are needed before a final categorization of silent myocardial ischemia can be made.

Day-to-day variability of ischemic episodes

Just as spontaneous variability of ventricular arrhythmias can affect evaluation of antiarrhthmic drugs, spontaneous day-to-day variability of myocardial ischemic episodes may affect the results of Holter studies, which monitor antiischemic therapy. In a previous investigation, Deanfield and coworkers [32] performed 4 days of monitoring to 30 patients and found marked day-to-day variability in ischemic parameters; in this study, however, no attempt was made to define the optimal duration of monitoring for evaluation of myocardial ischemia in daily practice. We conducted recently a study in 20 patients with chronic stable angina pectoris [33]. All had a positive treadmill stress test and angiographic evidence of significant coronary disease (>70% stenosis of at least one major coronary artery). All patients had 3 consecutive 24-hour Holter monitoring periods during unrestricted everyday life. To ensure routine daily activities the monitoring was performed during weekdays only and the patients were asked to maintain similar daily routines during the 3 monitoring days. We found, that the number of ischemic episodes per 25 hours varied from 2–15 (mean = 6.5). The number of ischemic episodes per patient during the 72 hours of the Holter monitoring was 7–38 (mean = 19.5). The total number of ischemic episodes in the 20 patients was 389, 27.7% with chest pain and 73.3% silent. The duration of ischemia per day varied from 6 to 419 min (mean = 76 min). The maximal ST depression varied from 1 to 6 mm (mean = 3.4 mm). The mean variation in the number of ischemic episodes per 24 hours was 36%, in the duration 51%; in the maximal degree of ST depression 31%, but only 9% in the heart rate at beginning of ST depression. The day-to-day variability in the 7 patients who had less than ischemic episodes in 3 days and in the 13 patients with more than 15 episodes was similar in respect to the number of episodes (43% vs. 31%), to their duration (55% vs. 48%) and to the maximal degree of ST depression (33% vs. 30%); between differences statistically not significant. The day-to-day variations observed in the number and the duration of the silent and the symptomatic ischemic episodes were also similar. The 5 patients who were on antianginal therapy had similar severity of ischemic changes and had similar day-to-day variations, as the 15 patients who had no drug therapy. To assess the additional information obtained by adding the second and the third monitoring days, we analyzed the results of the 3 monitoring days, relative to the day, in which ischemic changes were most prominent. During the first day of monitoring an average of 78% of ischemic episodes were detected, while during the first or second day 94% were detected, when the day with the most episodes was taken as 100%. On the first day, 63% of the maximal duration of ischemia was detected, and on the first or second day 97%. On the first day 84% of maximal degree of ST depression was detected, and 91% on the first or the second days. The first day of monitoring detected with 96% accuracy the heart rate at which the ST depression started, taking the day with the lowest heart rate as 100%.

Thus, for clinical purposes Holter monitoring can be used for evaluation of ischemia for the same monitoring period (24 hours) as for clinical arrhythmia evaluation. The addition of a second monitoring day increases ischemia detection by 7–29%. This figure, though definitely not negligable, will not markedly affect the clinical profile of an individual patient. However, for research purposes especially for evaluation of anti-ischemic drugs, a second monitoring day seems to be very important, while adding a third monitoring day will add little clinical information, but it will enable to reduce the size of the population studies as the number and the duration of ischemic episodes studied will be increased.

Conclusions

Transient myocardial ischemia frequently occur during daily activities in patients with coronary artery disease. More than 70% of the ischemic episodes are silent. Therefore the true incidence and severity of the ischemic process can be better assessed by ambulatory ECG monitoring. The characteristics of silent and symptomatic ischemic episodes is similar and therfore they seem to represent a similar severity of the ischemic process. Several studies have indicated that in high risk unstable angina patients these silent ischemic changes are associated with worse prognosis. Preliminary reports indicate that this may be true also in patients with stable ischemic heart disease. Therefore the aim of antiischemic therapy should be to abolish not only the symptomatic but also the silent ischemic episodes. Holter monitoring during everyday activities seems more and more to be needed for the estimation of the severity of the ischemic heart disease, for the evaluation of the therapy and for assessing prognosis.

References

1. Holter NJ (1961) New method for heart studies continuous electrocardiography of active subjects. Science 134:1214–20

2. Norland CC, Semlar HJ (1964) Angina pectoris and arrhythmias documented by cardiac telemetry. JAMA 190:115
3. Corday E, Bazika V, Lang TW, Pappelbaum S, Gold II, Bernstein H (1965) Detection of phantom arrhythmias and evanescent electrocardiographic abnormalities. JAMA 133:417
4. Hinkle Jr L, Meyer J, Stevens M, Carver ST (1967) Taperecordings of the ECG of active man. Circulation 36:752
5. Stern S, Tzivoni D (1972) The reliability of the Holter-Avionics system in reproducing the ST-T segment. Am Heart J 84:427
6. Stern S, Tzivoni D (1974) Early detection of silent ischemic heart disease by 24-hour electrocardiographic monitoring of active subjects. Br Heart J 36:481
7. Stern S, Tzivoni D, Stern Z (1975) Diagnostic accuracy of ambulatory ECG monitoring, as validated by coronary arteriography. Circulation 52:1045
8. Allen RD, Gettes LS, Phalan C, Avington MD (1976) Painless ST-segment depression in patients with angina pectoris. Chest 69:467–73
9. Schang SJ, Pepine CJ (1977) Transient asymptomatic ST segment depression during daily activity. Am J Cardiol 39:396–402
10. Linhart JW (1972) Atrial pacing in coronary artery disease, including pre-infarction angina and postoperative studies. Am J Cardiol 30:603
11. Guazzi M, Polese A, Fiorenti C, Magrini F, Olivari MI, Bartorelli C (1975) Left and right heart hemodynamics during spontaneous angina pectoris. Comparison between angina with ST segment depression and angina with ST segment elevation. Br Heart J 37:401
13. Biagini A, l'Abbate A, Maseri A (1982) Vasospastic ischemic mechanisms of frequent asymptomatic transient ST-T changes during continuous ECG monitoring. Am Heart J 103:13
14. Chierchia S, Brunelli C, Simonetti I, Lazzari M, Maseri A (1980) Sequence of events in angina at rest: primary reduction in coronary flow. Circulation 61:759
15. Deanfield JE, Shea M, Ribiero P, De Landsheere CM, Wilson RA, Horlock P, Selwyn PA (1984) Transient ST-segment depression as a marker of myocardial ischemia during daily life. Am J Cardiol 54:1195
16. Cohn PF, Brown EJ, Wynne J, Halman BL, Atkins HL (1983) Global and regional left ventricular ejection farction abnormalities during exercise in patients with silent myocardial ischemia. J Am Cardiol 1:931
17. Deanfield JE, Shea M, Ribiero P, De Landsheere C, Wilson RA, Horlock P, Selwyn AP (1984) Transient ST-segment depression as a marker of myocardial ischemia during daily life. Am J Cardiol 54:1195–1200
18. Tzivoni D, Benhorin J, Gavish A, Stern S (1985) Holter recording during treadmill testing in assessing myocardial ischemic changes. Am J Cardiol 55:1200–1203
19. Selwyn AP, Shea M, Deanfield JE, Wilson R, Horlock P, O'Brian HA (1986) Character of transient ischemia in angina pectoris. Am J Cardiol 58:21B
20. Pepine CJ (1986) Clinical aspects of silent myocardial ischemia in patients with angina and other forms of coronary heart disease. Am J Med 80 (suppl 4C):25
21. Weiner DA, Ryan TJ, McCabe CH, Chaitman BR, Sheffield LT, Ferguson JC, Fisher LD, Tristani F (1984) Prognostic importance of a clinical profile and exercise test in medically treated patients with coronary artery disease. J Am Coll Cardiol 3:772
22. Bonow RO, Kent KM, Rosing DR, Lan KKG, Lakatos E, Borer, JS, Bacharach SL, Green MV, Epstein SE. Exercise-induced ischemia in mildly symptomatic patients with coronary-artery disease and preserved left ventricular function: identification of subgroups at risk of death during medical therapy. N Engl J Med 311:1339
23. Weiner DA, Ryan TJ, McCabe CH, Fisher LD, Chaitman BR, Sheffield LT, Tristani FE (1985) Value of exercise testing in three-vessel coronary disease (CASS Registry). Circulation 72 (suppl III):III–463 (abst)

24. Cecchi AC, Dovellini EV, Marchi F, Pucci P, Santoro GM, Fazzini PF (1983) Silent myocardial ischemia during ambulatory electrocardiographic monitoring in patients with effort angina. J Am Cardiol 1:934
25. Campbell S, Barry J, Rocco MB, Nabel EG, Mead WK, Rebecca GS, Selwyn AP (1986) Features of the exercise test that reflect the activity of ischemic heart disease out of hospital. Circulation 74:72–80
26. Tzivoni D, Gavish A, Benhorin J, Karen A, Stern S (1986) Myocardial ischemia during daily activities and stress. Am J Cardiol 58:47B–50B
27. Stern S, Gavish A, Weisz G, Benhorin J, Tzivoni D (1986) Characteristics of silent and symptomatic myocardial ischemia during everyday activity (abstract). Circulation 74-II:57
28. Nademanee K, Intarachot V, Singh PN, Josephson MA, Singh BN (1986) Characteristics and clinical significance of silent myocardial ischemia in unstable angina. Am J Cardiol 58:26B
29. Gottlieb SO, Weisfeldt M, Ouyang P, Mellits DE, Gerstenblith G (1986) Silent ischemia as marker of unfavourable outcomes in patients with unstable angina. N Engl J Med 314:1214
30. Gavish A, Tzivoni D, Zin D, Karen A, Benhorin J, Banai S, Stern S (1986) Prognostic significance of ischemic episodes on Holter monitoring during daily activities: 2 years follow-up of 356 patients (abstract). J Am Coll Cardiol 9:240 A
31. Kannel WB, Abbott RD (1984) Incidence and prognosis of unrecognized myocardial infarction. Based on 26 years follow-up on the Framingham study. In: Rutishauser W, Roskamm H (eds) Silent myocardial ischemia. Berlin: Springer Verlag, pp 131–237
32. Deanfield JE, Selwyn AP, Cherchia S, Meseri A, Ribiero P, Kriller S, Morgan M (1983) Myocardial ischemia during daily life in patients with stable angina: its relation to symptoms and heart rate changes. Lancet 2:753–8
33. Tzivoni D, Gavish A, Benhorin J, Banai S, Karen A, Stern S (In press) Day-to-day variability of myocardial ischemic episodes in coronary artery disease. Am J Cardiol

8. Holter ECG and the evaluation of pacemakers

M. HÖHER[1], E. VONDERBANK, H.W. VERHOEVEN,
T. EGGELING[2], M. KOCHS[1], V. HOMBACH[2] & H.H. HILGER[1]

[1]*Medical Clinic III, University Cologne;* [2]*Department of Cardiology-Angiology-Pneumology, University Hospital of Ulm, F.R.G.*

Introduction

Pacemaker patients have been reported to suffer from heart related symptoms in about 10 to 60% of cases after implantation [1–3]. For the differential diagnosis of arrhythmias or pacemaker dysfunctions as possible causes of such complaints, provocative tests and 24 h-Holter-ECG have been proposed [4–6]. Ambulatory longterm ECG recording allows the detection of infrequently occurring pacing events and the assessment of the spontaneous incidence and the severity of pacemaker dysfunctions inducible by provocative tests. This allows an estimation of the individual clinical relevance of very commonly provocable pacemaker reactions, such as inhibition of the pacemaker spike delivery caused by isometric muscle contraction which has been reported in 11–77% of pacemaker patients [7–9]. Retrograde V-A conduction, a possible cause of tachycardias in dual-chamber devices, has been described in 47–95% of patients at the time of the pacemaker implantation [10, 11]. Beside detection of dysfunctions Holter-ECG allows the assessment of the underlying rhythms and background arrhythmias.

Using conventional Holter-ECG devices analysis of pacemaker recordings is difficult since the pacemaker spikes are often not visible, due to their high frequency current, low pass input filters, and the slow tape velocity of the recorders. This results in difficulties in the differentiation between paced beats and ventricular extrasystoles as well as in the detection of fusion beats. To overcome these problems special pacemaker-Holter-ECG systems has been developed, in which the pacemaker spikes are automatically detected and recorded as a marker signal on an additional tape track, in parallel to the ECG [12]. The analysis of the time intervals between the spike markers and the QRS complexes enables a semi-automatic analysis of pacemaker function in VVI-, AAI-, and DVI-systems.

V. Hombach, H. H. Hilger and H. L. Kennedy (eds), Electrocardiography and Cardiac Drug Therapy. ISBN 978-94-010-6976-2
© 1989, Kluwer Academic Publishers, Dordrecht –

The objectives of this study were to evaluate the persistent symptoms after pacemaker implantation as well as the pacemaker function or dysfunction in everyday life.

Patients and methods

In a group of 246 patients (mean age 60.8 ± 10.9 ys) a total of 320 long-term ECG recordings were analysed. The pacing modes of the pacemakers were: 219 VVI, 14 AAI, 39 DDD, 1 DDI, 16 DVI, 1 VAT, 11 VVI-TX (QT-triggered rate adaptive mode), 15 VVI with additional ventricular dynamic overdrive function, 3 VVI with antitachycardia ventricular burst function, 1 AAI with antitachycardia atrial burst function. The post-implantation period was 22.2 ± 1.5 months. The patients were intensively questioned about cardiac discomfort and clinically examined. Four Holter systems were used: Anatec (Ela Medical) $n = 102$, Pacerecorder (Del-Mar-Avionics) $n = 94$, Pathfinder II (Reynolds) $n = 66$, Surveyor (Reynolds) $n = 58$. The tapes were analyzed both visually and automatically.

Results

Cardiac symptoms

183/320 (57%) patients reported persisting heart related discomfort following pacemaker implantation (Table 1). Dizziness (28%) and dyspnoe (25%) were the most frequent symptoms. There was a relatively high

Table 1. Incidence of heart related symptoms in pacemaker patients ($n = 320$)

Cardiac symptoms	($n = 320$)
dizziness	28.1%
dyspnoe	24.7%
edema	17.2%
tachycardia	13.1%
angina pectoris	12.8%
palpitations	5.9%
eye flickering	5.9%
syncope	2.5%
total	57.2%

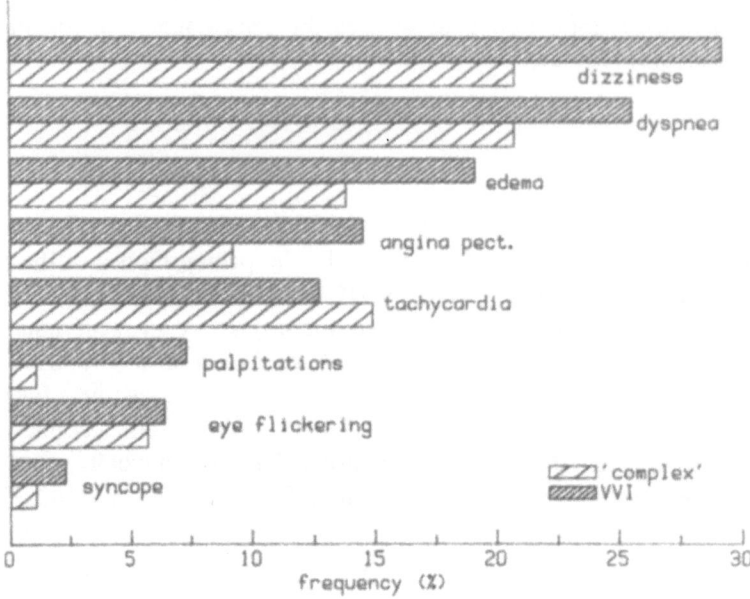

Figure 1. Frequency of heart related symptoms in patients with VVI pacemakers (*n* = 219) and in patients with more complex (dual chamber, rate adaptive, and antitachycardia) pacemakers (*n* = 87).

incidence of tachycardia of about 13%. Syncopes despite pacemaker implantation were reported by 8/320 (2.5%) patients, 5 with a VVI, 2 with a dual-chamber system, and 1 patient with an AAI pacemaker. Furthermore we compared the incidence of cardiac symptoms of patients with VVI implants and those with more complex systems, such as dual-chamber, rate adaptive, and antitachycardia devices (Figure 1). It was found, that dizziness, dyspnoe, and edema was more frequent in the VVI as compared to the complex pacemaker group. This may be caused at least in part by the about 10 years higher mean age of the VVI patients (64 ± 13 ys) compared to the complex pacemaker group (53 ± 14 ys).

Rate profile and underlying rhythm

24-hour Holter ECG revealed a mean of 69 ± 31% paced beats in our patient group. In 8 (2.5%) recordings no pacing event was found due to a sufficiently high spontaneous heart rate. In 72 (22%) recordings only paced

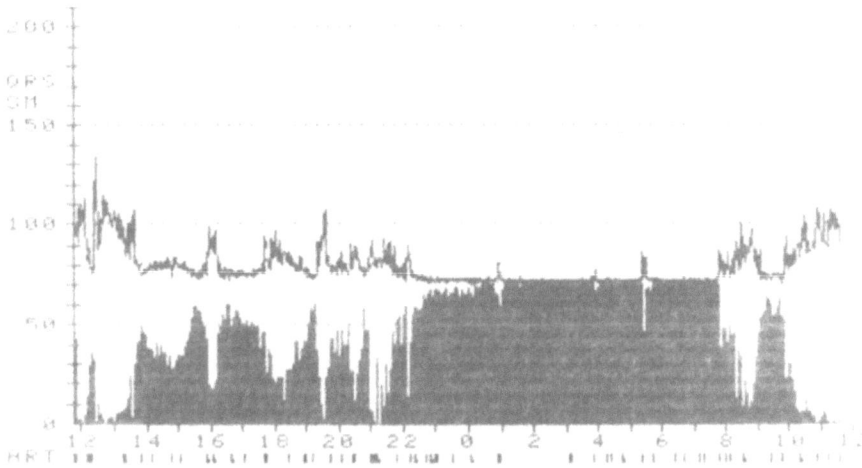

Figure 2. 24 hour profile of the spontaneous (bright) and paced (dark) beats in a 74 years old VVI patient suffering from brady- and tachyarrhythmias during atrial fibrillation. Pacemaker activity (51% paced beats) increases markedly during the night.

beats were found. The 24 h-heart rate profile in combination with a graph of the paced beats was very helpful in assessing the overall pacemaker function (Figure 2). Rate decreases below the programmed pacing rate indicating output-failures (see below) as well as pacemaker mediated and spontaneous tachycardias could easily be detected. This was especially useful in DDD pacemakers for the detection of pacemaker mediated tachycardias and in optimizing reprogramming of rate adaptive pace-makers. The underlying heart rhythm is an important parameter for choosing the correct pacing mode. The most common problems of underlying spontaneous rhythm during pacing are intermittent or persistent changes from sinus rhythm to atrial fibrillation. In an AAI pacemaker atrial fibrillation would cause ineffective atrial stimulation, most often in a fixed rate interference mode. In a DDD pacemaker atrial fibrillation often results in tachycardias due to atrial tracking. Therefore routine check of the underlying spontaneous rhythm in pacemakers with atrial sensing or stimulation is necessary. Conversion from sinus rhythm to atrial fibrillation may be spontaneous or caused by asynchronous pacing of the atrium as well. The importance of asynchronous atrial pacing recently has been shown by Belott [11], who found a conversion from sinus rhythm to atrial fibrillation in 7% during DVI, but only in 1% during DDD pacing. In our study patients with preserved spontaneous rhythm revealed sinus rhythm in 52% (166/320), continued atrial fibrillation in 17% (55/320), and intermittent atrial fibrillation in 5% (16/320).

Pacemaker dysfunctions

There are three basic forms of pacemaker dysfunction: failure to sense, failure to output and failure to capture.

Failure to sense. The pacemaker spike is delivered earlier than the pro-grammed escape interval after the last spontaneous beat. In this study failures to sense were seen in an unexpected high frequency of 50% (159/320) of the recordings, but in 50% of these recordings with sensing failures the incidence was less than 10/24 h. Frequent failures to sense of more than 30/h were found in 15/320 (4.7%) of the recordings. Figure 3 shows a graph of the detected pacemaker dysfunctions. The more frequent ones are marked as excised pie pieces. Failure to sense may be due to 3 mechanisms:

1) To avoid sensing of the deflection following the pacemaker spike, pacemaker sensing circuits are blocked for a certain time after spike delivery. This 'pacemaker refractory period' is often programmable and typically adjusted to 250–400 ms. If a spontaneous beat arises within this

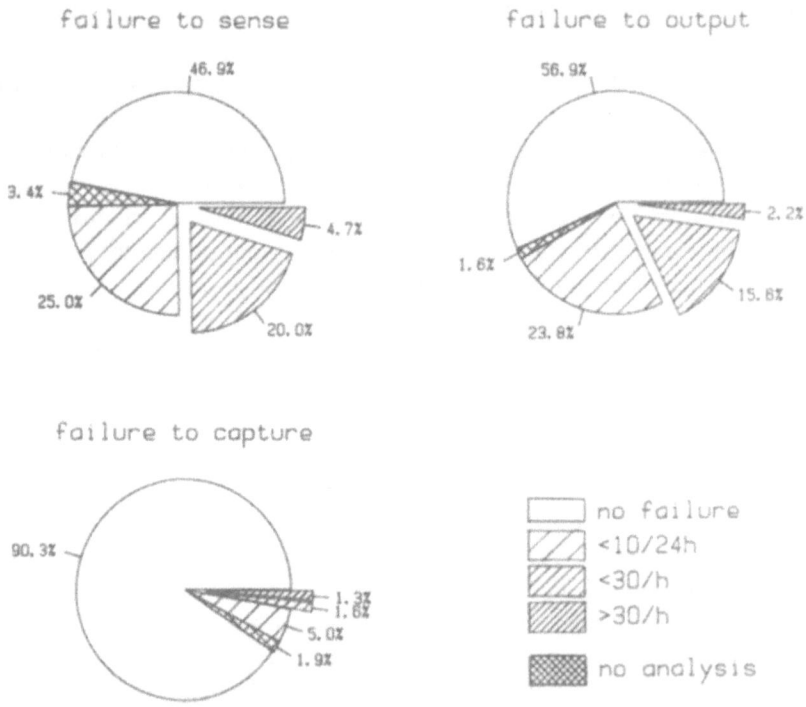

Figure 3. Incidence of pacemaker dysfunctions in 320 pacemaker Holter recordings. For details see text.

period, it will not be detected by the pacemaker sensing circuit and therefore the next pacemaker spike will be delivered at the correct escape interval after the last but one beat. This type of sensing failure typically occurs in patients with tachyarrhythmias and close coupled extrasystoles (Figure 4).

2) Oversensing. The pacemaker senses other than the cardiac signals, it is designed to detect. In case of sensing such wrong signals just before a spontaneous beat, the latter will fall into the pacemaker refractory period and will not be sensed. Oversensing is most often due to skeletal muscle potentials. Other causes are electromagnetic interferences, sensing of the atrial signal in the ventricle (and vice versa), and voltage changes produced by hairline fractures or loose connections of a pacemaker lead with inter-mittent contact (made-break signals). Sensing failures induced by over-sensing typically have no such constant interval between the last but one beat and the premature occurring pacemaker spike as discussed above. Oversensing of continuing interference signals such as myopotentials does not only result in failures to sense but also in pacemaker inhibition (failure to output) or activation of an asynchronous interference mode available in most pulse generators [13].

3) Undersensing of the cardiac signal due to a reduced signal amplitude or slope (e.g. tissue scarring from microinfarctions, rejection after heart transplant [14]), insulation defects or disruption of the pacemaker leads, and false programming of the pacemaker sensitivity.

Occasionally pseudofusion beats are misdiagnosed as sensing failure. In contrast to a fusion beat which is the simultaneous activation of the

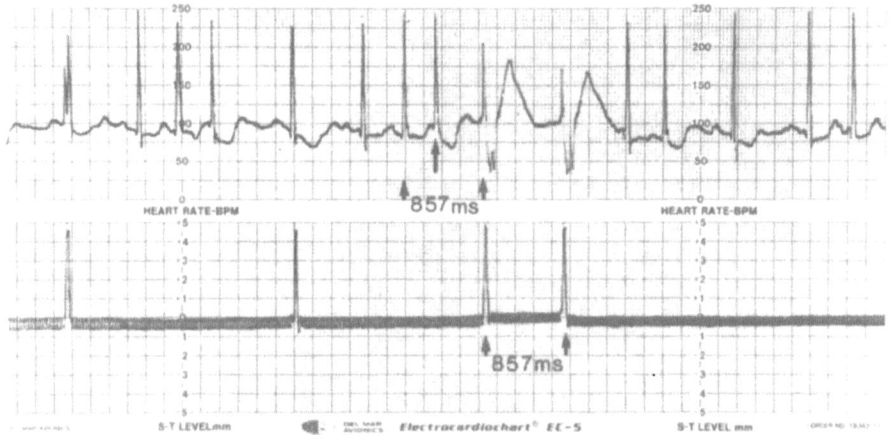

Figure 4. ECG (above) and pacemaker marker channel (below) showing failure to sense during supraventricular tachyarrhythmia due to the intrinsic beat occurring within the tech-nical pacemaker refractory period. VVI 70 ppm.

94

ventricle by the intrinsic impulse and the pacemaker stimulus, pseudofusion means a pacemaker spike delivery within an intrinsic QRS complex due to late arrival of the cardiac depolarisation at the electrode site. Especially in patients with right bundle branch block pseudofusion beats with pacemaker spikes even in the ST segment occur, which are not sensing failures.

Failure to output. Missing delivery of the pacemaker spike at the programmed escape interval causes pauses of variable length. In this study failures to output were detected in 133/320 (41.6%) of the recordings resulting in pauses of 1730±622 ms (960–4300 ms). In 76/113 (57.1%) of these recordings the frequency of output failures was less than 10/24 h. Frequent output failures of more than 30/h were found in 7/320 (2.2%) of the recordings. The most common cause of failure to output was oversensing of muscle potentials (Figure 5). Other reasons are triggering of the T-wave, which results in a marked decrease of the pacing rate but without significant pauses, and technical failures of the pulse generator. There was no significant correlation between the occurrence of output failures and reported symptoms such as vertigo or syncope, which may be due to the relatively short duration of the pauses with a mean value of less than 2 seconds. Even during longer lasting myopotential interference, cardiac pauses were most often limited by spontaneously occurring ventricular escape beats or by conversion of the pacemaker into the asynchronous interference mode.

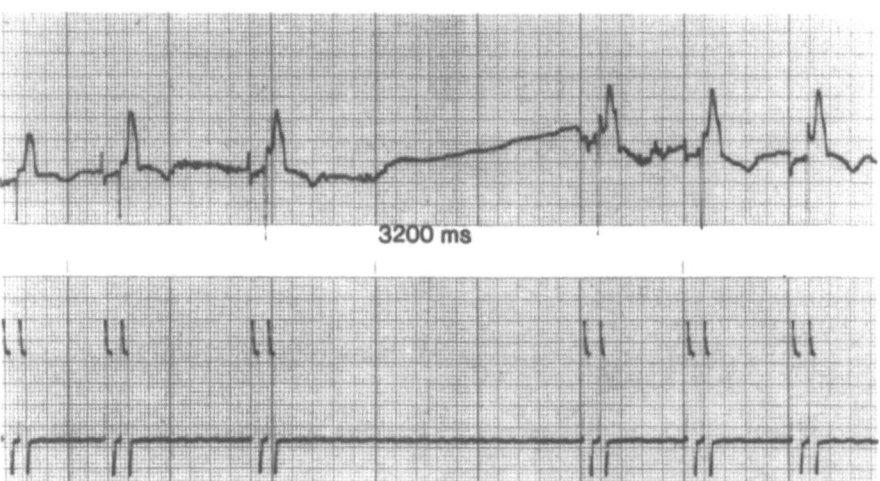

3200 ms

Figure 5. Failure to output due to oversensing of muscle potentials resulting in a pause longer than 3 sec in a committed mode DVI pacemaker (60 ppm, AV-delay 155 ms).

Failure to capture. The pacemaker spike is delivered outside of the ventricular refractory period but not followed by a cardiac depolarisation. Capture failures were much more rare than the other pacemaker dysfunctions and were found in 25/320 (7.8%) of the recordings. 4/320 (1.3%) of the patients had frequent capture failures with more than 30 events per hour. Automatic analysis of capturing was possible only in the ventricular pacing devices whereas controlling of atrial capturing required visual analysis. Possible causes of capture failures are lead dislodgement, defective lead insulation and/or wire fracture, increased stimulation threshold due to infarction and/or fibrosis at the electrode site, power source depletion, and inappropriate programming of the pacemaker output voltage or pulse width. Whereas lead dislodgement and wire fracture cause combined capture and sensing failure, increased stimulation threshold due to microinfarctions and/or microdislodgement at the electrode site most often results in failure to capture despite of an intact sensing function of the pacemaker (Figure 6).

Assessing both, the number as well as the clinical importance of detected pacemaker dysfunctions, this study revealed a normal pacemaker function in 221/320 (69.1%) of the recordings. Dysfunctions less frequent than 10/24 h and resulting in only minor arrhythmias were included in this group. Suspect pacemaker findings requiring further control were found in 37/320 (11.6%) of the recordings. In 40/320 (15.0%) of patients, reprogramming of the pacemaker due to dysfunctions first detected by Holter monitoring was necessary. In 14/320 (3.4%) repetition of the recording was recommended due to pacemaker unrelated technical problems such as

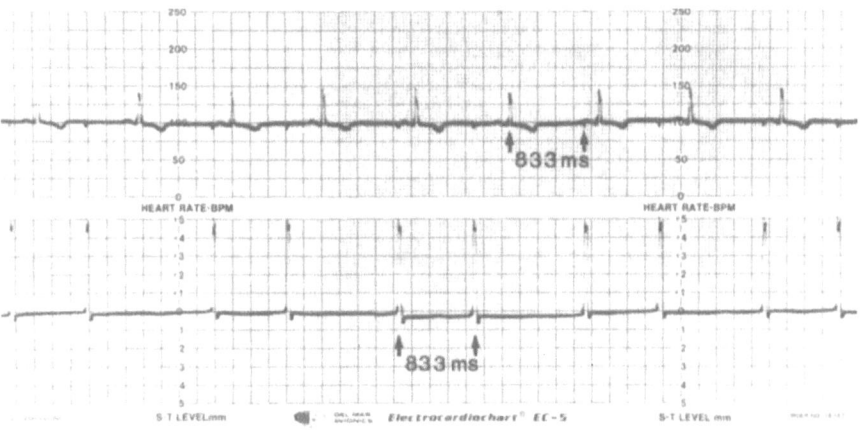

Figure 6. Failure to capture despite of preserved sensing function in a VVI pacemaker (72 ppm) during sinus rhythm.

incorrect triggering of the pacemaker spike, or bad quality of the electrograms.

Dual chamber pacemakers

Within each sensing or pacing circuit dual chamber pacemakers display in principle the same dysfunctions as mentioned before, but due to the atrial tracking function and some special algorithms for upper rate limiting these dysfunctions result in more different electrocardiographic patterns than in single chamber devices.

DVI. In DVI mode the pacemaker senses only the ventricle but is capable of stimulating both the atrium and the ventricle. In case of no sensed ventricular activity an atrial stimulus is delivered at the end of an atrial escape interval, followed by a ventricular stimulus at the completion of an additional AV-delay. The sum of the atrial escape interval and the AV-delay defines the pacing rate. There are three types of AV-coupling in DVI (as well as in DDD) pacing called committed, uncommitted, and semi-committed mode. In the committed mode, the atrial stimulus is always followed by a ventricular spike delivery, regardless of ventricular activity during the AV-delay. In the uncommitted mode the ventricular spike will be inhibited by sensed activity, and during semi-committed mode ventricular sensing within the AV-delay results in ventricular spike delivery after a shortened AV-delay.

Inconstant atrial cycle length: Sensing of ventricular activity within the AV-delay during committed or semi-committed DVI pacing results in shortening of the atrial stimulation interval by the time difference the ventricular signal occurred earlier than the programmed AV-delay. Depending on the length of the AV-delay this causes changes of the atrial stimulation rate of about 10–15 bpm [15].

Pseudo-pseudofusion: Since in DVI mode the pacemaker is sensing solely in the ventricle, the atrial spike will not be inhibited by a simultaneously occurring spontaneous beat. Therefore there might occur a pseudo-pseudofusion of the atrial spike and the spontaneous QRS complex [16]. During committed mode this pseudo-pseudofusion will be followed by a ventricular spike delivery within the ventricular refractory period, eventually within the vulnerable period. Induction of ventricular tachycardia has been demonstrated due to such stimulations [17]. In this study ventricular echobeats and in 1 patient initiation of a non-sustained ventricular tachycardia of 9 beats were seen due to ventricular pacing in the vulnerable period as a consequence of pseudo-pseudofusion.

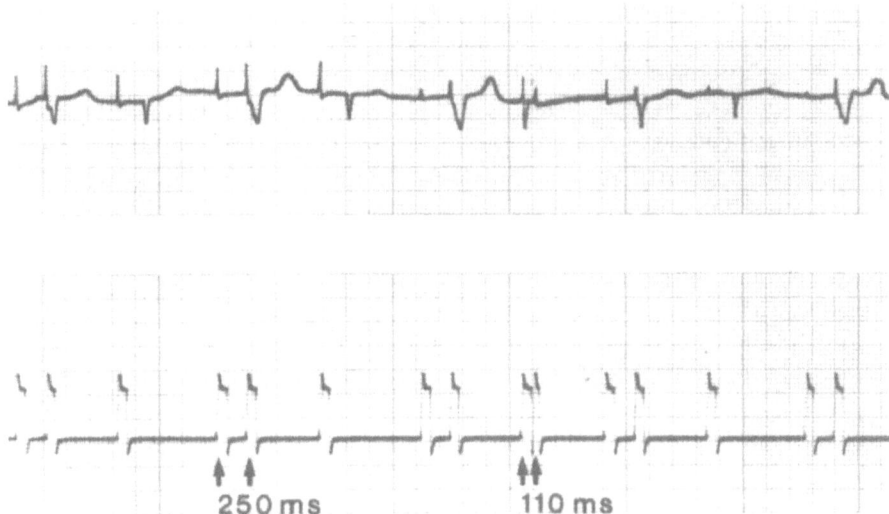

Figure 7. Semi-committed DVI pacemaker showing shortening of the AV-delay from 250 ms to 110 ms due to ventricular sensing during the AV-delay after the ventricular blanking period (*no* pacemaker dysfunction).

Change of the AV-delay: To prevent such arrhythmia induction DDI pacemakers most often are used in the semi-committed mode. Ventricular sensing within the AV-delay will shorten the given AV-delay to a 'non-physiologic' AV-delay of about 100 ms [18]. Pacemaker Holter ECG typically reveals two distinguishable AV-delays (Figure 7).

DDD. Due to the atrial tracking function, DDD pacemakers display some additional phenomena.

Upper rate response: The upper rate response of DDD pacemakers is controlled by the ventricular upper rate limit and the technical atrial refractory period, which determines the highest atrial rate sensed by the pacemaker [19]. If this maximum sensed atrial rate is programmed below the upper rate limit, atrial sensing is the limiting factor for upper rate response. If the spontaneous atrial rate exceeds this sensing limit, 2:1 block will occur. In contrast, if the maximum sensed atrial rate exceeds the ventricular upper rate limit, the pacemaker will increase the programmed AV-delay to match the upper rate limit resulting in a Wenckebach like rhythm. The purpose of this Wenckebach type of response is to protect against sudden changes in ventricular pacing rates in relation to sensed rapid atrial rates.

Pacemaker mediated tachycardia: Retrograde VA conduction has been demonstrated in 47–95% of patients at the time of pacemaker implantation

[10, 11]. Atrial sensing of the VA conduction with consecutive ventricular spike delivery can result in an endless loop tachycardia, which is the most important dysfunction in DDD pacemakers detected by Holter ECG [20]. Such pacemaker mediated tachycardias have been demonstrated in about 60% of patients with first generation DDD pacemakers [11]. In our study pacemaker mediated tachycardias were found in 11/39 (28.2%) of DDD recordings. Most often such episodes are asymptomatic and self-terminating. Pacemaker mediated tachycardias are often induced by ventricular extrasystoles or sensing failures. For prevention of such endless loop tachycardias modern DDD pacemakers are equipped with some protective mechanisms such as programmable atrial refractory period, post-extrasystolic prolongation of the atrial refractory period, and automatic AV block after a certain number of atrial tracked beats pacing at the upper rate limit (Figure 8). Differential diagnosis of such mechanisms from pacemaker dysfunctions by Holter-ECG requires detailed information about the special algorithms as well as the programmed pacing parameters.

Atrioventricular crosstalk: Ventricular sensing of the atrial pacemaker stimulus with consecutive inhibition of the ventricular spike delivery [21]. In the uncommitted DDD (or DVI) mode, this results in a dangerous self-inhibition of the pacemaker with solely atrial pacing. In such cases the electrogram will often reveal a PQ interval, which exceeds the programmed AV delay. Another sign indicating crosstalk is an increase of the atrial pacing rate with a stimulation interval exactly reduced by the programmed AV delay. During semi-committed DDD pacing crosstalk is characterized

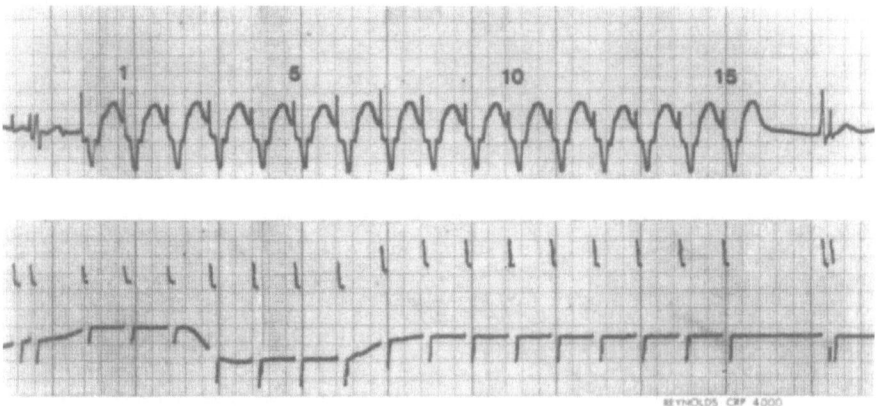

Figure 8. Pacemaker mediated tachycardia (spike markers below) in a DDD pacemaker (AV-delay 180 ms, upper rate limit 120 ppm, atrial refractory period 380 ms, ventricular refractory period 120 ppm). Due to a special termination algorithm, the 16. sensed event is AV-blocked resulting in an interruption of the 'endless loop' tachycardia.

by an unexpected occurrence of the non-physiologic AV delay without any interference potentials [22].

Technical limitations of automated analysis

Since today available Holter devices are not able to detect P-waves or to differentiate between ventricular and atrial pacemaker stimuli, an automated analysis of pacemaker function was possible only in VVI, AAI, VAT, and DVI pacemakers. Out of these, only VVI and DVI pacemakers were completely analysed, whereas in AAI and VAT devices only the ventricular response of the atrial pacemaker functions could be assessed. The quality of the automated pacemaker analysis depends on the correct pacemaker spike recognition as well as sufficient triggering of the QRS complexes. In the systems used in this study, spike recognition was sufficient only in unipolar pulse generators. The most frequent error in automated analysis were false positive sensing failures due to false spike detection, missing QRS triggering or pseudofusion beats. Reasons for false pacemaker spike detection within the tape recorders were a bad signal quality of the ECG, electrostatic disorders, and myopotential interferences. The difficulties arising from QRS-triggering were similar to conventional Holter analysis, but QRS-triggering was complicated by the marked differences in signal amplitude between paced and non-paced beats. Since analysis of pacemaker function depends on relatively short intervals an exact adjustment of the tape velocity and the recording leads is necessary.

Discussion

For diagnosis of bradycardias and indication for pacemaker therapy most often ambulatory Holter monitoring is performed. Consequently, it is logical to control the effect of pacemaker therapy by the same method, especially in patients with persisting symptoms despite of pacemaker implantation. Although Hoffman and Bleifer [1, 23] have demonstrated an unexpected high incidence of heart related symptoms in pacemaker patients, there is only few data about the type and frequency of such complaints. In this study group of 246 consecutive patients from our pacemaker ambulance, 57% of the patients reported heart related symptoms and there was a remarkable high incidence of dizziness (28%) and tachycardias (13%). Pacemaker interference especially by myopotentials is well known since many years [7]. Although syncopes due to myopotential inhibition have been described, the clinical symptoms in such patients are most often unspecific. Also in this study, there was no statistical correlation between the type or frequency of reported symptoms and pacemaker dysfunctions detected by Holter ECG. Intensive provocative testing has been proposed for recognition of pacemaker dysfunctions [5, 6]. This data are complemented by ambulatory Holter ECG which allows the assessment of the spontaneous incidence and the clinical relevance of such provocatable pacemaker dysfunctions during everyday life.

Pacemaker dysfunctions including rare and less relevant dysfunctions were found in about 70% of the recordings. 26% of the recordings revealed a suspect or abnormal pacemaker function, requiring for reprogramming. This relatively high percentage emphasizes the need for intensive follow-up of pacemaker patients. Studies in patients with multi-programmable pacemakers have shown that the use of multiprogram-mability is often limited to the pacing rate [24]. This may be due, at least in part, to a lack of detailed information about the pacemaker function, which may be provided by ambulatory Holter monitoring.

In more sophisticated physiological systems such as dual chamber and rate adaptive pacemakers, which are intended to emulate the normal heart rate profile during stress, pacemaker Holter ECG offers information about the general function as well as the occurrence of specific dysfunctions such as pacemaker mediated tachycardias, which is necessary for optimizing the pacemaker adjustment. Although several authors reported a higher rate of pacemaker dysfunctions in dual chamber as compared to single chamber pacemakers [25, 26], our data revealed no such difference. On the contrary, in VVI pacemakers we found slightly more sensing and output failures than in the more complex devices. But this reached statistical significance only in the very rare occurring dysfunctions of less than 10/24 h and might be due to the higher sensitivity of the automated VVI-analysis in relation to the visual analysis of the DDD recordings.

The main disadvantage of pacemaker Holter ECG is the time consuming procedure (30 min up to 5 h). Even if the automated analysis was used, which was restricted to VVI, AAI, VAT, and DVI pacemakers, the high incidence of false positive findings required an additional visual control of all detected events. Nevertheless, the spike marker channel was very useful during visual analysis as well. Technical improvements of the Holter systems with respect to pacemaker controlling are necessary and should include a combined pacemaker and arrhythmia analysis, an automated analysis of DDD pacemakers (which requires a differentiation between atrial and ventricular pacing stimuli [27]), and the analysis of consecutive rhythm patterns instead of single intervals.

References

1. Hoffman A, Jost M, Pfisterer M, Burkart F (1984) Persistent symptoms despite permanent pacing. Incidence, causes and follow-up. Chest 85:207
2. Gross-Fengels W, Schilling G, Neumann G, Funke HD, Simon H (1982) Ambulantes 24-Stunden-EKG bei symptomatischen Schrittmacherpatienten. Herz/Kreislauf 7:404–408
3. Fischer JD, Escher DJW, Hurzeler P et al. (1978) Recurrent syncope or dizziness after pacemaker implantation. Clin Res 26:231a
4. Ward DE, Camm AJ, Spurrell R (1977) Ambulatory monitoring of the electrocardiogram: An important aspect of pacemaker surveillance. Biotelemetry 4:109
5. Furman S (1985) Pacemaker follow-up. In: Barold SS (ed.) Modern cardiac pacing, Mount Kisco, NY: Futura, pp 889–918.
6. Strathmore NF, Mond HG (1987) Noninvasive monitoring and testing of pacemaker function. PACE 10:1359–1370.
7. Wirtzfeld A, Lampadius M, Ruprecht EO (1972) Unterdrückung von Demand-Schrittmachern durch Muskelpotentiale. Dtsch med Wschr 97:61
8. Gaita F, Asteggiano R, Bocchiardo M, Commodo E, Leo di M, Gobbi G, Grande A, Rosettani E, Brusca A (1984) Holter monitoring and provocative maneuvers in assessment of unipolar demand pacemaker myopotential inhibition. Am Heart J 107:925
9. Piller LW, Kennelly BM (1977) Myopotential inhibition of demand pacemakers. Chest 66:418
10. Hayes DL, Furman S (1983) Atrio-ventricular and ventriculoatrial conduction times in patients underoing pacemaker implant. PACE 6:38
11. Balott PH (1985) Clinical experience with over 250 DDD pacemakers. In: Barold SS (ed.) Modern cardiac pacing. Mount Kisco, NY: Futura, pp 439–481
12. Kelen GJ, Bloomfield DA, Hardage M, Gomes JA, Khan R, Gopalaswamy C, El Sherif N (1980) A clinical evaluation of an improved Holter monitoring technique for artificial pacemaker function. PACE 3:192–197
13. Irnich W (1987) Muscle noise and interference behavior in pacemakers: A comparative study. PACE 10:125–132
14. Markewitz A, Kemkes B, Reble B, Osterholzer G, Reichart B, Puricelii C, Feruglio G, Sternotti G, Behrenbeck DW (1987) Particularities of dual chamber pacemaker therapy in pateints after orthotopic heart transplantation. PACE 10: 326–332
15. Barold SS, Falkhoff MD, Ong LS, Heinle RA (1980) Characterization of pacemaker arrhythmias due to normally functioning AV demand (DVI) pulse generators. PACE 3:712
16. Barold SS, Falkhoff MD, Ong LS, Heinle RA (1981) Interpretation of electrocardiograms produced by a new unipolar multiprogrammable "committed" AV sequential (DVI) pulse generator. PACE 4:692
17. Luceri RM, Ramirez AV, Castellanos A (1983) Ventricular tachycardia produced by normally functioning AV sequential demand (DVI) pacemaker with "committed" ventricular stimulation. JACC 1:1177
18. Levine PA, Mace RC (1983) Normal rhythms associated with atrioventricular sequential (DVI) pacing. In: Pacing therapy: A guide to cardiac pacing for optimum hemodynamic benefit. Mount Kisco, NY: Futura, p 105
19. Furman S (1985) Dual chamber pacemakers: Upper rate behavior. PACE 8:197–214
20. Furman S, Fisher JD (1982) Endless loop tachycardia in an AV universal (DDD) pacemaker. PACE 5:486–489

21. Furman S, Reichter-Reiss H, Escher DJW (1973) Atrioventricular sequential pacing and pacemakers. Chest 63:783
22. Barold SS, Ong LS, Falkoff MD, Heinle RA (1985) Crosstalk or self-inhibition in dual-chambered pacemakers. In: Barold SS (ed.) Modern cardiac pacing. Mount Kisco, NY: Futura, pp 615–623
23. Bleifer SB, Bleifer DJ, Hansmann DR, Sheppard JJ, Karpman HL (1974) Diagnosis of occult arrhythmias by Holter electrocardiography. Prog Cardiovasc Dis 16:569–599
24. Hayes DL, Maloney JD, Meridith J, Holmes JDR, Gersh B, Broadbend JL, Osborn MJ, Fetter J. (1981) Initial and early follow-up assessment of the clinical efficacy of a multiprogrammable pulse generator. PACE 4:416–431
25. Dreifus LS, Zinberg A. Puziak A, Hurzeler P, Grant S, Morse DP (1985) Long term monitoring of 21.750 patients with implanted cardiac pacemakers. JACC 5:507 (abstract)
26. Griffin JC, Schuenemeyer TD, Hess KR, Glaeser D, Anderson BJ, Romans E, Jenkins MA, Nielsen AP (1986) Pacemaker follow-up: its role in the detection and correction of pacemaker system malfunction. PACE 9:387
27. Feldman CL, Hubelbank M (1983) Analysis of ambulatory ECG's for patients with dual chamber pacemakers. IEEE Computers in Cardiology: 97

9. ECG telemetry and ambulatory ECG: role in cardiac rehabilitation

NANETTE K. WENGER

Emory University School of Medicine, Cardiac Clinics, Grady Memorial Hospital, Atlanta, Georgia, U.S.A.

ECG telemetry and ambulatory ECG; role in cardiac rehabilitation

ECG telemetric monitoring and ambulatory ECG recording enable the assessment of disturbances of cardiac rhythm and/or abnormalities associated with the occurrence of myocardial ischemia that may occur during cardiac rehabilitative physical activity and/or during occupational or recreational activities. The challenge to the clinician is the selection of patients who are likely to benefit from these testing and surveillance modalities, in view of their cost and the requirement for trained personnel.

ECG telemetry in rehabilitative physical activity

In the early years of exercise rehabilitation for patients recovered from myocardial infarction there was very limited availability of ECG telemetry. However, most patients began their rehabilitative physical activity no earlier than several months following infarction, and the patients enrolled in exercise rehabilitation programs were predominantly those with an uncomplicated clinical course.

With the increasing availability of this new technology, comparisons of patient safety were made in medically supervised cardiac exercise classes with and without continuous ECG monitoring; there was concern that the increased myocardial oxygen demand of exercise might trigger arrhythmic sudden death or myocardial infarction. The reported occurrence of major cardiovascular complications of exercise rehabilitation of coronary patients in the medical literature of the 1970s varied from absent [1, 2] to reasonably frequent [3, 4].

A retrospective questionnaire survey of cardiac exercise programs in the

V. Hombach, H. H. Hilger and H. L. Kennedy (eds). Electrocardiography and Cardiac Drug Therapy. ISBN 978-94-010-6976-2
© 1989. Kluwer Academic Publishers, Dordrecht –

U.S.A. and Canada reported by Haskell in 1978 [5] delineated the nonfatal and fatal cardiovascular complications among 13 570 participants who exercised in supervised classes at 103 centers for a total of 1 629 634 patient-hours. The data reflected the experience between 1960 and 1977 and showed 1 fatal complication per 116 402 exercise hours. One cardiac arrest occurred per 32 593 patient-hours, and one myocardial infarction every 232 809 patient-hours of participation. Although the risk of exercise-related ventricular tachycardia or ventricular fibrillation was low, complication rates were lower in exercise programs with continuous ECG monitoring; this applied both to the total experience and to the more recent experience (since 1970). However, it was not able to be ascertained whether the differing intensities of exercise, the closer medical supervision, or the ECG monitoring per se was the determinant of the apparent increase in patient safety.

More recent data [6] compiled by Van Camp and Peterson were based on questionnaire responses from 167 supervised outpatient cardiac rehabilitation programs and concerned the period 1980–1984. The patient-hours of supervised exercise that were summarized totaled 2 351 916. The risk of cardiovascular complications was substantially lower, with one-fourth the number of cardiac arrests and one-seventh the fatality rate previously described. One cardiac arrest occurred per 111 996 patient-hours and one myocardial infarction per 293 990 patient-hours, resulting in one fatality for 783 972 hours of patient participation. Additionally, there was no difference in the frequency of major cardiovascular complications related to the application or extent of ECG monitoring; ECG telemetry was characterized as provided continuously, intermittently or as graduated monitoring. Potential explanations for the improved safety of exercise included better patient selection, concurrent medical or surgical therapies, and better patient education and exercise prescription. The conclusion of the authors was that the *routine* use of ECG telemetry monitoring offered no safety advantage, particularly since the occurrence of life-threatening arrhythmias was not greatest in proximity to an acute coronary episode [7], and that routine telemetry entailed an unwarranted substantial cost and requirement for trained personnel.

There are, however, subgroups of coronary patients who appear at excess risk of ischemic and arrhythmic complications during exercise; interim guidelines have been developed to identify patients with ischemic heart disease for whom unsupervised exercise rehabilitation appears unwise and for whom ECG telemetric monitoring should probably be recommended [8] to minimize the risk of exercise training. These include patients with a markedly reduced maximal functional capacity, less than 6 METS; with several depressed left ventricular function (left ventricular ejection fraction below 35%, cardiomegaly, an S3 gallop); patients who develop angina pectoris or objective signs of myocardial ischemia at exercise testing at a heart rate less than 120 beats/minute or at an exercise workload less than 6 METS (low exercise intensities); those with an abnormal hemodynamic response to exercise, particularly exercise-induced hypotension or a decrease in exercise ejection fraction; those with complex ventricular arrhythmias, Lown class III or IV; patients with QT prolongation; those unable to self-monitor their exercise heart rates and those who habitually exceed their prescribed training heart rate range; and survivors of ventricular fibrillation not associated with an episode of myocardial infarction [9]. Another subset of coronary patients at increased risk of cardiac arrest, even remote from an acute coronary episode, is characterized by an above average exercise performance, absence of exercise-induced angina, markedly ischemic ST segment responses during exercise testing, and frequent exercising at intensities beyond their prescribed heart rate range [7]. Self-efficacy scales [10] have been shown to identify with reasonable accuracy the patients prone to dangerous exercise overexertion.

The optimal duration and intensity of ECG telemetry for these high-risk patients are not known; more information is needed to formulate guidelines for decreasing or terminating ECG telemetry during their exercise rehabilitation.

Ambulatory ECG recording, transtelephonic ECG transmission

The use of ambulatory ECG recording during exercise and more recently the use of intermittent transtelephonic ECG transmission [11, 12] and portable heart rate monitors have been described to encourage adherence to a program of exercise rehabilitation, as well as to provide reassurance and encouragement in exercising for low-risk patients, particularly those living in areas remote from exercise centers.

Heart rate monitors, as well as telephone ECG transmitters, have been described to help patients remain within their prescribed training heart rate range during a home exercise program designed for low-risk patients recovered from a clinically uncomplicated myocardial infarction. The home program was equally effective as supervised group exercise in improving functional capacity and the telephone contact was suggested to improve compliance with home exercise [13, 14]. The advantages cited were that exercise intensity could be gauged by the heart rate response and ECG complications readily documented.

The cost effectiveness of this approach in a clinical rather than a research setting remains to be ascertained.

Although ambulatory-ECG-documented arrhythmias, particularly ventricular ectopic complexes, are common in patients with coronary atherosclerotic heart disease, particularly following myocardial infarction, the correlation of ventricular ectopic activity so demonstrated with that provoked by exercise testing and/or that occurring during exercise training has not been systematically evaluated. It is not known whether simple ventricular ectopic activity documented by ambulatory ECG, with or without associated ventricular dysfunction, identifies a patient at increased risk of cardiovascular complications during exercise training.

Ambulatory ECG recording with ST segment analysis can document episodes of silent, as well as symptomatic, ischemia that may occur during rehabilitative exercise training or occupational or recreational activities. Many painless ischemic episodes are described to occur during very light activity, often without major increases in heart rate, and interspersed with symptomatic ischemic episodes [15, 16]. The prognostic value of silent ischemia so detected remains controversial; studies have not been done apropos of cardiac rehabilitative physical training.

Ambulatory ECG recording permits the correlation of ECG evidence of arrhythmia and/or manifestations of ischemia with work-related cardiovascular symptoms; it may serve to guide the vocational rehabilitation of high-risk coronary patients and/or those with marked functional limitations. The intensity of work-relatd activities can also be judged by the heart rate response; and any ECG abnormalities associated with emotional provocations can be identified. The metabolic demands of occupational work can be importantly influenced by environmental factors such as temperature and humidity, as well as the stresses of intellective function, excitement, anger and other emotions; where occupational capabilities fail to correlate with the physical work capacity estimated by exercise testing, the heart rate, arrhythmia and ST segment responses documented by ambulatory ECG may be of value; however, this has yet to be formally evaluated in a rehabilitation setting.

Also, exercise training has been suggested to decrease exercise-induced ventricular arrhythmias [17], but this has not been subsequently documented in patients with coronary heart disease. Finally, the response of arrhythmic or ischemic complications to drug therapy can be ascertained both throughout the day and during periods of exercise training.

Obviously these latter uses of ambulatory ECG recording should not be routine in the rehabilitation setting, but should be selectively applied to appropriate patient subgroups.

References

1. Sanne H (1973) Exercise tolerance and physical training of non-selected patients after myocardial infarction. Acta Med Scand (suppl) 551:1–124
2. Kentala E (1972) Physical fitness and feasibility of physical rehabilitation after myocardial infarction in men of working age. Ann Clin Res (suppl) 9:1–84
3. Hakkila J (1973) Complications during physical rehabilitation of coronary patients. G Ital Cardiol 3:632–636
4. Mead WF, Pyfer HR, Trombold JC, Frederick RC (1976) Successful resuscitation of near simultaneous cases of cardiac arrest with review of fifteen cases occurring during supervised exercise. Circulation 53:187–189
5. Haskell WL (1978) Cardiovascular complications during exercise training of cardiac patients. Circulation 57:920–924
6. Van Camp SP, Peterson RA (1986) Cardiovascular complications of outpatient cardiac rehabilitation programs. JAMA 256:1160–1163
7. Hossack KF, Hartwig R (1982) Cardiac arrest associated with supervised cardiac rehabilitation. J Cardiac Rehabil 2:402–408
8. Williams RS, Miller H, Koisch FP Jr, Ribisl P, Graden H (1981) Guidelines for unsupervised exercise in patients with ischemic heart disease. J Card Rehabil 1:213–219
9. Miller HS Jr (1984) Supervised versus nonsupervised exercise rehabilitation of coronary patients. In: Wenger NK (ed.) Exercise and the Heart, 2nd ed, Cardiovascular Clinics, Philadelphia: FA Davis, pp 193–200
10. Gillilan RE, Chopra AK, Kelemen MH, Stewart KJ, Ewart CK, Kelemen MD, Valenti SA, Manley JD (1984) Prediction of compliance to target heart rate during walk-jog exercise in cardiac patients by a self-efficacy scale. Med Sci Sports Exerc 16:115
11. Fletcher GF, Chiaramida AJ, LeMay MR, Johnston BL, Thiel JE, Spratlin MC (1984) Telephonically-monitored home exercise early after coronary artery bypass surgery. Chest 86:198–202
12. DeBusk RF, Houston N, Haskell W, Fry G, Parker M (1979) Exercise training soon after myocardial infarction. Am J Cardiol 44:1223–1229
13. DeBusk RF, Haskell WL, Miller NH, Berra K, Taylor CB, in cooperation with Berger WE III and Lew H (1985) Medically directed at-home rehabilitation soon after clinically uncomplicated acute myocardial infarction: a new model for patient care. Am J Cardiol 55:251–257
14. Miller NH, Haskell WL, Berra K, DeBusk RF (1984) Home versus group exercise training for increasing functional capacity after myocardial infarction. Circulation 70:645–649
15. Schang SJ Jr, Pepine CP (1977) Transient asymptomatic ST segment depression during daily activity. Am J Cardiol 39:396–402
16. Deanfield JE, Shea M, Ribiero P, de Landsheere R, Wilson A, Horlock P, Selwyn AP (1984) Transient ST segment depression as a marker of myocardial ischemia during daily life. Am J Cardiol 54:1195–1200
17. Blackburn H, Taylor HL, Hamrell B, Buskirk E, Nicholas WC, Thorsen RD (1973) Premature ventricular complexes induced by stress testing. Their frequency and response to physical conditioning. Am J Cardiol 31:441–449

10. Ambulatory blood pressure

EDWARD BERNARD RAFTERY

Cardiology Department, Northwick Park Hospital & Clinical Research Centre, Watford Road, Harrow, Middlesex, HA1 3UJ, U.K.

Key words: ambulatory blood pressure

Abstract

Indirect methods of recording blood pressure suffer from all the known methodological inaccuracies of the Riva Rocci-Korotkoff technique, are slow-moving and are difficult to use for repeated measurements. Nevertheless, the causal indirect blood pressure has powerful predictive value for cardiovascular disease in populations. It is not known if the same applies to individuals, but it is thought that repeated measurements of ambulatory subjects are more likely to provide accurate prognostic information. There are some indications that this may be true, but the most valuable information on blood pressure and its variation has been provided by the Oxford technique for direct intra-arterial recording of blood pressure. The application of coherent averaging to data from these studies has allowed the description of a circadian rhythm of blood pressure and its reversal in central and peripheral autonomic denervation. Studies in chronic stable angina have outlined the essential differences between 'spontaneous' and induced angina, and studies in congestive heart failure have directed attention to the heart as a central regulator of the circulation. Attempts to develop indirect techniques which can match the direct technique for accuracy and speed have not been very successful, but indirect techniques must be the ultimate object of the research and development in this field.

Introduction

The measurement of blood pressure as an integral part of the physical examination first began about the turn of the century, although it had been realised for many years that there was a relationship between life expectancy and the tension of the pulse [1]. The indirect method of the Riva-Rocci cuff and the Korotkoff sounds enabled physicians to express blood

V. Hombach, H. H. Hilger and H. L. Kennedy (eds), Electrocardiography and Cardiac Drug Therapy. ISBN 978-94-010-6976-2
© 1989. Kluwer Academic Publishers, Dordrecht –

pressure as numerical values, and the advent of Life Insurance lead to a search for those observations made during physical examination, which carried the greatest degree of prognostic information. It was natural that much actuarial attention should have focussed on the blood pressure since it is one of the few items of clinical observation which can be expressed quantitatively and is therefore amenable to mathematical processing. It became rapidly apparent that blood pressure was a powerful indicator of life expectancy [2] and could be used to assess the chances of cardio-vascular disease with a high degree of accuracy in populations. However, it was not clear whether the same accuracy applied to the individuals who made up those populations, and physicians remained sceptical about the value of an indirect reading of blood pressure.

The reasons for this are readily apparent. The indirect technique is known to embrace a number of methodological uncertainties which have never been properly resolved. Thus, the relationship between cuff size and arm circumference remains undecided, there is still no satisfactory explanation for the 'silent gap', and the recommended auscultatory point for diastolic pressure changes every few years, depending upon the prevailing mood of Committees [3]. Under the very best conditions, there can still be a systematic difference between intra-arterial and indirect blood pressure of ±30/20 mmHg. It is impossible to know to what extent such a possible error may apply to any one reading. Furthermore, the indirect technique is static and slow-moving; it can only respond to events over a finite period of time, and cannot take phenomena such as the 'alerting reaction' [4] into account.

It was partially this scepticism which set the scene for the Platt vs Pickering controversy of the 1950's [5]. Platt maintained that hypertension was a disease entity which could be identified by bimodel population frequency curves, while Pickering maintained that levels of causal blood pressure were evenly distributed by a unimodal curve with a slight skew to higher levels induced by entities such as renal and adrenal hypertension. Pickering won the debate and the continuous distribution of blood pressure is now generally accepted.

But if causal blood pressure is normally distributed in populations, how is the practising physician to assess the prognostic value of any one indirect measurement?

Multiple measurements

It is logical that a single measurement of indirect blood pressure is not representative of blood pressure over a period of time. Repeated measurements are more likely to provide a representative mean reading and have a powerful appeal for the practising physician [6]. Most authorities [7] recommend that readings should be repeated at regular intervals on at least three occasions before any decisions are made, despite the lack of evidence that such a mean level contains any more (or less) prognostic information than the first causal reading.

Another approach to the same problem is typified by the work of Smirk and his co-workers [8]. They measured the blood pressure repeatedly under conditions of sedation and sensory deprivation and defined the lowest reading obtained in any one individual as the Basal blood pressure. The difference between this and the causal reading was defined as the Supplemental blood pressure. They produced evidence in a small number of patients [9] that the Basal blood pressure contained more prognostic power than the Supplemental, thereby introducing the idea that the time of day might have a significance in determining both the level and the prognostic importance of a blood pressure reading.

Ambulatory recording

The most significant advance in the direction of multiple recordings came with the development of indirect ambulatory blood pressure recording by Sokolow and his co-workers in San Franscisco [10]. They developed a portable recorder which utilised a microphone over the brachial artery and a manual inflate/deflate mechanism for a cuff around the arm. The Remler semi-automatic machine is the direct linear descendant of the Sokolow instrument, and has been supplemented by many other similar instruments, such as the Avionics and the Squibb instruments.

Using this semi-automatic instrument, Sokolow and his co-workers [11] produced evidence that the ambulatory blood pressure was a better predictor of target organ damage than the casual clinic blood pressure. It is noteworthy that they also found ambulatory and office pressures to be equal as predictors of future events; by the time they made this observation it was clear that active intervention could be effective in reducing the incidence of the cardio-vascular complications of hypertension, and it was no longer ethically reasonable to withhold treatment in order to test a scientific hypothesis. It is not likely that the superiority of ambulatory blood pressure, if it exists, will ever be clearly demonstrated.

And it is surprising that the Sokolow experiment produced the result that it did. All the available indirect ambulatory techniques use the same basic principles as the Riva Rocci-Korotkoff technique and must be open to the same inaccuracies. Furthermore, all indirect techniques involve the cessation of physical and mental activity during recording, and seldom give an accurate measurement of blood pressure during sleep.

Careful independent evaluations [12, 13] have shown that the Remler and Avionics systems are no more accurate than home recorded blood pressures. Furthermore [14], they are no better at replicating the results of continuous intra-arterial recordings, and may show some potentially serious deviations in directional movement of blood pressure. Attempts to devise a 'better' indirect technique in my own Department have met with little success. Despite the plethora of non-invasive reports [15] the unhappy truth is that these non-ivasive ambulatory techniques have lagged behind the invasive methods in precision and accuracy of results, and are likely to do so for some time.

Direct intra-arterial recordings

In contrast, direct methods of blood pressure recording have developed rapidly in sophistication and accuracy, but their invasive nature has precluded wide-spread application in clinical studies of blood pressure. Hence the significance of the method for direct ambulatory blood pressure recording developed by Scott and his co-workers [16] in the laboratories of Sir George Pickering at Oxford University in the 1960's. This technique has been developed and refined at Northwick Park Hospital and Clinical Research Centre, and is currently in routine use at three centres in the U.K., two centres in Italy, and one each in Australia and New Zealand. The technique is essentially a research tool, but has provided powerful patho-physiological information on blood pressure which was never previously available. Many studies have outlined the way in which blood pressure responds to the activities of daily life [17, 18], but the most important observations have stemmed from the application of statistical methods to the plethora of data obtained from such studies.

Blood pressure variability

One such study involved the application of coherent averaging to hourly means of systolic and diastolic blood pressure and heart beats in normal and hypertensive subjects which appeared to confirm the presence of a long-suspected circadian rhythm of blood pressure, with highest readings in the morning and the lowest during the night (Figure 1) [19]. The only signifi-

112

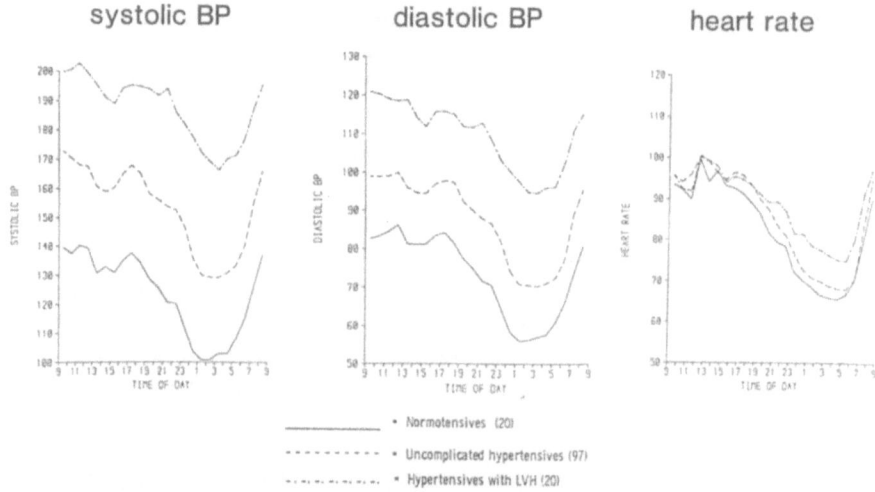

Figure 1. Circadian variation of blood pressure and heart rate in normotensive and hypertensive subjects, displayed by the technique of coherent averaging of hourly means. Note the two peaks of blood pressure and the rise before the hour of awakening. By way of contrast, heart rate peaks once, at a different time, and does not change until the time of awakening.

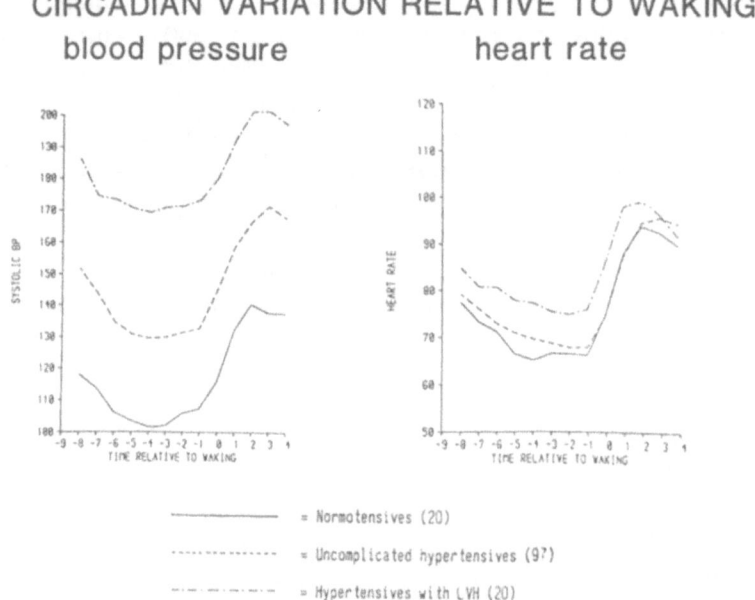

Figure 2. The same data as in Figure 1 orientated around the hour of awakening. Note that the rise of pressure is still present, but heart rate does not begin to change until the hour of awakening.

cant difference between the hypertensive and normal groups was a relative failure of the blood pressure to fall at night. Crucial to this description was the finding of a slow rise in pressure between the nadir at 03.00 hours and the rapid rise around the hour of awakening. Regrouping the data around the documented hour of awakening confirmed that this rise is a true event, and drew a sharp distinction between the behaviour of blood pressure and heart rate, which continues to fall throughout this time (Figure 2). Further observations confirmed that the rhythm of blood pressure is not a simple alternation of activity and inactivity [20] and recordings in patients with fixed-rate pacemakers [21] confirmed the divergence in behaviour of blood pressure and heart rate. These observations fit well with other evidence

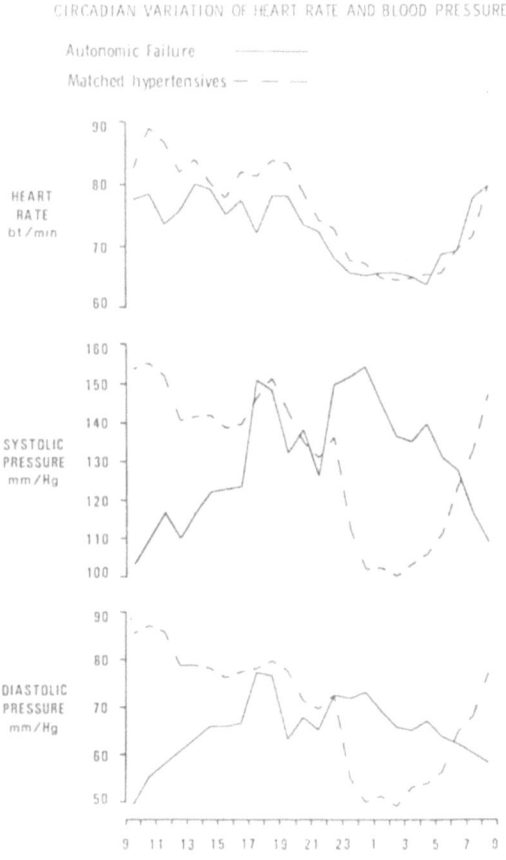

Figure 3. The circadian rhythm in a group of patients with Shy-Dragers Syndrome (central automatic denervation), compare with an age- and sex-matched group of hypertensive subjects. Note the complete inversion of the rhythm.

114

RHYTHMS OF BLOOD PRESSURE

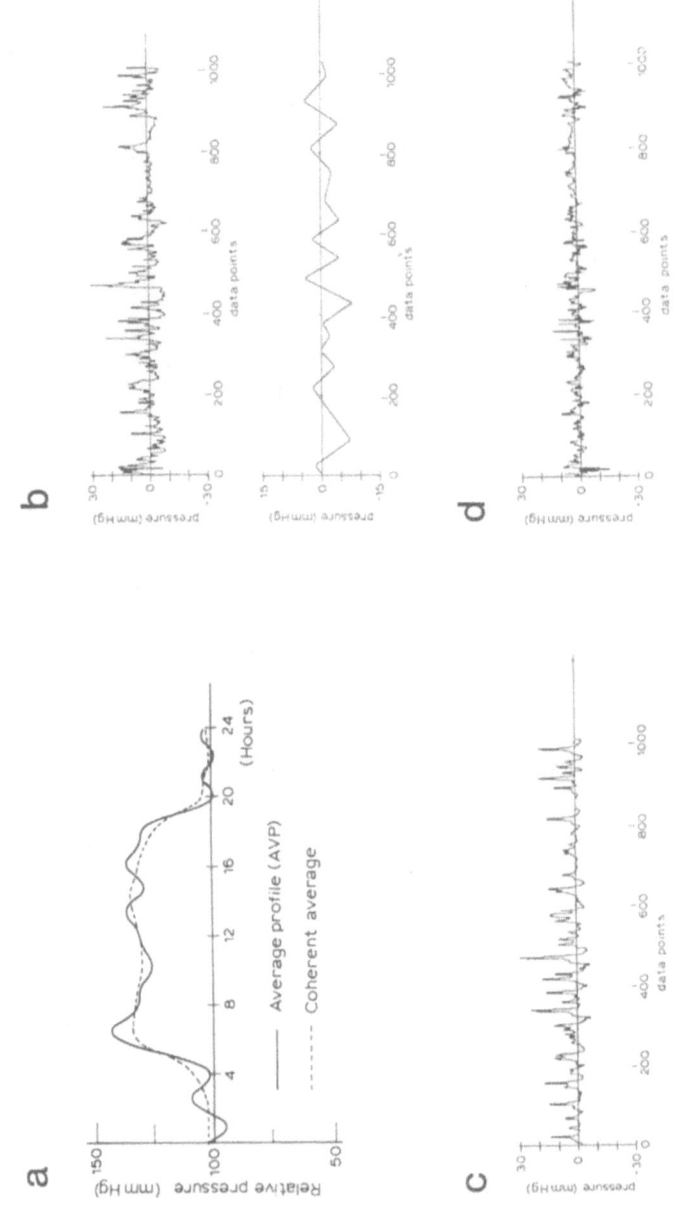

Figure 4. The four basic rhythms of blood pressure which have been described: *a* = circadian; *b* = slow baseline drift; *c* = rapid transients; *d* = vasomotor components.

[22] of increased sympathetic activity during the morining and have focussed attention upon the possibility that blood pressure may be reflecting a series of physiological events which might be responsible for the increased incidence of stroke [23] and myocardial infarction [24] at this time of day.

This conclusion was supported by the finding that central and peripheral sympathetic denervation produces a reversal of this rhythm [25], with highest pressures during the night and lowest during the day (Figure 3). This suggests that the sympathetic nervous system is imposing a rhythm upon the body which is a complete reversal of what would otherwise happen. The same effect has been reported in patients after heart transplant, which raises the interesting possibility that the drive for this sympathetic activity may be originating in the heart itself.

More sophisticated analysis [26] of 24-hour ambulatory intra-arterial studies has shown that four basic rhythms can be defined (Figure 4):

1. The 24-hour circadian rhythm;
2. Slow baseline fluctuations;
3. Rapid transients;
4. Cyclic variations due to respiration and baro-receptor adjustments.

The physiological significance of these rhythms and the role they play in the pathogenesis of cardiovascular disease remains to be defined.

Which blood pressure?

For the practising clinician, the question of prognosis still remains the most important issue in deciding the correct management for an individual patient. It has been repeatedly emphasised [27] that blood pressure alone is not the only factor to be considered in assessing the risk of cardio-vascular disease in an individual. Other factors such as smoking habits and blood cholesterol levels play an important part in such an assessment, but at the end of the day the blood pressure is still a powerful and independent predictor. However, there are indications that the number and the timing of recordings may increase predictive accuracy. A recent study [28] of the predictive accuracy of causal and 24-hour intra-arterial blood pressure recordings for target organ damage and cardio-vascular events over a one-year period has confirmed the power of causal blood pressure readings, but has also shown that the 24-hour mean blood pressure increases this power dramatically (Figure 5). The most interesting part of this study is the suggestion that the 24-hour mean is a better predictor of developing morbid events than the causal pressure. Breakdown of the 24-hour cycle

116

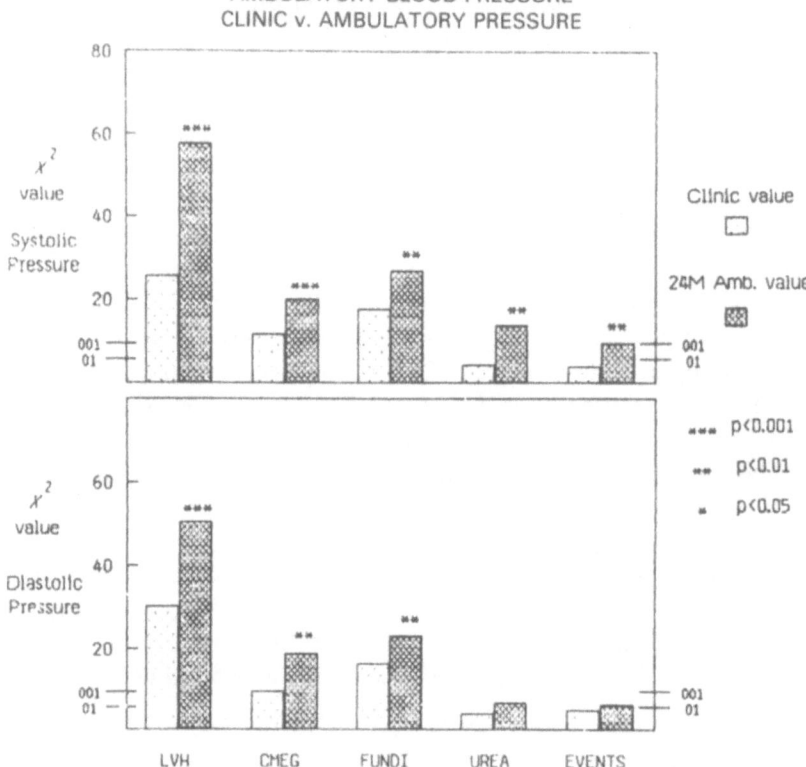

Figure 5. The predictive value of the causal and 24-hour intra-arterial blood pressure for target organ damage and morbid events. Note the power of the causal blood pressure, but the much greater power of the intra-arterial 24-hour mean pressure.

into four six-hour periods has shown that most of this predictive power resides in the mean pressures between 00.00 and 00.06 hours and 00.06 hours and 00.12 hours. This data supports the work of Smirk in stressing the importance of nocturnal blood pressure and must provide a powerful stimulus to the efforts to produce a method of accurately recording blood pressure at these times of day. This study is too small to be considered as aynthing but a 'pilot' but the findings are powerful enough to provoke a bigger and most intensive investigation; which has now been mounted.

Ischaemic heart disease

The technique of direct recording of ambulatory blood pressure has also been applied to studying the mechanisms of angina and silent myocardial

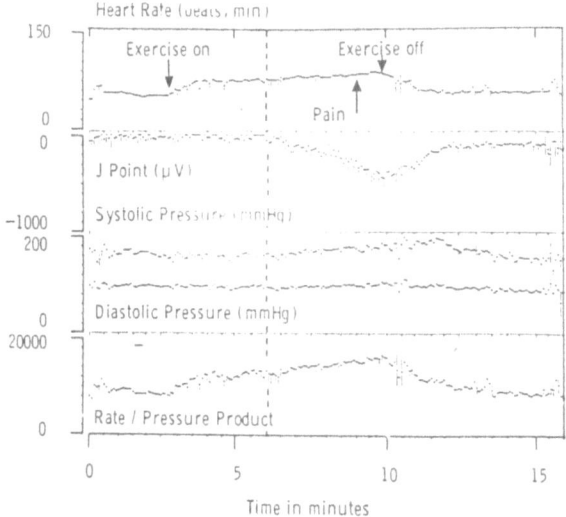

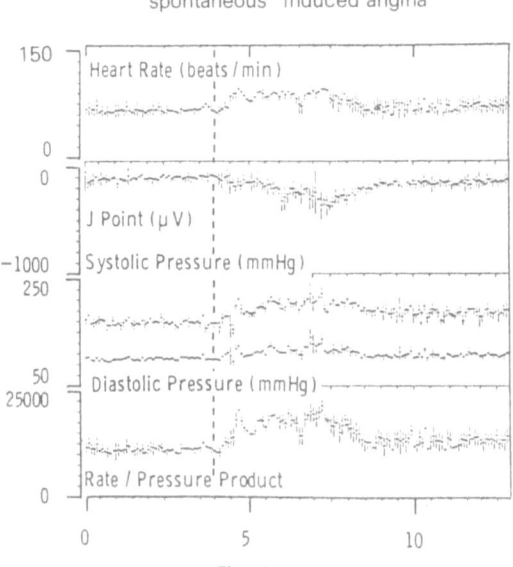

Figure 6. Trends of blood pressure, heart rate, ST segment and double product during exercise-induced and 'spontaneous' angina. Note that all the haemodynamic changes start after the onset of ST depression in 'spontaneous' angina.

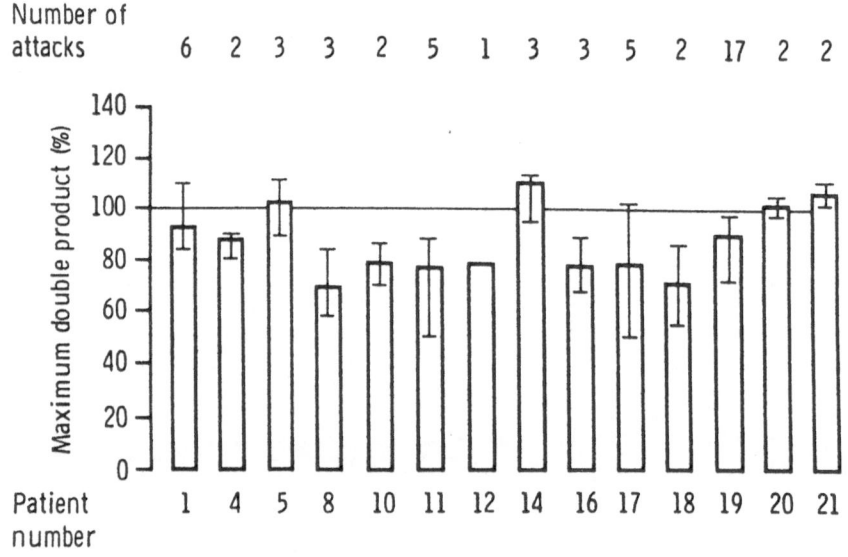

Figure 7. Maximal double product during 'spontaneous' angina expressed as a proportion of the double product during exercise-induced angina. The 'spontaneous' double product is usually less than the exercise induced value.

ischaemia [29]. A system for accurate simultaneous recording of the ST-segment of the electrocardiogram and systemic blood pressure on the same recorder has been devised and used to record the haemodynamic changes during exercise-induced and 'spontaneous' ischaemic episodes in patients with obstructive coronary artery disease. This study has clearly shown that the development of ischaemia in the two situations is very different (Figures 6 and 7). During exercise-induced angina, ST segment depression does not occur until significant changes in heart rate, blood pressure, and 'double product' are well established. During 'spontaneous' angina, none of these changes occur until after the ST segment has become depressed. Further-more, the peak double-product during 'spontaneous' angina is lower than during exercise-induced angina, and there are no significant differences between silent and painful episodes of ST-segment depression.

All of which indicates that the classical 'supply-and-demand' theory of obstructive coronary heart disease does not tell the whole story. Other mechanisms such as coronary spasm must also be at work, and these are bound to have important therapeutic implications for the management of ischaemic heart disease.

Heart failure

Similar studies of ambulatory blood pressure in patients with documented chronic heart failure due to ischaemic heart disease have clearly shown that the nocturnal fall in blood pressure is abolished under these circumstances. Coherent averaging imaging reveals a remarkably flat 24-hour cycle with little variation in blood pressure or heart rate. Furthermore, there is a significant relationship between the degree of myocardial damage, as measured by the resting ejection fraction and pulmonary capillary wedge pressure, and all the indices of blood pressure variability which have been devised to date (unpublished data). These findings lend strong support to the concept of the heart as a powerful central organ with a significant part to play in the regulation of the circulation. Recent attention to the endocrine function of the heart [30] points in the same direction.

Conclusions

The causal indirect blood pressure has undoubted power in the prediction of morbid cardiovascular events in populations, but there is considerable doubt about its value when applied to individuals. These doubts centre upon the known inherent inaccuracies of the technique and the feeling that the sample is not big enough to be 'representative'. There are indications that repeated ambulatory measurements give better prognostic information in individuals, but all the indirect methods of recording that have been described to date suffer from the inherent inaccuracies of the Riva Rocci-Korotkoff technique. The only accurate method available is the Oxford technique for ambulatory intra-arterial blood pressure recording. This has been successfully applied to normal and hypertensive subjects to describe the circadian rhythm of blood pressure and the changes produced by disease states.

Long term studies are emphasising the importance of nocturnal and morning blood pressures in the pathogenesis of cardiovascular disease states. The technique has also been applied to studies of angina and silent myocardial ischaemia which have highlighted the differences between ischaemia induced by exercise and that which occurs 'spontaneously' in a natural environment. Studies in heart failure have produced evidence which points to the heart as a central regulating organ in the circulation and not just a pump which responds to outside controlling influences. Despite the considerable contribution which the direct technique has made, it remains a research tool for application in only a few centres and strictly controlled conditions. The search for an equally accurate indirect method has not been very fruitful, but must go forward since the need for such a technique is self-evident.

References

1. Sigerist HE (1955) A History of Medicine. Vol. 1. Oxford: Oxford University Press, pp 311 and 329
2. Metropolitan Life Insurance Co (1961) Blood Pressure: Insurance experience and its implications, New York
3. Gould BA (1982) An evaluation of indirect methods of ambulatory blood pressure recording. M.D. Thesis, University of London, pp 54–55
4. Pickering GW (1968) High blood pressure. London: J & A Churchill Ltd., pp 15–17
5. Swales JD (1985) Platt vs Pickering: published by Keynes Press (BMA publication)
6. Raftery EB (1985) Hypertension: Who and when to treat. Update 155–158
7. Miall WE (1982) Screening for hypertension. British Journal Hospital Med: 592–594
8. Alam GM, Smirk FH (1943) Causal and basal blood pressures in British and Egyptian Men. British Heart J 5: 152–155
9. Smirk FH (1964) Observations on the mortality of 270 treated and 199 untreated grade 1 and 2 hypertensive patients followed in all instances for 5 years. New Zealand Medical J 63:413–443
10. Kain H, Hinman AT, Sokolow M (1964) Arterial blood pressure measurements with a portable blood pressure recorder in hypertensive patients. Circulation 30:882–892
11. Perloff D, Sokolow M, Cowan R (1983) The prognostic value of ambulatory blood pressures. Journal of the American Medical Association 249:2792–2798
12. Gould BA, Hornung RS, Kieso HA, Altman DG, Cashman PMM, Raftery EB (1984) Evaluation of the Remler M2000 Blood Pressure Recorder. Hypertension 6:209–215
13. Gould BA, Hornung RS, Cashman PMM, Altman D, Raftery EB (1986) An evaluation of the Avionics Pressurometer III 1978 at home and in hospital. Clinical Cardiology 9:335–343
14. Gould BA, Hornung RS, Keiso H, Cashman PMM, Raftery EB (1986) An evaluation of home-recorded blood pressures during drug trials. Hypertension 8:267–271
15. Fitzgerald DJ, O'Malley K, O'Brien ET (1983) Abulatory Blood Pressure in Non-monotensive and Hypertensive Subjects. In: Magometschrigg D, Hitzerbenger G (eds) Blood Pressure Variability. Vienna: Uhlen, pp 75–84
16. Bevan AT, Honour AJ, Stott FM (1969) Direct arterial blood pressure recording in unrestricted man. Clinical Science 36:329–344
17. Wertheimer L, Bandul I, Amarasinghe S (1977) Blood Pressure in normal subjects. Proc. Second International Symposium on Ambulatory Monitoring. London: Academic Press, pp 143–148
18. Littler WA, Honour AJ, Sleight P (1974) Direct arterial pressure, pulse rate, and electrocardiogram during micturation and defaecation in unrestricted man. American Heart J 88:205–210
19. Millar Craig MW, Bishop CN, Raftery EB (1978) Circadian variation of blood Lancet 1:795–797
20. Mann S, Millar Craig MW, Melville D, BalaSubramanian V, Raftery EB (1979) Physical activity and the circadian rhythm of blood pressure. Clinical Science 57:Suppl. 5, 375s–377s

21. Davies AB, Gould BA, Cashman PMM, Raftery EB (1984) Circadian rhythm of blood pressure in patients dependent on ventricular demand pacemakers. British Heart J 52:93–98

22. Turton MB, Deegan T (1974) Circadian variations of plasma catecholamines, cortisol, and concentrations in Supine subjects. Clinical Chim Acta 55:389–397

23. Bock KD, Kreuzenbeck W (1966) Spontaneous blood pressure variations in hypertension: the effect of anti-hypertensive therapy and correlations with the incidence of complications. In: Gross F (ed.) Anti-hypertensive therapy. Principles and Practice. Berlin: Springer, pp 224–228

24. Myers A, Dewar HA (1975) Circumstances attending 100 sudden deaths from coronary artery disease with Coroners Necropsies. British Heart Journal 37:1133–1143

25. Mann S, Altman D, Raftery EB, Bannister R (1983) Circadian variation of blood pressure in autonomic failure. Circulation 68:477–483

26. Sayers BMcA, Cicchiello LR, Raftery EB, Mann S, Green H (1982) The assessment of continuous ambulatory blood pressure records. Medical Informantics 7:2, 93–108

27. Kannel WB (1987) Current concepts of coronary risk factors. American College of Cardiology Learning Centre Highlights 2, No. 3

28. Mann S, Millar Craig MW, Raftery EB (1985) Superiority of 24-hour measurement of blood pressure over clinic values in determining prognosis in hypertension. Clinical and Experimental Hypertension 7:279–281

29. Davies AB, BalaSubramanian V, Cashman PMM, Raftery EB (1983) Simultaneous recording of continuous arterial pressure, heart rate, and ST segment in ambulant patients with stable angina pectoris. British Heart Journal 50:85–91

30. Rudolf EL, Unger T, Ganten D (1987) Atrial Natriuretic Peptide: a New Factor in Blood Pressure Control. Journal of Hypertension 5:255–272

11. Ambulatory recording of cardio-respiratory disorders: sleep apnea syndrome

JÖRG HERMANN PETER & PETER VON WICHERT

Medizinische Poliklinik, Zeitreihenanalyse, Baldingerstraße, D-3550 Marburg, F.R.G.

Introduction

The specific importance, which nocturnal disturbances of the respiratory regulation have for the wide range of cardiopulmonary and cardiovascular diseases, is only recently being recognized, although some of the pathophysiological interrelations indicating such a connection have long been familiar to physicians and researchers. It can be assumed that technical difficulties in obtaining continuous recordings of respiration—problems which could only recently be solved—were largely responsible for the delayed development in this field of research.

As early as 1917, Osler described the so-called Pickwickian Syndrome [1], and almost 40 years later, Burwell established this syndrome in the framework of internal medicine by describing it in terms of a combination of alveolar hypoventilation, cardiac insufficiency, hypertension, adipositas per magna, and hypersomnia [2]. It took the better part of a decade, until Jung and Kuhlo recognized sleep apnea as the principal mechanism in the development of the Pickwickian Syndrome [3]. Another ten years later, Coccagna described the hemodynamic changes in both circulatory systems during apnea [4]. In 1979, the American Society of Sleep Disorders Centers (ASDC) introduced a classification of the sleep/wake disorders, making the principal distinction between 'Difficulties of Excessive Sleepiness (DOES)' and 'Difficulties of Initiating and Maintaining Sleep (DIMS)' [5]. In 1982, Coleman reported first results of multi-center epidemiological studies, obtained by means of the ASDC classification [6]. It came as a surprise, that DOES were more frequent than DIMS, and that the most frequent cause for DOES was sleep apnea. In the meantime, many further studies have documented an increased general morbidity and mortality associated with nocturnal disturbances of the respiratory regulation, such as sleep apnea and snoring. As a consequence, internal medicine had to come to grips with the problem of to what extent sleep apnea and other sleep-

V. Hombach, H. H. Hilger and H. L. Kennedy (eds), Electrocardiography and Cardiac Drug Therapy. ISBN 978-94-010-6976-2
© 1989, Kluwer Academic Publishers, Dordrecht –

related breathing disorders had to be considered in the differential diagnosis of patients with wide-spread complaints such as essential hypertension, cardiac insufficiency, cardiac arrhythmias, obesity, polyglobulism, ventilatory insufficiency, and many more. Apart from technical difficulties regarding the measurement and recording of the relevant parameters, problems of definition constituted a severe obstacle for the inclusion of sleep-related breathing disorders in the diagnostic routines in internal medicine [7]. Concepts and definitions concerning snoring, for instance, are still widely divergent, although it is now an accepted view that snoring is a serious cardiovascular risk factor.

Sleep apnea: the clinical picture

Definitions

There are today universally accepted definitions and unequivocal descriptions of patterns characterizing the picture of sleep apnea [8, 9]. Three basic patterns of sleep apnea can be distinguished:

- *central sleep apnea* is characterized by complete cessation of muscular respiratory activity in thorax and abdomen as well as the absence of nasal airflow;
- *obstructive sleep apnea* is distinguished by obstruction of the upper airways and, in consequence, the absence of effective airflow and ventilation in spite of sustained respiratory efforts;
- *mixed apnea*, the most frequent form of sleep apnea, and almost the only one which is found in non-geriatric internal patients, is composed of both types, characteristically with an initial phase of central apnea, followed by a longer phase of the obstructive type.

Sleep Apnea Syndromes (SAS) include, by definition, all clinical pictures characterized by symptoms and clinical features which can be attributed to an elevated Apnea Index (Ai) and, vice versa, which can be reduced along with the therapeutical reduction of sleep apnea activity.

In terms of quantity, sleep apnea is defined according to the Apnea Index (Ai), i.e. the average number of apnea episodes of ≥ 10 s found in 1 h of sleep. Sleep apnea activity with an:

- $Ai < 5$ occurs in healthy persons and can be regarded as physiologically normal;
- $Ai \leq 5 < 10$ must be regarded as elevated sleep apnea activity, bordering

on a pathological result. Careful consideration of accompanying clinical results and diagnostic checks at regular intervals are recommended;
- Ai ≥ 10 is clinically relevant sleep apnea activity with a high probability of internal complications and serious long-term effects.

Extreme results of Ai > 50 and an absolute number of apnea episodes exceeding 500 per night have been documented.

Symptoms and clinical findings

Sleep apnea is characteristically accompanied by symptoms of psychomental alterations as a consequence of sleep fragmentation. These symptoms are therefore not confined to sleep apnea alone, they can be the consequence of any events which constitute repeated and profound disturbances of the natural sleep structure [10]. These psychomental symptoms include depression, sexual dysfunction, difficulties in maintaining concentration, and difficulties of daytime somnolence. The only symptom in the field of general internal medicine is cardiac insufficiency. In a study of 60 patients with sleep apnea, including right heart catheterization, Podszus found elevated pulmonary artery pressure values under exertion in every second patient. These findings could neither be explained on the basis of lung function test results, nor left ventricular function findings [11].

The characteristic clinical findings in patients with sleep apnea are arterial hypertension as well as cardiac arrhythmias during the night. Obesity and polyglobulism have also been reported as characteristic findings. According to our experiences, however, their frequency seems to be overrated [7]. Motz and coworkers [12] found a significantly high proportion of dilatative hypertrophy in patients with systemic hypertension and sleep apnea, while Wittig, in his doctoral dissertation [13], found an elevated apnea index in 40% of patients with dilatative cardiomyopathy. High coincidence rates between nocturnal cardiac arrhythmias and sleep apnea have also been reported [14].

Therapy

If diagnosed early enough, sleep apnea can today be successfully treated, and all symptoms and results originating in apnea activity can be completely reversed. The treatment of choice in cases of pronounced sleep apnea is nasal continuous positive airway pressure (nCPAP) therapy. With this form of treatment, normal room air is continuously administered to the patient during sleep via a tight-fitting nose-mask at a pressure of 5–15 mbar. The stimulus exerted by this airflow is sufficient to eliminate the disturbances of the respiratory regulation and their consequences [15].

Table 1. List of therapeutical steps and options in the treatment of sleep apnea

A. Influencing the patient's behavior	1. Weight reduction
	2. Avoidance of sleep loss
B. To be avoided	1. All Medication reinforcing sleep-related breathing disorders
	2. Medication increasing inclination of falling asleep
	3. Medication accelerating the process of falling asleep
	4. Alcohol before going to bed
	5. Substances amplifying myocardial insufficiency and lowering heart rate
C. Medication	1. Theophyllines
	2. Methyl-progesterone
	3. Protriptylin
D. Surgical treatment	1. Oropharyngeal surgery (tonsillectomy etc.)
	2. Tracheostomy
E. Effective conservative treatment	Nasal continuous positive airway pressure therapy (nCPAP)

Table 1 summarizes the therapeutical options, which range from behavioral advice to the patient to surgical intervention and nCPAP therapy, which can today be regarded as the most effective form of treatment. Thus, Mayer was able to show that apnea-related blood pressure elevations can be reversed by nCPAP therapy, including not only acute pressure increases during the night, but also presenting daytime pathological changes in terms of essential systemic arterial hypertension [16]. Under aspects of prevention and therapy, the relationship between sleep apnea and essential hypertension will surely be of primary importance to the cardiologist [17].

Figures reported on the prevalence of sleep apnea still vary in the literature. Depending on the individual approach, prevalence rates of increased sleep apnea activity between 1% and 10% among males have been documented [7].

Diagnostics

Indications for diagnostic recordings

The necessity of timely recognition of sleep apnea follows from the high prevalence of this clinical picture and its connection with severe cardiovascular and cardiorespiratory sequelae, on the one hand, and from the fact that it is basically treatable if diagnosed early enough. The indications for diagnostic recordings are listed in Table 2.

126

Table 2. Catalogue of indications for apnea diagnostics

A. For differential diagnosis in cases of
   systemic arterial hypertension;
   - chest pains or cardiac insufficiency without apparent cause;
   - cardiac arrythmias, predominantly occurring at night;
   - nocturnal sinus arrhythmia;
   - polycythemia;
   - overweight;
   - psychomental impairments (decline in performance and capacities); fatigue;
   - nocturnal dyspnea;
   - nocturnal seizures;
   - loud and irregular snoring.
B. In search of a factor liable to complicate actual state, development, and therapy in
   - all cardiovascular diseases;
   - cardiorespiratory diseases.

The portable 4-channel recorder

As sleep laboratory polysomnography is too complicated and expensive for early diagnostics, we looked for a more flexible approach in 1981, developing a portable unit for ambulatory use in the wide range of internal medicine. Equipped with an Oxford-Medilog-4-24-Recorder, it permits synchronized recordings of ECG, thoracic and abdominal respiratory activities by means of inductive plethysmography, and partial arterial O_2-tension, measured transcutaneously and recorded together with a clock on the fourth channel [18, 19]. The diagnostic unit combines safe recognition of sleep apnea with the advantages of long-term recording under home care conditions.

A diagnostic unit based on ECG and breathing sounds analysis

According to the manufacturers of medical equipment, the continuous transcutaneous recording of blood gases which we employed in our 4-channel recorder was too complicated for routine applications and wide-scale screening. We therefore developed a less complicated screening device based on recordings of heart rate, which is automatically calculated beat-to-beat, and of laryngeal breathing sounds, facilitating the recording of characteristic snoring sounds by means of appropriate frequency filters. The analysis of these two parameters permits the detection of sleep apnea [20]. Figure 1 shows a sample recording, illustrating the characteristic peaks in low frequent sounds which are associated with the onsets and the termination of obstructive apnea episodes, and the characteristic ups and

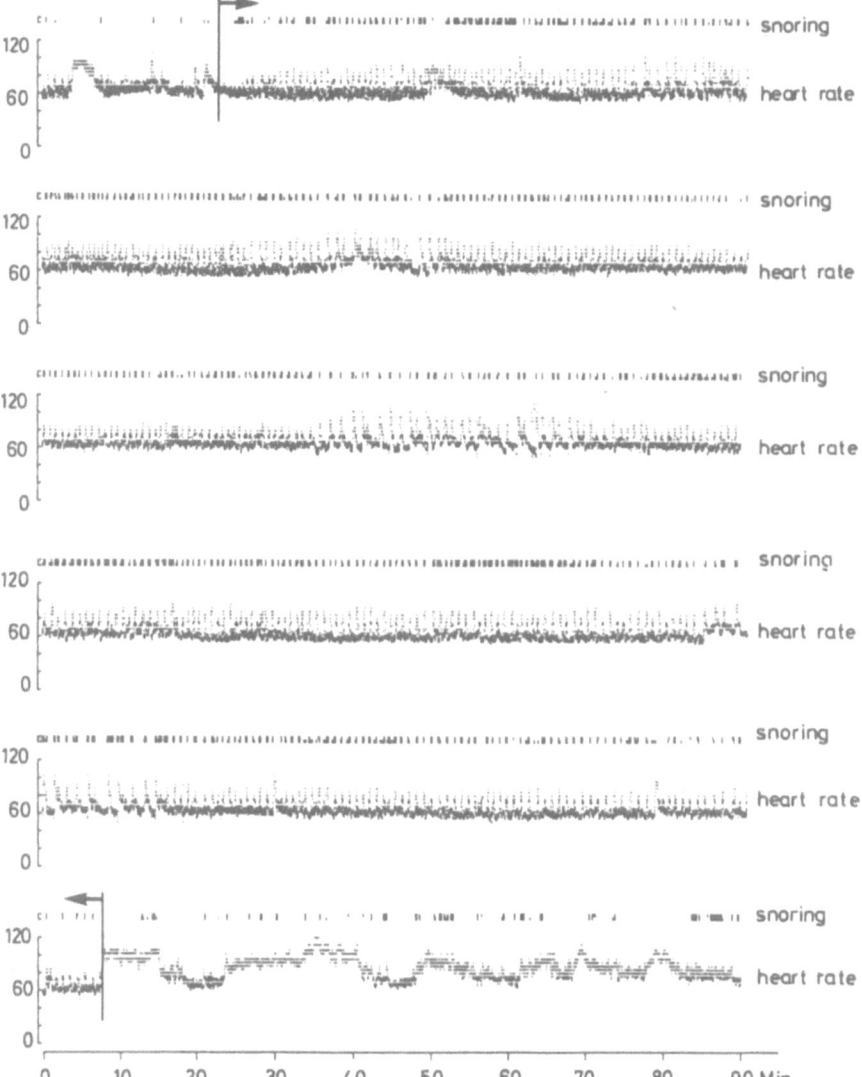

Figure 1. Example of a recording made with the newly developed diagnostic unit combining recordings of snoring and beat-to-beat heart rate variability: full disclosure record of a patient with pronounced sleep apnea. Peaks in heart rate synchronized with bursts of snoring indicate sleep apnea. Onset of sleep and of wakefulness are indicated.

downs in heart rate which are synchronized with the pattern of apnea and intermittent compensatory respiration, while Figure 2 shows a detail from the same recording. In combination with an anamnestic questionnaire, this new technique is the first method to permit successful apnea screening on a

128

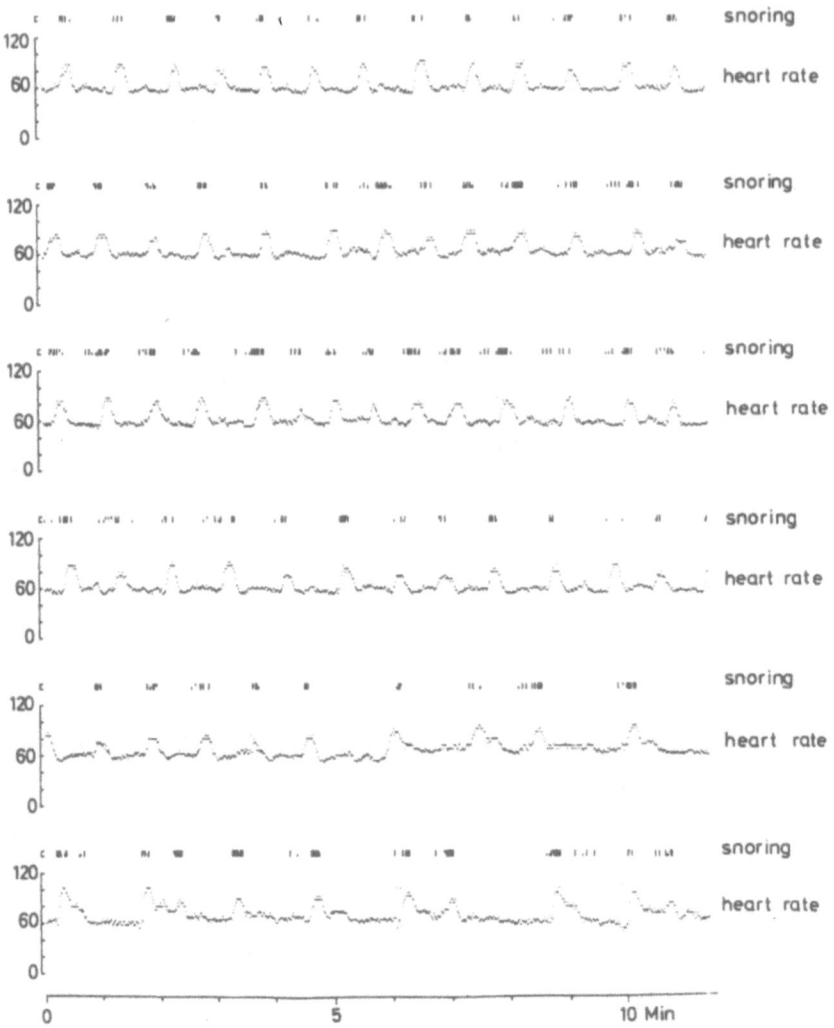

Figure 2. Excerpt from a recording similar to the one in Figure 1, illustrating extreme heart rate variability and repetitive heavy snoring. Snoring filter signal and heart rate variability permit safe apnea recognition.

large scale [21]. The standardized questionnaire includes items regarding altered sleep/wake behavior during day and night, the main sequelae, as well as relevant data for differential diagnosis. The questionnaire has by now been passed as an official instrument of inquiry by the German Society of Pneumology and Tuberculosis [22].

Table 3. Diagnostic parameters in a hierarchical scheme of extended sleep apnea diagnostics, including a standardized anamnestic inquiry, ambulatory apnea recording, and clinical examinations

A) Sleep/wake behavior	Patient's report (questionnaire), including time in bed; reported sleep period; vigilance and performance during the day;
B) Breathing	Patient's report (questionnaire); Number and type of apneas; Hypoventilation; Duration of these events; Pattern of intermittent breathing; Respiratory rate; Thoraco-abdominal motion/(de-)synchronized breathing); Snoring (obstructive)
C) Standardized risk factor profile	History (anamnestic questionnaire); Standardized clinical investigations: Risk factor screening (bodyweight, blood lipids, blood sugar, uric acid, general laboratory status); ECG at rest and during exercise; Long-term ECG; Echocardiography; Right heart catherization, if indicated; Lung function test; Blood gases during the day; ENT examinations; Neuropsychiatric examination.

Extended diagnostics

Both the ambulatory diagnostic unit and the questionnaire form part of a hierarchical diagnostical scheme, the main steps of which are listed in Table 3.

It is only in cases of problems of differential diagnosis which can not be reliably solved on the basis of these easy-to-use diagnostic instruments, that classical full-scale polysomnography in the sleep laboratory becomes necessary. The new techniques of ambulatory non-invasive cardiorespiratory monitoring offer a chance to cardiologists, pneumologists, and general internists to consider the nocturnal disturbances of the respiratory regulation within the framework of their diagnostic routines in a way which, for the first time, reflects their actual epidemiological and pathogenetic relevance.

130

References

1. Osler W (1918) The principles and practice of medicine. Eighth edition. New York: Appleton
2. Burwell CS, Robin ED, Whaley RD, Bickelmann AG (1956) Extreme obesity associated with alveolar hypoventilation—A Pickwickian syndrome. Am J Med 21:811–818
3. Jung R, Kuhlo W (1965) Neurophysiological studies of abnormal night sleep and the Pickwickian syndrome. Progr Brain Res 18:140–159
4. Coccagna G, Mantovani M, Brignani F, Parchi C, Lugaresi E (1972) Continuous recording of the pulmonary and systemic arterial pressure during sleep in syndromes of hypersomnia with periodic breathing. Bull Physiopathol Respir 8:1159–1172
5. Association of Sleep Disorder Centers (1979) Diagnostic classification of sleep and arousal disorders. Sleep 2:1–137
6. Coleman RM, Roffwarg HP, Kennedy SJ (1982) Sleep-wake disorders based on a polysomnographic diagnosis. A national cooperative study. JAMA 247:997–1003
7. Peter JH (1984) Klinik der Hypersomnien. Internist 25:547–551
8. Guilleminault C, Dement WC (1978) Sleep apnea syndrome and related sleep disorders. In: Williams R, Karacan I (eds) Sleep Disorders: Diagnosis and Treatment, New York: Wiley, pp 9–28
9. Strohl KP, Saunders NA, Sullivan CE (1984) Sleep apnea syndromes. In: Saunders NA, Sullivan CE (eds) Sleep and Breathing. New York: Dekker, pp 365–402
10. Lavie P (1980) Sleep disturbances in industrial workers. Sleep Res 9:209–221
11. Podszus T, Becker H (1987) The prevalence of increased pulmonary arterial pressure among sleep apneics. In: Peter JH, Podszus T, V. Wichert P (eds) Sleep Related Disorders and Internal Diseases. Berlin – Heidelberg – New York: Springer, pp 241–247
12. Motz W, Bethge C, Klepzig M, Blanke H, Strauer BE (1987) Echocardiographic findings in sleep apnea. In: Peter JH, Podszus T, V. Wichert P (eds) Sleep Related Disorders and Internal Diseases. New York – Heidelberg: Springer, pp 326–329
13. Wittig G (1987) Schlafapnoe bei Patienten mit echokardiographisch gesicherter, erheblicher Kontraktilitätsstörung des Herzens. Inaugural-Dissertation, Marburg.
14. Köhler U, Becker H, Borrmann R, Faust M, Himmelmann H, Liesendahl K, Peter JH, V. Wichert P (1987) Das EKG bei Patienten mit schlafbezogenen Atemregulationsstörungen—Seine Stellung in Diagnostik und Therapie. Prax Klin Pneumol (im Druck)
15. Becker H, Figura M, Himmelmann H, Köhler U, Peter JH, Retzko R, Schwarzenberger F, Weber K, V. Wichert P (1987) Die nasale 'Continuous Positive Airway Pressure' (nCPAP)—Therapie—Praktische Erfahrungen bei 54 Patienten, Prax Klin Pneumol (im Druck)
16. Mayer J, Becker H, Köhler U, Penzel T, Peter JH, Weber K, V. Wichert P (1987) Variabilität von arteriellem Blutdruck und Herzfrequenz bei Schlafapnoe. Prax Klin Pneumol (im Druck)
17. Peter JH (1986) Hat jeder dritte Patient mit essentieller Hypertonie ein undiagnostiziertes Schlafapnoe-Syndrom? DMW 111: 556–559
18. Peter JH, Becker I, Fuchs E, Meinzer K, V. Wichert P (1982) Ambulante transkutane Langzeitregistrierung von arterieller Sauerstoffspannung und Herzrhythmusströungen bei Patienten mit Schlaf-Apnoe-Syndrom. Verh Dt Ges Inn Med 88:390–394
19. Peter JH (1985) Holter monitoring technique in a comprehensive approach: Ambulatory monitoring of sleep apnea. In: Hombach V, Hilger HH (eds) Holter monitoring technique. Stuttgart – New York: Schattauer, pp 127–149
20. Peter JH, Fuchs E, Hügens M, Köhler U, Meinzer K, Müller U, V. Wichert P, Zahorka M

(1987) An apnea-monitoring device based on variation of heart rate and snoring. In: Peter JH, Podszus T, V. Wichert P (eds) Sleep Related Disorders and Internal Diseases. Berlin – Heidelberg – New York: Springer, pp 140–146

21. Penzel T, Amend G, Peter JH, Podszus T, V. Wichert P, Zahorka M (1987) Objective monitoring of therapeutical success in heavy snorers: a new technique. Proceedings of 1st International Congress on Chronic Rhonchopathy, Paris, July (forthcoming)

22. Siegrist J, Peter JH, Himmelmann H, Geyer S (1987) Erfahrungen mit einem Anamnesebogen zur Diagnostik der Schlafapnoe. Prax Klin Pneumol (im Druck).

12. Long-term spontaneous variability of simple and complex ventricular ectopy

GEORG SCHMIDT, KURT ULM[1], LISELOTTE GOEDEL-MEINEN, GABRIELE JAHNS, PETRA BARTHEL, BERND STIEF & ULRICH SCHAUDIG

Department of Cardiology, 1st Department of Internal Medicine, and [1]Institute for Epidemiology and Biomedical Statistics, Technische Universität München, F.R.G.

Introduction

Spontaneous variability in the frequency of single and complex forms of ventricular arrhythmia has long been considered a major problem in evaluating long-term antiarrhythmic drug efficacy [1].

Most of the calculations in so far published studies are based on the results of two or three Holter-ECGs, recorded either successively or separated by several days. In the present article, the influence of the period of time between two Holter ECG registrations (i.e. the control interval CI) on the spontaneous variability (SV) and on the criteria calculated to assess the effect of antiarrhythmic treatment is systematically studied.

Patients

A total of 444 Holter ECGs were obtained from 59 male and 21 female patients with a mean age of 55.8 ± 12.1 years. The underlying heart disease was CHD in 43 (left ventricular ejection fraction $45 \pm 15\%$) and dilative cardiomyopathy in 47 patients (LVEF $35 \pm 12\%$). 16 patients had a history of syncope and 7 patients had undergone cardiopulmonary resuscitation. 35 patients had a history of myocardial infarction, 10 had had an operation for a coronary artery bypass graft. The mean hourly frequency ($\pm$SD) of ventricular arrhythmia was 345.6 ($\pm$390.2) for single VPCs, 17.7 ($\pm$35.4) for CPLs and 4.3 ($\pm$19.5) for Salvos.

38 patients received no antiarrhythmic treatment at all over the whole observation period. 52 patients were treated with antiarrhythmic drugs for severe hemodynamic complications such as syncopes, because they had a history of cardiopulmonary resuscitation, or because they participated in a clinical drug trial. Control Holter ECGs in these patients were registered

V. Hombach, H. H. Hilger and H. L. Kennedy (eds), Electrocardiography and Cardiac Drug Therapy. ISBN 978-94-010-6976-2
© 1989, Kluwer Academic Publishers, Dordrecht –

both prior to treatment and in drug-free states during follow-up (the interval between final drug administration and control was at least 5 days). 23 patients were on β-blocker therapy prior to the study and remained on this medication. All patients were controlled by ambulatory Holter monitoring during regular outpatient visits. Patient follow-up consisting of 3-12 Holter-ECGs (mean 4.2) was carried out over an average of 181 ± 297 days.

Methods

24-hour Holter monitoring was done with the ICR-7200 recorder; the tapes were automatically analyzed by the ICR 6201-G-3 arrhythmia computer, a device that had been shown to have a sensitivity of >96% and a predective accuracy of >94% in detecting single and repetitive VPCs [2]. In addition, all recordings were printed out in a miniature form and subjected to exact manual counts.

Calculation of spontaneous variability

In each recording the degree of arrhythmia was expressed by the mean hourly VPC, CPL and Salvos rate. The variability between two Holter ECGs was defined as the logarithm of the quotient: mean hourly frequency day 2 $(n + K)$ over mean hourly frequency day 1 $(n + K)$. The constant K added was 1 for VPCs and 0.01 for CPLs and Salvos. Variability quotients close to 0 thus indicate stable ectopy rates at the two different days, while quotients far from 0 indicate unstable rates, i.e. high spontaneous variability.

The spontaneous distribution of variability quotients was defined separately as the mean ± 2 standard deviations (SD) for each of four ranges of control intervals, from 0 to 6 days, 7 to 89 days, 90 to 364 days and over 364 days. For each range of control intervals we separately calculated the criteria required to distinguish antiarrhythmic drug effects from spontaneous variation.

In determining the per cent change (C) in VPC, CPL and salvos frequency necessary to secure an effective reduction (R) at a given probability margin of 95%, we used the formula:

$$CR(\%) = 100 - 10^{-2SD} \cdot 100$$

whereas the per cent change necessary to prove aggravation (A) of

134

arrhythmia was assessed by the formula:

$$CA(\%) = 100 + 10^{+2SD} \cdot 100.$$

Results

The overall arrhythmia rate remained unchanged in the whole group; this was indicated by the fact that the sum of all variability quotients was almost 0 over the whole observation period.

Spontaneous variability between two recordings was strongly influenced by the length of the control interval. Figures 1–3 show the different results for single VPCs, CPLs and Salvos. With short control intervals the spontaneous variability of VPC and CPL counts was rather small, but increased continuously with longer control intervals. The area of confidence became larger and higher changes in arrhythmia counts were thus necessary to establish antiarrhythmic or proarrhythmic drug effects.

Table 1 shows the criteria for the validation of antiarrhythmic drug effects at different control intervals. Antiarrhythmic treatment is considered to be effective during the first week if VPCs ar reduced at least by 63% and CPLs by 90%. However, control intervals between one week and three months require reductions of 81% and 96%, respectively, intervals between three months and one year require 93% and 99%, intervals over 1 year 98% and 100%.

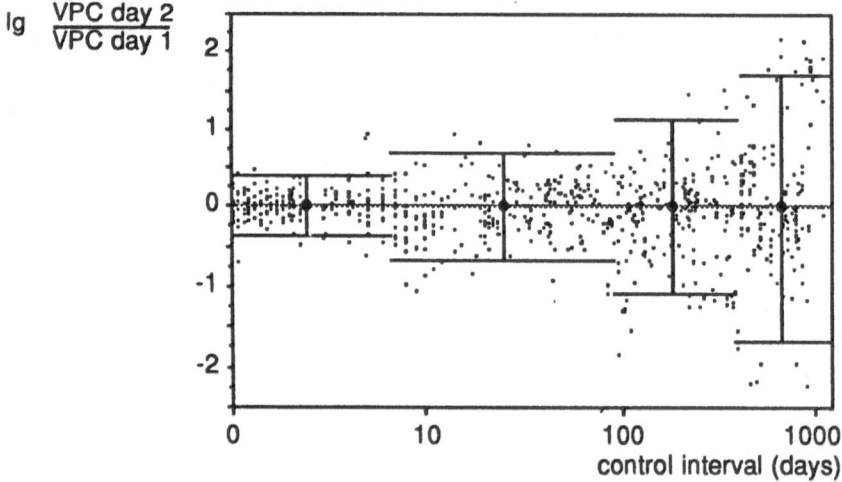

Figure 1. Spontaneous variability of single VPCs as detected at different control intervals. Data points mark the log quotient of the mean hourly frequency at day 2 $(n+1)$ over day 1 $(n+1)$.

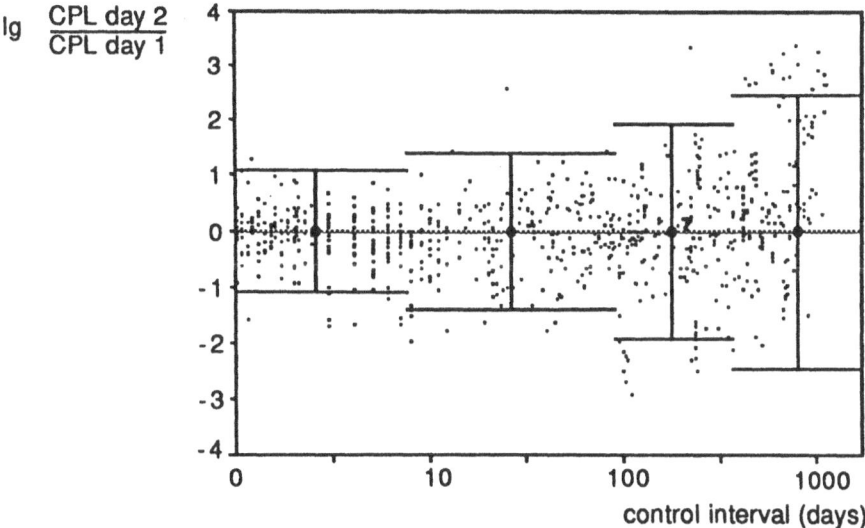

Figure 2. Spontaneous variability of CPLs as detected at different control intervals. Data points mark the log quotient of the mean hourly frequency at day 2 ($n = 0.01$) over day 1 ($n + 0.01$).

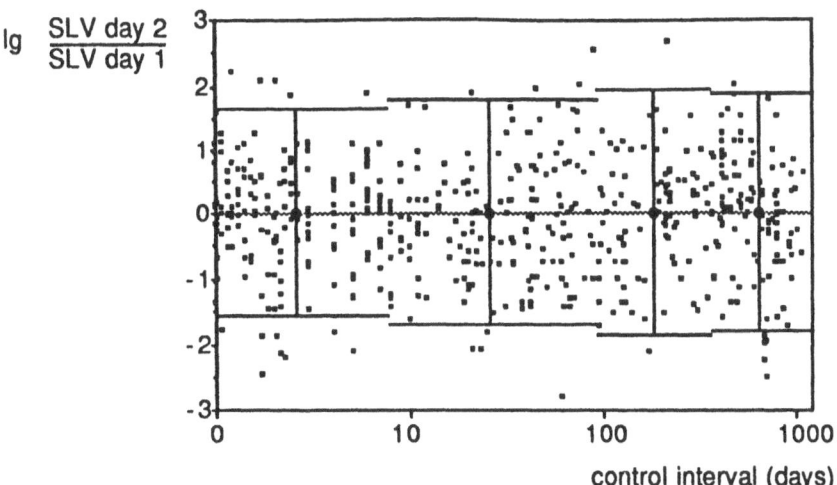

Figure 3. Spontaneous variability of salvos as detected at different control intervals. Data points mark the log quotient of the mean hourly frequency at day 2 ($n + 0.01$) over day 1 ($n + 0.01$).

The percentage of VPC-count increase considered to be drug-induced has to be over 269% (1037%) during the first week and this margin increases continuously with longer control intervals, to 525% (2322%) from 1 week to 3 months, 1242% (8790%) from 3 months to 1 year and 5081% (24660%) over 1 year.

The results of the studies about ventricular salvos were somewhat different. Maybe for their lower frequency is the occurrence of salvos not equally strong influenced by the length of the control interval; the reduction (aggravation) required to prove a drug effect changed only slightly with the different control intervals: 98% at CIs of 0 to 6 and 7 to 89 days (4808 and 5808%), 99% at CIs of 90 to 364 and over 364 days (6982 and 6637%).

To determine the influence of the underlying heart disease on these observations, we separately studied the variability in patients with CHD and cardiomyopathy. We found no obvious differences between these groups at control intervals up to 3 months, but over longer control intervals the CHD group tended to have an even higher VPC and CPL count variability than the cardiomyopathy group.

Discussion

While spontaneous variability in short control intervals has repeatedly been the subject of intensive studies [3–7] it remains unclear how criteria derived from short term observations can be used for long term treatment. In a recently published article, Pratt et al. [8] studied 26 clinically stable patients during two periods of placebo treatment separated by 17 months and observed high spontaneous changes in the frequency of arrhythmia. It was concluded that investigators could thus be mislead regarding the evaluation of antiarrhythmic drug efficacy but no definite recommendations concerning adequate criteria were made.

Based on our data we have for the first time been able to calculate criteria for the evaluation of chronic antiarrhythmic drug effects at different times after initiating the treatment. Our data support the presumption that spontaneous variability increases extensively and that criteria for the evaluation of drug effects become more rigid with longer control intervals. Not unexpectedly, we could see a higher influence of the CI on the variability of single VPC and CPL frequency than on the variability of ventricular salvos. In our patient group the frequency of salvos in 24 hour Holter ECGs changed strongly no matter how long the period of time between two registrations was. A total suppression of ventricular salvos was thus required to distinguish drug effects from spontaneous variation at all control intervals. Spontaneous variability of single

Table 1. Criteria for the evaluation of antiarrhythmic drug efficacy; reductions (RQ) and aggravations (AQ) (in per cent of a baseline recording) required to distinguish drug effects from spontaneous variability at different control intervals

Control interval (days):		0–6	7–89	90–364	≥365
RQ(%)	for VPCs:	−63	−81	−93	−98
	for Cpl:	−90	−96	−99	−100
	for Slv:	−98	−98	−99	−99
AQ(%)	for VPCs:	+269	+525	+1242	+5081
	for Cpl:	+1037	+2322	+8790	+24660
	for Slv:	+4808	+5808	+6982	+6637

VPCs and CPLs increased with the length of the CI and the per cent reduction required to prove a drug effect changed from 63% (90% for CPLs) at intervals between 0–6 days to 81% (96%), 93% (99%) and 98% (100%) at longer intervals; similar patterns could be found for the assessment of drug induced aggravations (Table 1). While we arrived at the four divisions of the control intervals arbitrarily, several considerations speak strongly for this scheme. First, the intervals one week, three months, one year and over one year roughly correspond with common clinical patterns. More importantly perhaps, a curve delineating the range of the data points over time can be best approximated by the divisions we chose (as seen in the figures).

However, any selected division does not affect the absolute distribution of the data points, but rather serves only to simplify clinical application of these observations.

We consider the results of our study to be of major clinical interest, for they mean that it is extremely difficult to evaluate drug effects in a majority of patients after more than three months and almost impossible after one year of therapy. This has to be considered in clinical practice as well as in the design of future drug trials dealing with chronic antiarrhythmic drug efficacy. Our data indirectly support the call for regular reassessments of baseline arrhythmia in order to prove chronic efficacy. When the effect of drugs with long half lives (e.g. Amiodarone) is evaluated, accurate evaluation might even be impossible after duration of therapy over more than 3 months.

References

1. Winkle RA (1978) Antiarrhythmic drug effect mimicked by spontaneous variability of ventricular ectopy. Circulation 57:1116–1120

2. Schmidt G, Goedel-Meinen L, Weixel G, Jahns G, Ulm K (1986) Analysegenauigkeit des Holter-Systems ICR 6201-G3. Z Kardiol 57:211–214
3. Michelson EL, Morganroth J (1980) Spontaneous variability of complex ventricular arrhythmias detected by long-term electrocadiographic recording. Circulation 61:690–695
4. Morganroth J, Michelson EL, Horowitz LN, Josephson ME, Pearlmann S, Dunkman B (1978) Limitation of routine long-term electrocardiographic recording to assess ventricular ectopic frequency. Circulation 58:408–414
5. Sami M, Kraemer H, Harrison DC, Houston N, Chimaski S, DeBusk RF (1980) A new method for evaluating antiarrhythmic drug efficacy. Circulation 62:1172–1179
6. Schmidt G, Ulm K, Goedel-Meinen L, Jahns G, Barthel P, Klein G, Wirtzfeld A, Baedeker W (1986) Z Kardiol 75:156–160
7. Andresen D, Leitner R v, Wegscheider K, Schröder R (1984) Neue Methode zur Beurteilung eines antiarrhythmischen Therapieerfolges und eines paradoxen arrhythmogenen Medikamenteneffekts beim Einzelpatienten. Z Kardiol 73:492–497
8. Pratt CM, Slymen DJ, Wierman AM, Young JB, Francis MJ, Seals AA, Quinones MA, Roberts R (1985) The changing baseline of complex ventricular arrhythmias: A new consideration in assessing long-term antiarrhythmic drug therapy. Am J Cardiol 56:66–72

Part III: High Resolution Electrocardiography

13. Detection of his bundle potentials

RICHARD VINCENT

Department of Cardiology, Royal Sussex County Hospital, Eastern Road, Brighton BN2 5BE, U.K.

Abstract

Conducting system potentials were first recovered from the body surface in dogs in 1973 using a sequence of high-gain amplification and filtering followed by digital signal averaging. Subsequent application of similar methods to man by more than 18 research groups world-wide have shown it feasible to record His Purkinje signals non-invasively in about 75% of subjects studied. Surface signals are of the order of 0.5–2.0 μV in amplitude. In 70–100% of cases they correlate well in time with the simultaneous internal His bundle electrogram but the pattern of surface signals varies from patient to patient. Their appearance fails to correlate with any specific underlying pathological change in AV conduction and is affected both by lead position and as a result of filtering. "High resolution" recordings made without signal averaging have been achieved in a few centres but with greater technical difficulty and a lower rate of signal recovery.

Patients most suitable for investigation by commercially available devices for surface His bundle electrocardiography are those with a prolonged PR interval or who are receiving drugs that depress His Purkinje conduction. The surface recording of His Purkinje signals is unlikely to become a widely used and routine technique until further technical improvements can be made in its methodology.

Introduction

The detection of His bundle potentials from the body surface presents a challenge to the engineer and cardiologist alike. The technical challenge is to recover microvolt signals of unknown shape, timing, and vector from overwhelming background noise is substantial; the clinical contribution, to

V. Hombach, H. H. Hilger and H. L. Kennedy (eds), Electrocardiography and Cardiac Drug Therapy. ISBN 978-94-010-6976-2
© 1989, Kluwer Academic Publishers, Dordrecht –

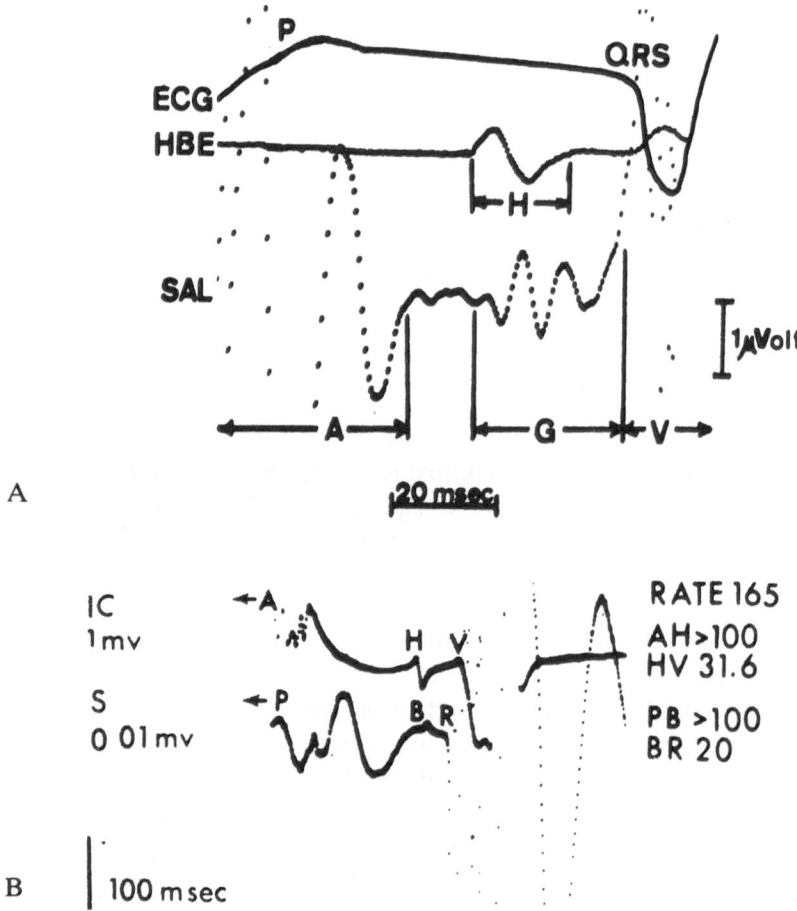

Figure 1. Recordings of electrical activity in the PR segment in dogs by the groups of Berbari (panel A) [1] and of Flowers (panel B) [2] (Panel A is reproduced by permission of the American Heart Association Inc., and Panel B by permission of the Editor of the American Journal of Cardiology).

make sense of the surface PR segment deflections in relation both to conventional records and to the underlying clinical condition is no less daunting.

The possibility of recording His-Purkinje activity from the body surface was raised first by two independent groups in animal experiments performed during 1973 [1, 2] (Figure 1). Attempts to record surface conducting system activity in man were reported also in the same year by Lazzara in the US [3] and by Stopczyk in Poland [4]. The methodology in all cases comprised a sequence of analog high-gain amplification, filtering, and

143

digital signal averaging to recover surface electrical activity during the PR segment that could be attributed to His Purkinje depolarisation.

Verification of the source of surface PR segment activity relied on showing its close temporal association with the His bundle deflection recorded by internal electrodes, an association that was stable in spite of both varying rates of atrial overdrive pacing and the use of drugs to alter selectively the components of artio-ventricular conduction.

Methodology

Modelled on the early experiments of 1973/4 most investigations have followed the methodology outlined in Figure 2. Signals from the chest surface have been subjected to high-gain amplification, analog filtering, and digital signal averaging with or without post-average processing. Since the average incorporates ECG cycles occurring successively in time, the technique is known also as "temporal" averaging and requires an accurately-defined time-reference or "fiducial point" within each cardiac cycle, for its correct alignment in the average.

In the past 15 years, research in cardiac micropotentials has been based on averaging systems developed in individual laboratories or on commercial devices of which the most successful has been the MAC-1 (Marquette Electronics Inc.) [5]. A handful of investigators have attempted to recover His Purkinje signals *without* averaging. Their results have not always been easy to evaluate, but Hombach [6] on the basis of an unusual oesophago-apical or oesophago-sternal lead, and Xiansheng [7] using a

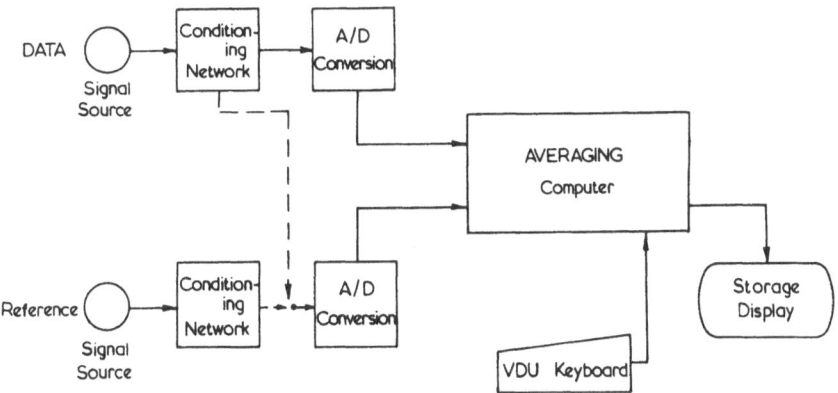

Figure 2. Outline system diagram for the recovery of surface 'His' deflections by signal averaging[3].

144

"cross-correlation" method have demonstrated traces little different to those obtained by signal averaging. Signal recovery on a beat-to-beat basis has also been possible with or without a Faraday cage using either special electrodes or spatial averaging in which several *simultaneous* but spatially separate ECG signals are summed for noise cancellation [8, 9, 10]. But conditions favourable for obtaining clear deflections occur in only a small proportion of patients.

Results

During the past 13 years studies by more than 18 groups in over 500 patients have led to over 85 publications addressed to surface His Purkinje recording. (See for example [11, 12, 13]). The key observations derived from these studies are now described.

In most studies deflections attributable to His Purkinje activity have been recorded in more than 50% of cases though in some recovery rates have been as low as 30%. Failures have resulted from excessive residual noise, inappropriate lead placement, poor triggering, filter artifact, and overlap with atrial activity—but some remain unexplained. Most surface 'His' deflections after satisfactory noise reduction, are of 0.5 μV to 2.0 μV in amplitude; ideally, cases require noise reduction to less than 0.2 μV for adequate signal resolution.

The timing of surface PR segment signals is compatible with an origin in the His Purkinje system. Close correlation of their onset with that of the spike of a simultaneous intracavity His bundle electrogram has been reported in 70–100% of cases. But both theoretical and practical considerations make it unlikely that the internal and external 'HV' interval

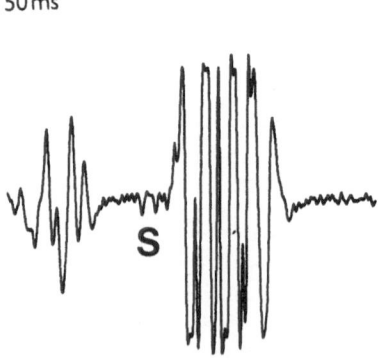

50 ms

S

Figure 3. PR segment activity recorded by signal averaging. 1. Recording of a dual 'spike'. (S)

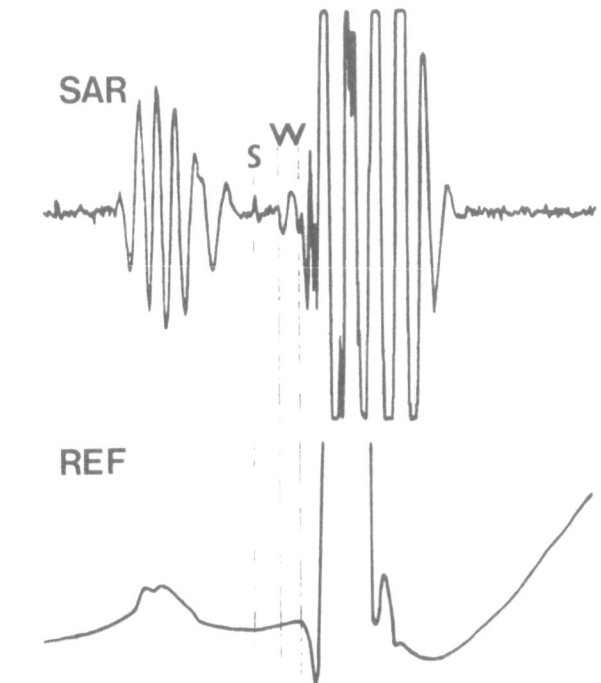

Figure 4. PR segment activity recorded by signal averaging. 2. A different pattern of deflection showing a spike (S) and a later slower waveform (W). SAR—Surface averaged recording. REF—reference ECG at conventional gain.

would be identical, or that the waveforms of internal and surface signals morphology would be similar even in optimum non-invasive recordings.

The pattern of PR segment activity varies considerably from patient to patient: a 'spike' corresponding to the His bundle activation is common—and still seems the most attractive form to the Cardiologist. But a dual spike (Figure 3), a spike with later lower frequency waves (Figure 4), or the commonly-found continuous undulations throughout the period of His Purkinje activation (Figure 5) are also well recognised. Late PR segment activity is likely to come from bundle branch activation but there is no easy method by which this may be proved. Unfortunately, the form of surface PR segment activity does not seem to be influenced in any systematic manner by the presence of known AV conduction abnormalities, left anterior hemiblock, left or right bundle branch block. '

Lead position invariably alters the form of surface conducting system signals (Figure 6) [14] but inter-patient variability is observed irrespective of lead configuration and comparison between studies is hindered by the lack of any standardised lead set.

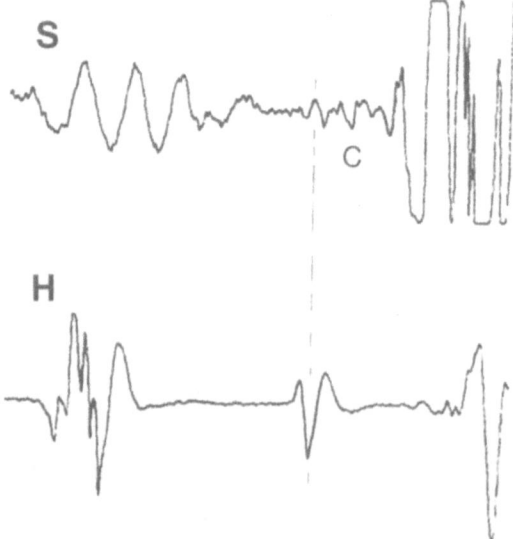

Figure 5. PR segment activity recording by signal averaging. 3. Continuous surface activity (C) appearing during H–V conduction time. S—surface averaged recording; H—internally recorded His bundle electrogram.

Filtering has an important effect on the clarity and form of PR segment activity [14]. High-pass filtering is required to flatten the PR segment but attenuates the low frequency information now judged to be present in His bundle signals. In addition prolongation of the atrial signal by non-linear phase effects (or filter 'ringing') has always threatened recovery of His Purkinje activity especially where the PR interval is short. This problem has prompted a gradual swing from preprocessing that includes high-gain amplification and narrow passband analog filtering to early digitisation of a lower gain broad spectrum signal with subsequent digital amplification and filtering. Digital filtering has brought greater flexibility and control especially where Finite Impulse Response (FIR) filters have been used to retain phase linearity and limit 'ringing' to a programmable duration. But without filter ringing interference from atrial activity remains a troublesome reason for loss of clear external 'His' deflections.

In the averaging process itself triggering stability is critical for satisfactory signal recovery; allowable trigger jitter appears to be in the range of 1–2 ms being achieved in most systems by the use of a QRS template matched to the incoming reference signal by cross-correlation, mean squared error, or more sophisticated techniques.

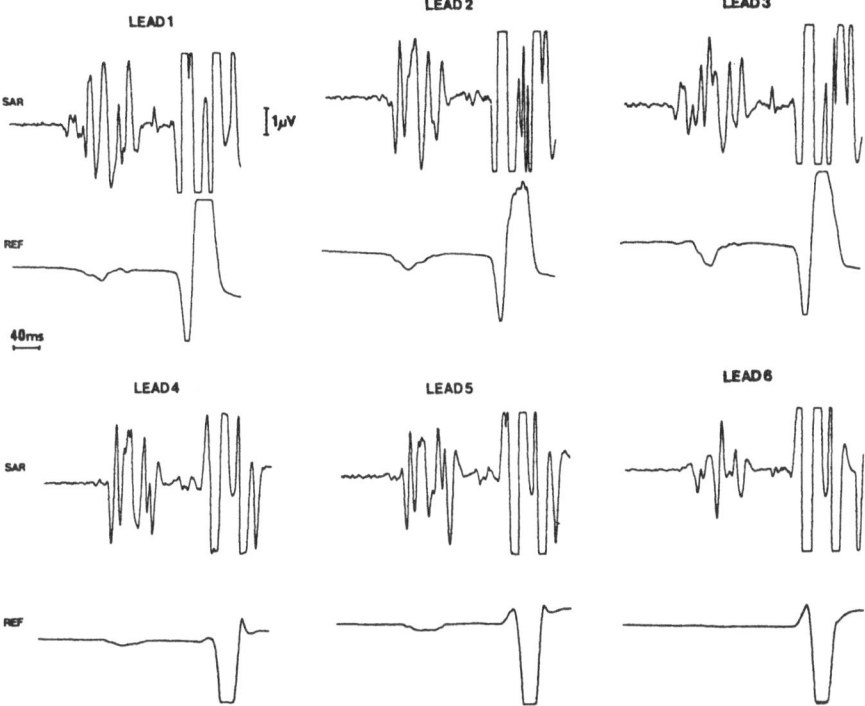

Figure 6. The effect of lead position on the form of PR segment deflections. Each lead has a different bipolar orientation. Lead 1 is an anteroposterior lead at the level of the fourth intercostal space. Other leads are from the anterior and left lateral chest surface. SAR—surface averaged recording. REF—reference trace at conventional gain.

Present position and future developments

In spite of many successful recordings in experimental and early commercial systems the interest in external His bundle electrocardiography evident in the decade from 1973 seems now to be fading. The technique has not become established as a routine clinical tool. Contributory reasons include a lack of a straightforward and standardised technique, failure to record satisfactory signals in spite of 'optimum' recording conditions, uncertainty over the delineation or interpretation of the surface deflections (especially where preceding atrial activity obscures the onset of the 'His' deflection), lack of beat-to-beat information in the signal averaged traces, and doubt over the value of the HV interval as a prognostic marker.

Improving microvolt signal recovery, especially on a beat-to-beat basis,

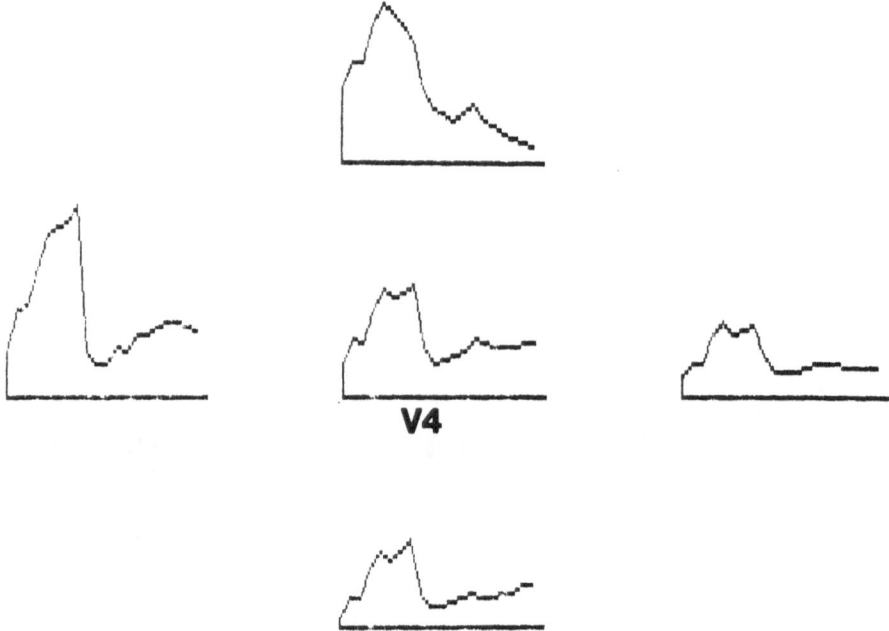

Figure 7. Relative amplitude of a His signal at orthogonal positions on the chest surface with a 4 cm lead separation from the V4 position determined by digital modelling.

requires further technical innovation. The most promising directions for development include spatial averaging, a more rigorous derivation of the optimum lead set, and development of more complex digital filtering. Spatial averaging requires that the desired signals—but *not* the noise—retain coherence between the leads contributing discrete information to the final average. Noise coherence is lost with increasing electrode separation but the signal may also thereby be diminished (Figure 7).

Digital filtering has already shown advantages over its analog counterparts for the recovery of cardiac micropotentials. Further merit will be found in filtering systems that incorporate in their algorithm for improving signal-to-noise ratio an estimate of the noise characteristics of the individual patient together with a detailed model of the expected signal.

The varying filtering [15] (a modification of the Weiner a posteriori estimation filtering) [16], and adaptive filtering have been found effective in the recovery of surface His bundle signals and offer hope for further system enhancement. The contribution of advanced filtering with spatial averaging may allow satisfactory signal recovery on four to sixteen beat temporal average, or at best on a beat-to-beat basis [17].

Conclusions

With present technology external His bundle elctrocardiography is unlikely to become a technique that is used widely. But currently available commercial equipment can recover PR segment activity in about three quarters of patients to whom it is applied, and with experience many of the recordings obtained can provide an estimate of HV interval of clinical value. Patients most suitable for study are those with a prolonged PR interval since in these the effects of atrial overspill will be minimised and in this group the HV interval will be especially relevant. Serial application to patients receiving drugs affecting HV conduction forms a second important application of present devices.

Enthusiasm for widespread use application of this technique will be engendered if technical improvements lead to reliable beat-to-beat registration in more than 80% of cases and if further guidelines can be established for the clinical interpretation of PR segment activity.

References

1. Berbari EJ, Lazzara R, Samet P, Scherlag BJ (1973) Noninvasive technique for detection of electrical activity during the P-R segment. Circulation 48:1005–1013
2. Flowers, NC, Hand RC, Orander PC, Miller KB, Walden MD, Horan, LG (1974) Surface recording of electrical activity from the region of the bundle of His. Am J Cardiol 33:384–389
3. Lazzara, R, Campbell R, Berbari EJ, Scherlag BJ, Myerburg RD (1973) Electrocardiogram of the His-Purkinje system in man. Circulation 48:Suppl IV:IV–22 (abstract)
4. Stopczyk MJ, Kopec J, Zochowski RJ, Pieniack M (1973) Surface recording of electrical heart activity during the P-R segment in man by a computer averaging technique. International Research Communication Systems 11:21–2 (abstract)
5. Rozanski JJ, Castellanos A (1980) Clinical evaluation of an improved high-resolution ECG cart for recording the His bundle electrogram non-invasively. PACE 3:479–484
6. Hombach V, Behrenbeck DW, Hilger HH (1977) Oesophagosternale und osophagospikale ableitungen zur resigtrierung von oberflachen-His-potentialen. (Oesophagosternal and oesophagoapical leads for registration of surface His bundle potentials.) Zeitschrift fur Kardiologie, 66:565
7. Xiengsheng W (1980) Correlation and its application in His bundle electrocardiograms. Chinese Medical Journal 93:239–250
8. Flowers NC, Shvartsman V, Kenneily BM, Sohi GS, Horan LG (1981) Surface recordings of His Purkinje activity on an every beat basis without digital averaging. Circulation 63:948–957
9. El-Sherif N, Mehra R, Gomes JAC, Kelen G (1983) Appraisal of a low noise electrocardiogram. J Am Coll Cardiol 1:456–467
10. Hombach V, Kebbel U, Hopp H-W, Winter U, Hirche H (1984) Noninvasive beat-by-beat registration of ventricular late potentials using high resolution electrocardiography. Int J Cardiol 6:167–183

11. Berbari EJ, Scherlag BJ, Lazzara R (1977) A computerised technique to record new components of the electrocardiogram. Proc IEEE 65:799–802
12. Wajszczuk WJ, Stopczyk MJ, Moskowitz MS, Zochowski RJ, Bauld T, Dabos P, Rubenfire M (1978) Noninvasive recording of His-Purkinje activity in man by QRS triggered signal averaging. Circulation 58:95–102
13. Vincent R (1984) His bundle electrocardiography from the body-surface. MD Thesis, University of London
14. Vincent R, Werneck S, English MJ, Woollons DJ, Chamberlain DA (1983) Influence of recording techniques and cardiac rhythm on the surface recording of conducting system activity. In: Feruglio GA (ed.) Cardiac Pacing—Electrophysiology and Pacemaker Technology Padova: Piccin Medical Books, pp 175–180
15. De Weerd JPC (1981) A posteriori time-varying filtering of averaged evoked potentials. I. Introduction and conceptual basis. Biol Cybern 41:211–222
16. Walter DO (1969) A posteriori 'Wiener filtering' of averaged evoked responses. Electroencephalogr Clin Neurophysiol Suppl 27:61–70
17. Lander PT (1986) Computer processing methods for the recovery of low-amplitude ECG signals. D Phil thesis, University of Sussex UK

14. Detection of ventricular late potentials with signal averaging

EDWARD J. BERBARI, BENJAMIN J. SCHERLAG &
RALPH LAZZARA

University of Oklahoma Health Sciences Center, Department of Medicine, Division of Cardiology, and Veterans Administration Medical Center, Oklahoma City, Oklahoma, U.S.A.

Introduction

High resolution electrocardiography (HRECG) implies the use of techniques which will enhance the ECG to identify potentials not normally seen with standard ECG machines. This can involve increased time and voltage resolution as well as computer processing to improve the signal-to-noise ratio (SNR). Two applications of the HRECG have been to record, noninvasively, the signals from the His-Purkinje system and from diseased regions of the heart involved with arrhythmogenesis. In the latter case it has been shown with direct epicardial and endocardial recordings that viable tissue is present within regions of a myocardial infarction. Slow conduction within the infarct labyrinth is reflected in electrogram recordings as having low amplitude, multiphasic high frequency content, i.e. fractionation. This activity can extend beyond the end of the QRS and has become the focus of HRECG techniques in recent years. Both animal [1–4] and human [5, 6] studies have demonstrated the relationship of these late potentials recorded directly from the myocardium with arrhythmias following myocardial infarction. The focus of this paper will be on the methods and technology for recording the late potentials from the body surface and will not concentrate on the clinical application. Other chapters of this volume will review the clinical application of the HRECG.

The clinical usefulness of late potential analysis is being established by many investigators, but specific goals which could be used to optimize the technology have not been formally elucidated. For example, one goal which will be emphasized in this paper is the determination of the latest moment of ventricular depolarization. Only a few animal studies [7, 8] and human studies [9] have looked at this issue by comparing the surface recording of late potentials with direct epicardial or endocardial recordings. These studies demonstrated that the body surface recordings of late poten-

V. Hombach, H. H. Hilger and H. L. Kennedy (eds), Electrocardiography and Cardiac Drug Therapy. ISBN 978-94-010-6976-2
© 1989, Kluwer Academic Publishers, Dordrecht –

tials did not always coincide with the direct recordings. However, there was no attempt to optimize the recording technology in order to reconcile these observed differences. Lead position, signal processing, and automatic detection algorithms all play a role in identifying late potentials. These factors will be examined in this study as they pertain to identifying the termination of the late potentials. No correlations will be made with invasive recordings as future studies will examine this in more detail.

Review of methods

The most common approach for recording late potentials is to record bipolar XYZ leads. One method of lead placement is based on anatomically orthogonal leads with the heart at the origin. The left mid-clavicular line is the Y axis. The negative Y electrode is in the subclavicular space along this line and the positive Y electrode is in the lower left abdominal region, also along this line. The positive Z electrode is placed between the 4th and 5th intercostal space on the Y axis. The negative Z electrode is placed on the back at the reflection of the anterior Z electrode. The positive X electrode is in the left midaxillary line at the level of the $Y-Z$ axis intersect. The negative Y electrode is on the right midaxillary line at this same level. A reference electrode is usually placed in the lower right abdominal region. The current hardware/software system is based upon an IBM PC/AT (Corazonix Corporation, Oklahoma City, OK) and has been previously described [10].

Figure 1A shows a 3 second rhythm strip of the XYZ leads obtained from a patient with an old myocardial infarction. The gain is in the normal range and minimal filtering (0.05–300 Hz) is used. Figure 1B is from the same patient but after increasing the sampling rate to 2 KHz to provide a 300 msec window. The gain was increased by a factor of five and a 200 beat signal average was performed. It is possible to see higher frequency deflections in the terminal portion of the HRECG QRS, but it is almost impossible to observe and quantify these signals in Figure 1A. These HRECG signals are usually high pass filtered and Figure 2 shows three different high pass filters applied to the XYZ leads of Figure 1. In panel A a digital filter is applied in the same manner as would be done with electronic filters. The data are processed in the normal time sense (unidirectional) with a 25 Hz, 4th order Butterworth high pass filter. Note that the latest moment of ventricular depolarization is marked by an automatic algorithm [11] at 245 msec, relative to the origin in the Y lead. It is known that such filters (infinite impulse response) have a nonlinear phase response.

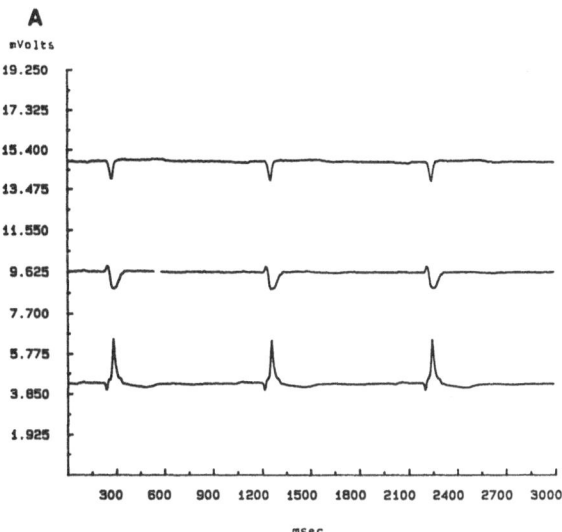

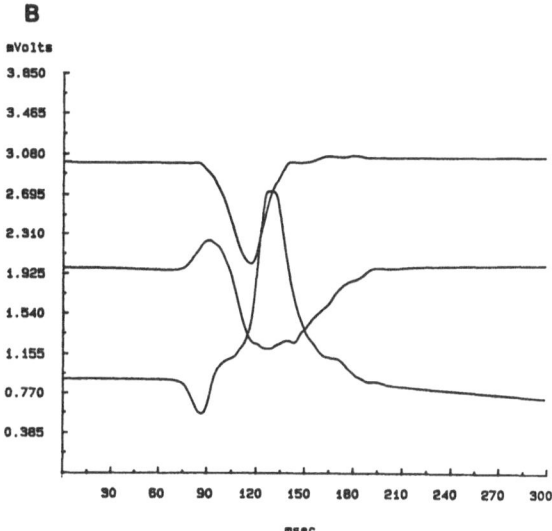

Figure 1. The top panel shows the *XYZ* (top to bottom) leads obtained prior to signal averaging and at normal gain settings. The 3 second duration of the rhythm strip corresponds to 200 Hz sampling rate per channel. The bottom panel was obtained after increasing the sampling rate to 2000 Hz, increasing the gain by 5, and signal averaging for 200 cardiac cycles.

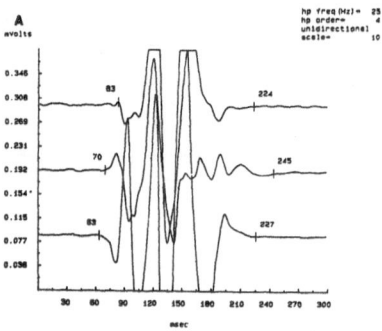

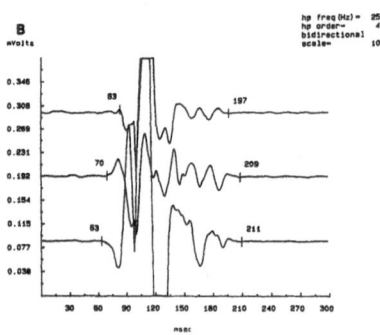

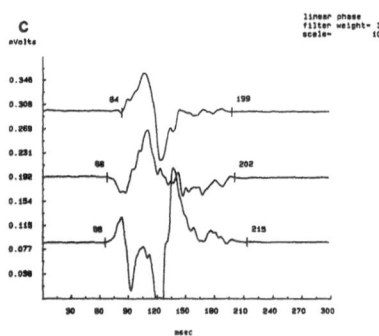

Figure 2. The filtered version of the averaged *XYZ* leads of Figure 1. The top panel is a 25 Hz unidirectional filter, the middle panel is a 25 Hz bidirectional filter, and the bottom panel is linear phase, 8 term finite impulse response filter.

This results in a distortion of the terminal QRS region since the QRS energy is time shifted into this region. One solution to the problems caused by the nonlinear phase response was suggested by Simson [8, 11]. The same digital algorithm can be applied from each end of the data window and terminate at the peak of the QRS. The phase shift artifact affects only the central portion of the QRS complex. Figure 2B demonstrates this bidirectional filter applied to the XYZ leads. Note that the the latest moment of ventricular depolarization appears in the Z lead at 211 msec after the reference point. Not only is there a significant time difference in the endpoint of 34 msec, but the lead in which the longest duration is measured is also different. Another approach to this problem of filter artifact is to use a class of filters known as finite impulse response (FIR) filters which were designed to have a linear phase response [12]. These filters do not simulate electronic filter designs as in the case for the Butterworth filter, but can be described as a form of numerical differentiation operating in a unidirectional model. The frequency response of such filters can be calculated, but characteristics such as cut-off frequency, and roll-off are not the usual design criteria. An example of an eight term filter (filter weight = 3) applied to the test XYZ recordings is shown in Figure 2C. Note that the QRS onsets and offsets are similar to those of the bidirectional filter with only a few milliseconds difference. The Z lead also shows the latest moment of ventricular depolarization.

A common approach which attempts to simplify the late potential measurement problem is to combine the filtered XYZ leads into a vector magnitude defined as $M = \sqrt{X^2 + Y^2 + Z^2}$. This is the length of a vector in 3 dimensional space. An alternate vector magnitude would be $M = |X| + |Y| + |Z|$ which is just the sum of the absolute values of the XYZ leads. This latter method when used to analyze late potentials [10, 13] has no geometric basis, but is computationally efficient. It is presumed all late potential information may be garnered from the vector magnitude. Figure 3 shows the corresponding transformation of the individual panels of Figure 2 into the filtered vector magnitudes of panels 3A, 3B, and 3C, respectively. Note again the prolonged QRS measurement in Figure 3A compared to Figures 3B and 3C.

There is great desire by many investigators to have an automatic algorithm which defines the appropriate characteristics of the terminal QRS region. Both time domain [11, 13–15] and frequency domain [16] approaches have been described. Frequency domain approaches are prone to a myriad of technique dependent factors and will not be the focus of this report. The time domain characteristics have been primarily duration and amplitude measurements. Exactly how these measurements are made is

156

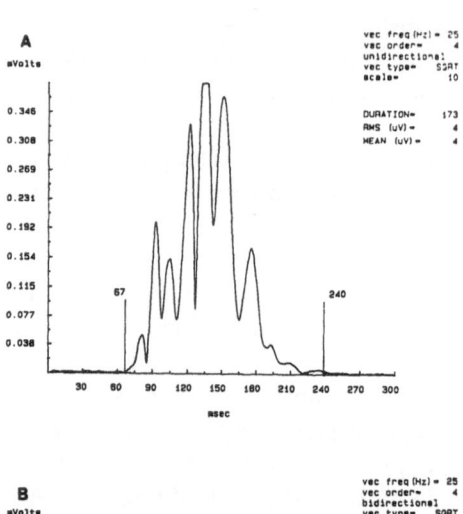

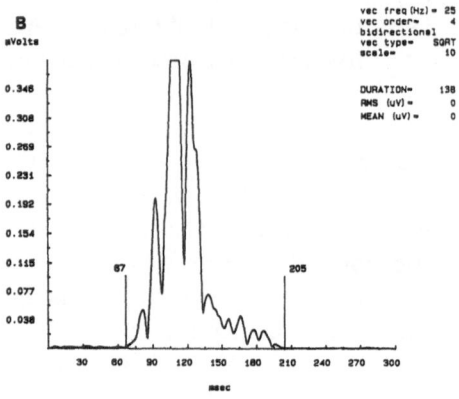

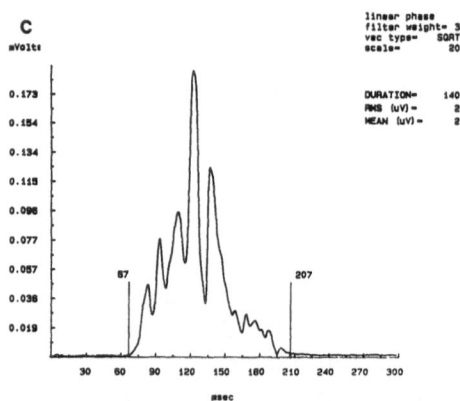

Figure 3. The filtered vector magnitude transformation of Figure 2 with each panel respectively transformed.

crucial to accepting the accuracy of the results desired from many studies published thus far. For example, the author's early work with noninvasive His-Purkinje recordings [17] demanded that repeated averages be obtained to rule out artifact and ensure the reproducibility of the observations. Analysis of repeated averages is recommended for identifying waveform in any signal averaging study.

The work of Breithardt et al. [18, 19], in the long-term follow-up of patients following myocardial infarction relied upon dual readers to visually identify the late potentials. In this case the late potential was considered to be an appendage to the QRS complex. The significant influence of Simson's work [11] in this field essentially eliminated this concept by not classifying the late potential as a separate entity, but merely part of the total QRS duration observed in high resolution. This seems at first to be just a semantic difference but it does relieve the reader from choosing a third point between the onset and offset to be defined as the QRS endpoint and the beginning of the late potential. Simson [11] has also described an automatic algorithm for selecting the QRS duration from the filtered vector magnitude. Briefly, this approach is applied to the beginning and end of QRS. It is based on calculating two adjacent moving averages placed at the end of the data window. If the mean of the leading moving average exceeds the mean of the trailing moving average by 3 standard deviations then the inflection point (onset or offset) is chosen. Otherwise, the windows are shifted one point closer to the QRS complex and the calculation repeated. Variables for these algorithms are the duration of the moving averages and the number of standard deviation by which the two means differ. The measurement points in Figures 2 and 3 were based upon this approach. An algorithmic approach for identifying late potentials [20] as a separate entity after the QRS has also been described. Comparison of repeated averages is not part of any algorithm for analyzing late potentials and the authors feel this is a weakness in current approaches.

Other parameters have also been obtained from the late potentials, which are decidedly dependent on the choice of the QRS endpoint. The root mean square (rms) of the terminal 40 mrsec (V40) and the duration of the terminal QRS segment which is below 40 μ Volts (LAS) are two such parameters. Both are measured from the filtered vector magnitude. The choice of the filter frequency and type of filter can significantly alter these measurements. Four sets of published criteria [11, 13–15] for defining late potentials in patients with inducible ventricular tachycardia are summarized in Table I. Each set of criteria was derived from the individual data set obtained by each research group. Multicenter studies using each set of criteria or comparing these criteria has yet to be performed.

158

Table 1. Late potential criteria

Authors	Filter	Vector	QRSd		V40		LAS
Simson [11]	25 Hz bidir.[1]	SQRT[3]	>110 ms	and	<25 uV		–
Kuchar [15]	40 Hz bidir.	SQRT	>120 ms	or	<20 uV		–
Gomes [14]	80 Hz bidir.	SQRT	>107 ms	or	<17 uV		–
Nalos [13]	100 Hz unidir.[2]	ABS[4]	>120 ms		–	and	≥30 ms

[1]4th order Butterworth bidirectional digital filter; [2]1st order unidirectional analog filter; [3]SQRT $= \sqrt{X^2 + Y^2 + Z^2}$; [4]ABS $= |X| + |Y| + |Z|$.

Analysis of methods

Identifying the latest moment of ventricular depolarization was one goal set forth to optimize the recording methods for late potential analysis. However, without a 'gold standard' for evaluating performance, it is only possible to point out the inconsistencies present in the current techniques. Examined below are problems associated with selecting leads, signal processsing methods, and late potential parameters.

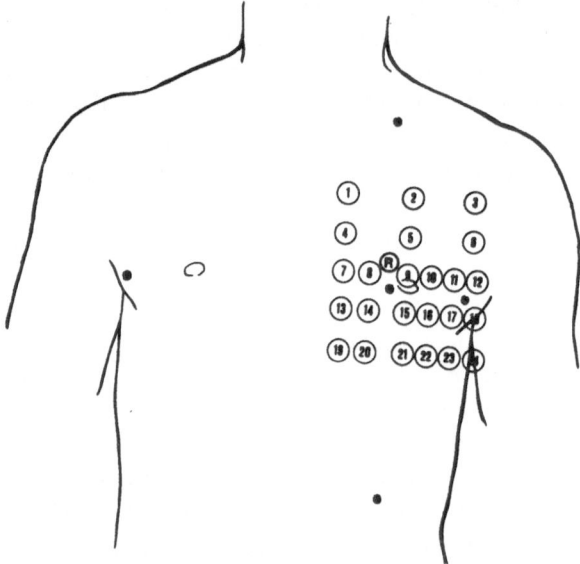

Figure 4. Approximate placement of the 24 precordial electrode sites used to obtain a map of signal averaged recordings.

Adequacy of XYZ Leads

Most investigators use an uncorrelated bipolar XYZ lead system. In order to test this approach a left precordial map from 24 sites was obtained. Each lead in this set was signal averaged for 400 cardiac cycles. Figure 4 shows the placement of the 24 electrodes on the torso. The solid dots are the positions of the XYZ lead electrodes. All of the electrodes were referenced to an anterior electrode, labeled R on the figure. Figure 5 shows the high pass filtered recordings obtained from each site shown in Figure 4. The QRS duration was determined by the automatic measurement algorithm. Figure 6 shows the filtered XYZ leads in panel A and the recordings from sites 9–10 (panel B) and 13–14 (panel C). The automatic algorithm selected a maximum duration from the XYZ set of 141 msec in the Z lead. The same algorithm found QRS duration at 145 and 149 msec in sites 13 and 9, respectively. The endpoints with respect to the data window origin show an even greater discrepancy. They are 197 msec, 209 msec, and 202 msec for the Z lead (panel A), site 9 (panel B), and site (panel C), respectively. Careful examination of Figure 5 indicates that late potentials may sppear at several other sites, but that the algorithm fails to detect them, e.g. sites 15 and 16. This may be due to the shortcomings of the automatic algorithm, but also points out that the distribution of the SNR on the precordium is not known. It also indicates that the XYZ lead set may not be sufficient for identifying the latest moment of ventricular depolarization. This was found to be the case in 4 of 18 patients from whom precordial maps were obtained [21].

The Vector Magnitude

After establishing that the XYZ leads may not be the optimum lead set for identifying late potentials another aspect of current approaches comes into question, specifically the vector magnitude. The standard vector magnitude is calculated by taking $\sqrt{X^2 + Y^2 + Z^2}$, so it is directly dependent on the XYZ leads. If a signal does not appear in the individual XYZ leads it will not appear in the vector magnitude. The problems of using the vector magnitude extend beyond this because it is possible that this nonlinear combination will act in a manner detrimental to late potential identification. Figure 7 is the filtered vector magnitude from the same patient whose XYZ leads were shown in Figure 4. Notice the automatic algorithm failed to detect the late potentials as the QRS duration is 114 msec and the rms value of the terminal 40 msec was 28 uV.

The vector magnitude loses its sensitivity for detecting late potentials

160

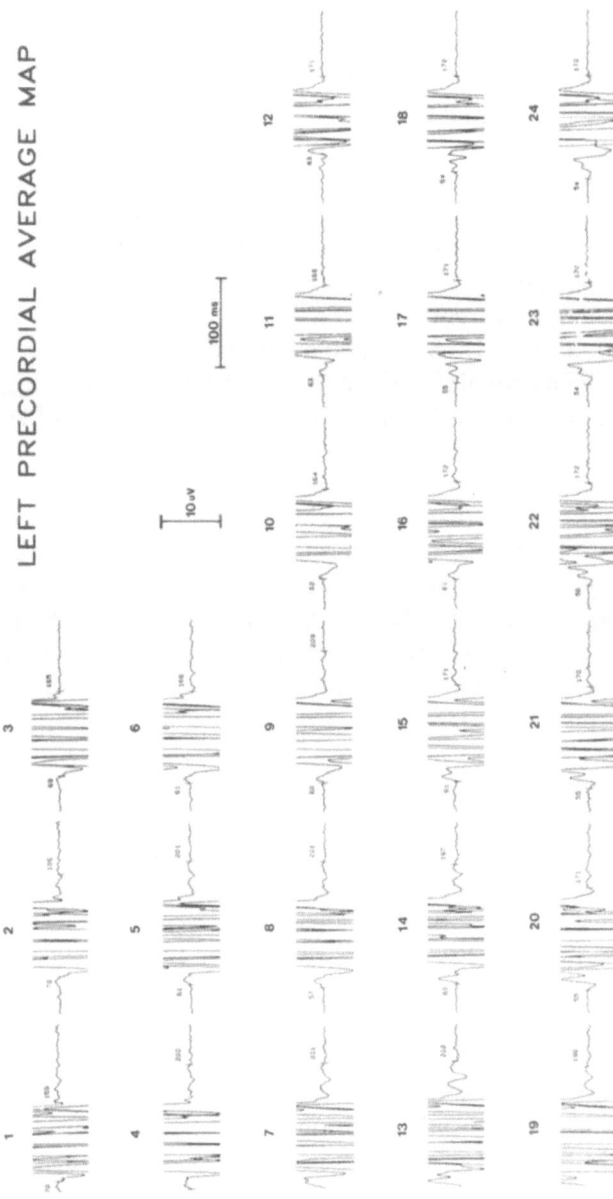

Figure 5. The averaged (400 beats) and bidirectional filtered recordings from the sites shown in Figure 4.

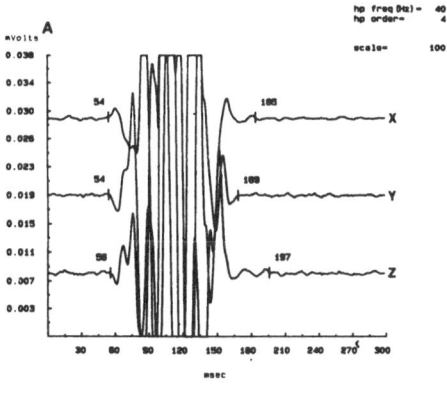

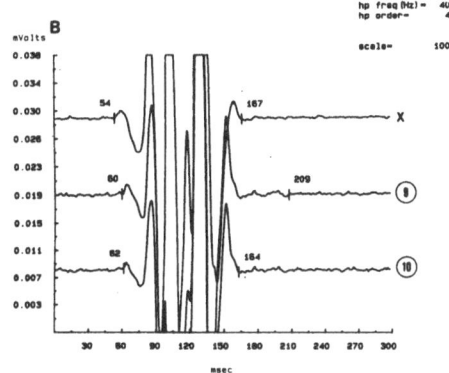

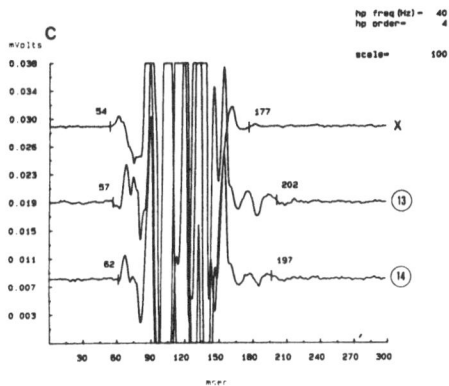

Figure 6. The *XYZ* leads in panel A from the subject whose left precordial map is shown in Figure 5. Panel B and C show, in higher resolution, the signals from sites 9, 10, 13, and 14. The longest duration QRS in the *XYZ* set is 141 msec in the *Z* lead. The longest duration in the precordial grid is 149 msec at site 9.

162

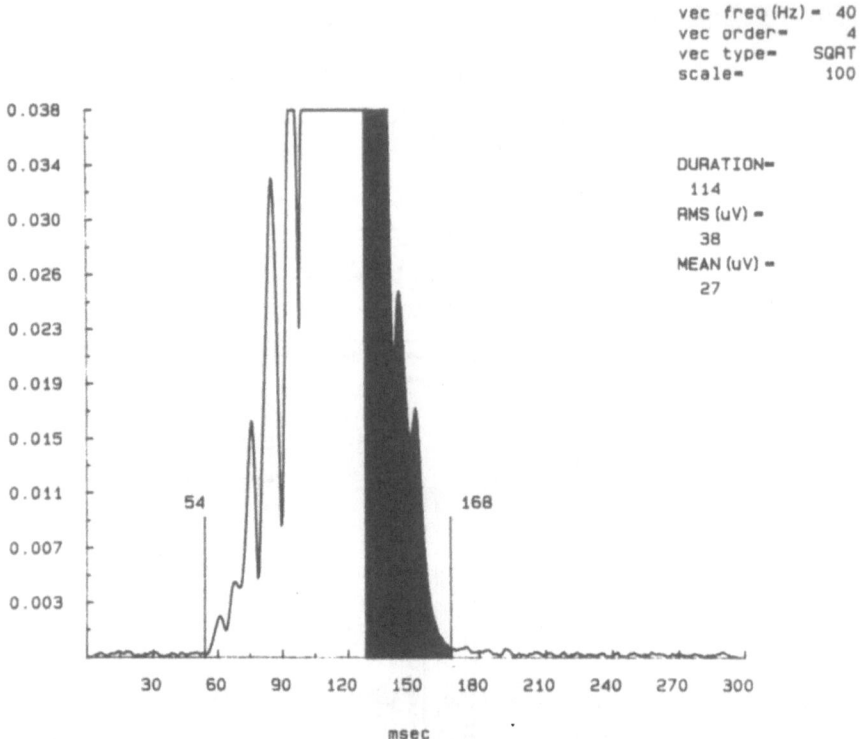

vec freq (Hz) = 40
vec order= 4
vec type= SQRT
scale= 100

DURATION=
114
RMS (uV) =
38
MEAN (uV) =
27

Figure 7. The filtered vector magnitude of the subject whose precordial map and *XYZ* recordings were shown in Figures 5 and 6. Note that the QRS duration is only 114 msec. The V40 region is shaded.

because the vector operation will always degrade the SNR of the lead which has the highest SNR prior to the vector operation. This conclusion was arrived at by a mathematical analysis and numerical simulation [22]. The degree to which this affects actual signal averaged data is still unknown. For studies which relied upon the vector magnitude it appears that their results could be improved by analyzing the individual *XYZ* leads providing an increased sensitivity for late potential identification.

Parameter Selection

Parameters defined as significant for characterizing the late potentials (see Table I) were generally based upon a specific set of test patients from individual laboratories. It is not always clear from such studies how specific decision values were derived. One solution to this is to generalize some of these parameters. The rms function [10, 23], is one such generalization of the V40 type of measurement. Once the QRS endpoints are determined, instead of calculating the rms value of the terminal 40 msec, the values of ... V39, V40, V41 ... can be calculated and displayed graphically. The top panel in Figure 8 shows a filtered vector magnitude with the V40 region shaded. The bottom panel is the rms function, calculated from the end of

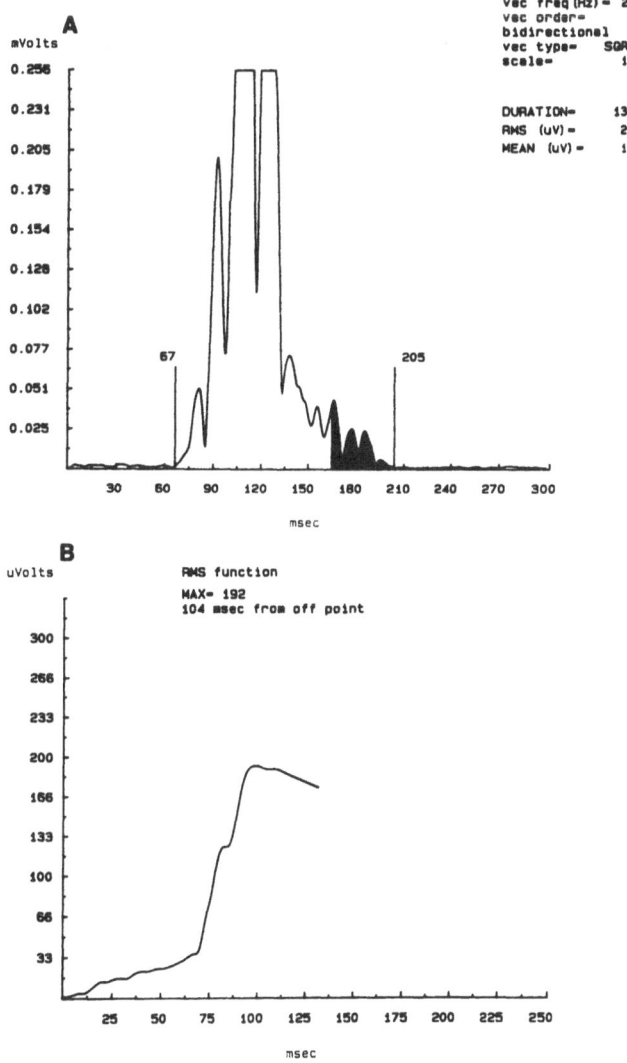

Figure 8. The filtered vector magnitude of the *XYZ* set shown in Figures 1–3 and the rms function in the lower panel. The V40 region is shaded in the top panel and can be read directly from the rms curve in the lower panel.

the QRS to the beginning of the QRS. For example, the value of V40 can be found by reading the voltage value on the ordinate specified for the 40 msec point on the abscissa. One further feature of this approach is that this new function has more recognizable characteristics compared to an individual voltage value.

Conclusions

The HRECG has established itself as a practical means for analyzing the ECG, particularly with regard to microvolt level potentials. The clinical data base of late potential information is rapidly increasing. From an engineering point of view specific goals need to be defined in order to optimize the late potential recording technology. Determining the latest moment of ventricular depolarization was chosen as one such goal. A critical overview of current approaches with respect to this goal was the basis of this report. The problems identified with lead selection, signal processing and parameter selection were examined with shortcomings pointed out. In some cases no final solution can be offered. No optimal lead set, short of a complete precordial map, can be recommended. However, approaches which rely on the vector magnitude should be re-examined with the prospect of improved late potential detection if individual XYZ leads are analyzed. High pass filtering seems to remain a necessary, but less desirable, signal processing method. No single filtering scheme will prove to be critical, but some approaches such as traditional infinite impulse response filters used in a unidirectional mode should be avoided. The variety of late potential parameters have been derived by individual groups without the benefit of a multicenter approach. More general approaches such as the rms function may simplify the parameter selection process but more work is needed to establish the usefulness of such approaches.

Acknowledgements

The authors would like to thank Pamela Tomey for her secretarial assistance in preparing this manuscript. Portions of this work were funded by NIH Grants HL27646 and a Veterans Administration Merit Review Grant.

References

1. Scherlag BJ, El-Sherif N, Hope RR, Lazara R (1974) Characterization and localization of ventricular arrhythmias due to myocardial ischemia and infarction. Circ Res 35:372–383

2. Hope RR, Williams DO, El-Sherif N, Lazzara R (1974) The efficacy of antiarrhythmic agents during acute myocardial ischemia and the role of heart rate. Circulation 50:507–514

3. Williams DO, Scherlag BJ, Hope RR, Lazzara R (1974) The pathophysiology of malignant ventricular arrhythmias during acute myocardial ischemia. Circulation 50:1163–1172

4. El-Sherif N, Scherlag BJ, Lazzara R, Hope RR (1977) Reentrant ventricular arrhythmias in the late myocardial infarction period. I. Conduction characteristics in the infarction zone. Circulation 55:686–702

5. Fontaine G, Guiraudon G, Frank R, Vedel J, Grossgogeat Y, Cabrol C (1978) Modern concepts of ventricular tachycardia. Eur J Cardiol 8:565

6. Josephson ME, Horowitz LN, Farshidi A (1978) Continuous local electrical activity: A mechanism of recurrent ventricular tachycardia. Circulation 57:658

7. Berbari EJ, Scherlag BJ, Hope RR, Lazzara R (1978) Recording from the body surface of arrhythmogenic ventricular activity during the ST segment. Am J Cardiol 41:697

8. Simson MB, Euler D, Michelson EL, Falcone RA, Spear JF, Moore EN (1981) Detection of delayed ventricular activation on the body surface in dogs. Am J Physiol 241:H363

9. Simson MB, Untereker WJ, Spielman SR, Horowitz LN, Marcus NH, Falcone RA, Harken AH, Josephson ME (1983) Relation between late potentials on the body surface and directly recorded fragmented electrograms in patients with ventricular tachycardia. Am J Cardiol 51:105–112

10. Berbari EJ, Ozinga L, Albert D (1986) Method for analyzing cardiac late potentials. In: Computers in Cardiology, IEEE Computer Society Press

11. Simson MB (1981) Use of signals in the terminal QRS complex to identify patients with ventricular tachycardia after myocardial infarction. Circulation 64:235–242

12. McClellan JN, Parks TW, Rabiner LR (1973) A computer program for designing optimum FIR linear phase digital filters. IEEE Trans. Audio Electroacoust. AU-21:506–526

13. Nalos PC, Gang ES, Mandel WJ, Ladenheim ML, Lass Y, Peter T (1987) The signal-averaged electrocardiogram as a screening test for inducibility of sustained ventricular tachycardia in high risk patients: A prospective study. JACC 9:534–548

14. Gomes JA, Horowitz SF, Millner M, Machac J, Winters SL, Barreca P (1987) Relation of late potentials to ejection fraction and wall motion abnormalities in acute myocardial infarction. Am J Cardiol 59:1017–1074

15. Kuchar DL, Thorburn CW, Sammel NL (1987) Prediction of serious arrhythmic events after myocardial infarction: Signal-averaged electrocardiogram, holter monitoring and radionuclide ventriculography. JACC 9:531–538

16. Denes P, Santarelli P, Hauser RG, Uretz EF (1983) Quantitative analysis of the high frequency components of the terminal portion of the body surface QRS in normal subjects and in patients with ventricular tachycardia. Circulation 67:1129

17. Berbari EJ, Lazzara R, Samet P, Scherlag BJ (1973) Noninvasive technique for detection of electrical activity during the P-R segment. Circulation 48:1005

18. Breithardt G, Becker R, Seipel L, Abendroth RR, Ostermeyer J (1981) Noninvasive detection of late potentials in man: A new marker for ventricular tachycardia. Eur Heart J 2:1–11

19. Breithardt G, Schwarzmaier J, Boggrefe M, Haerten K, Seipel L (1983) Prognostic significance of late ventricular potentials after acute myocardial infarction. Eur Heart J 4:487–495

20. Karbenn U, Breithardt G, Borggrefe M, Simson MB (1985) Automatic identification of late potentials. J Electrocardiol 18:123–134

21. Berbari EJ, DeCarlo L, Friday KJ, Jackman WM (1987) Methods and results of noninvasive detection of ventricular late potentials. In: Aliot E, Lazzara R (eds) Ventricular Tachycardia. Dordrecht: Martinus Nijhoff
22. Lander P, Lazzara R, Berbari EJ: The analysis of ventricular late potentials using orthogonal recordings. Submitted for publication
23. Berbari EJ, Ozinga L, Friday KJ, Jackman WM (1986) New methods for analyzing cardiac late potentials. Circulation 74:II–180

15. The influence of fibrinolytic therapy using streptokinase on the frequency and pattern of ventricular late potentials

L. GOEDEL-MEINEN, M. HOFMANN, G. SCHMIDT, G. JAHNS,
G. KLEIN, W. BAEDEKER & H. BLÖMER

I. Medizinische Klinik der TU München, Klinikum rechts der Isar, F.R.G.

Introduction

Streptokinase, given in high doses, is already considered one of the standard treatments for acute myocardial infarction. The goal of this method is the reduction of the size of the infarction through the earliest possible reperfusion. Infarcted tissue is known to be a frequent cause of impeded conduction which can be seen in the signal-averaged ECG as late potentials. We were interested in the question, whether the incidence of noninvasively measured late potentials is influenced by an intravenously given fibrinolytic therapy in the acute phase of myocardial infarction. Therefore we compared the frequency of late potentials in patients treated with streptokinase with their frequency in patients who remained untreated.

Patients

This study included 26 patients, 2 women and 24 men with a mean age of 57 years. 9 patients showed previous myocardial infarctions. The acute event was an inferior myocardial infarction in 14 patients and an anterior myocardial infarction in 10 patients, whereas 2 patients showed multiple infarction areas. Within the first days, left ventricular failure with pulmonary congestion occurred in 7 patients. A midbrain lesion appeared in 3 patients, one of whom died on the 10th day. The other two patients died some time after their last measurement.

Method

A fibrinolytic therapy using streptokinase was given in the cases of clinically evident infarction (confirmed by ECG) always inside of 4 hours after

V. Hombach, H. H. Hilger and H. L. Kennedy (eds), Electrocardiography and Cardiac Drug Therapy. ISBN 978-94-010-6976-2
© 1989, Kluwer Academic Publishers, Dordrecht –

168

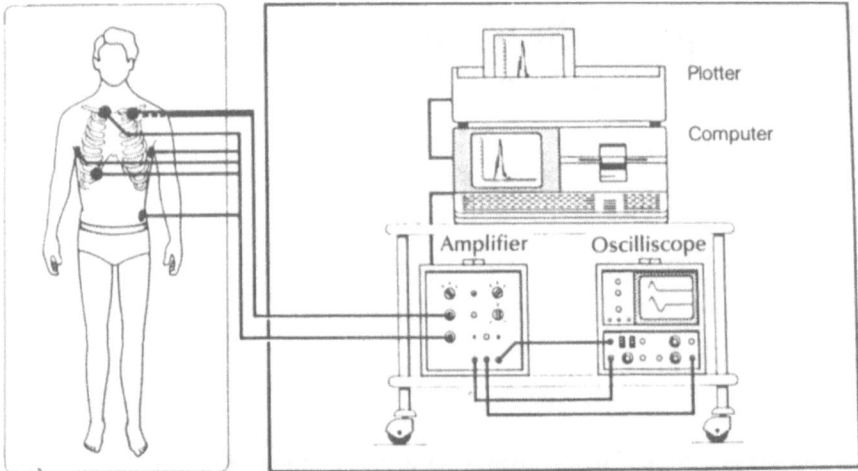

Figure 1. Recording set-up. Technical data: Amplification 2-5000; Low-pass filter 250 Herz; A/D Conversion to 12 bit accuracy at 1000 samples/sec; Bidirectional filter: 25 and 40 Herz; QRS recognition program.

the event. None of the patients had conditions adverse to streptokinase which was given at a rate of 1.5 million units per hour over a 2 hour period. Recording of the signal averaged ECG (after the method developed by Simson, modified by Karbenn (see Figure 1)) was carried out daily, from the day of the infarction until the 10th succeeding day. We collected the following computer measured data: duration and voltage of the filtered

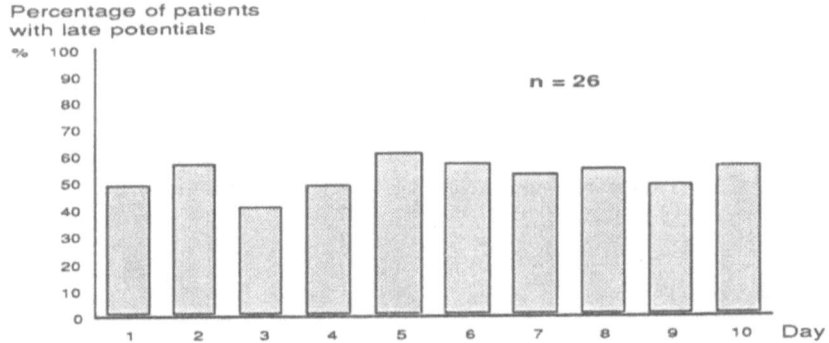

Figure 2. Incidence of late potentials in the overall group during the first 10 days of acute myocardial infarction.

QRS complex and the duration and voltage of any evidenced late potentials.

Results

The incidence of late potentials in the overall group during the first 10 days of acute myocardial infarction ranged between 40% on the third day and 60% on the fifth day. There was no clear increase or decrease of late potentials (see Figure 2). If we differentiate the patients according to the localisation of their infarction, we don't see any significant difference in the incidence of late potentials in patients with anterior myocardial infarction in comparison to those with inferior myocardial infarction (see Figure 3).

On the day of maximum levels of creatinine phosphokinase MB isoenzyme, 57% of our patients showed late potentials of which 14% had a duration of more than 40 msec. The frequency of late potentials on this day did not differ significantly from the incidence of late potentials on the other days of the study, (see Figure 4). Comparing the patients with fibrinolytic therapy and without fibrinolytic therapy, we found that the first group showed a slightly higher incidence of late potentials; however, the difference was not significant (see Figure 5).

In the 7 patients who developed left ventricular failure and pulmonary congestion in the acute phase of myocardial infarction, we noticed a significantly higher incidence of late potentials in comparison to the overall group (see Figure 6).

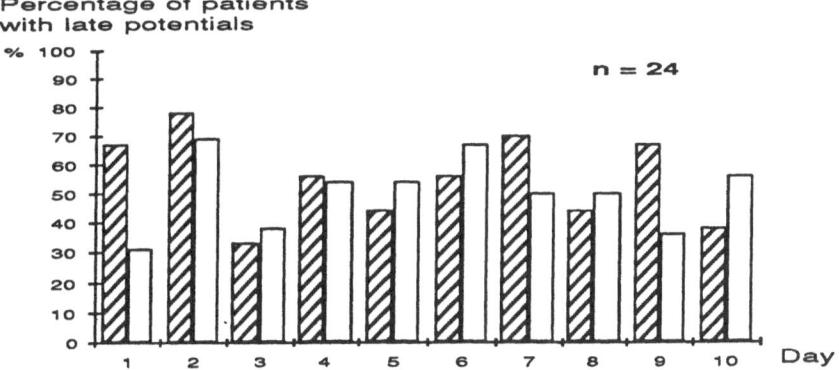

Figure 3. Incidence of late potentials in patients with anterior myocardial infarction ▨▨▨ and patients with inferior myocardial infarction ▭▭▭ The difference was not significant (Fisher-exact-Test).

170

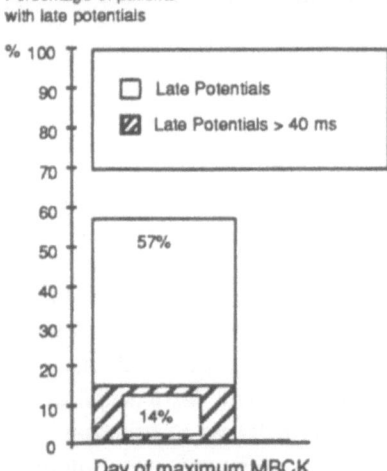

Figure 4. Incidence of late potentials on the day of maximum levels of the creatinine phosphokinase MB-isoenzyme. The frequency of late potentials on this day did not differ significantly from the incidence of late potentials on the other days of the study.

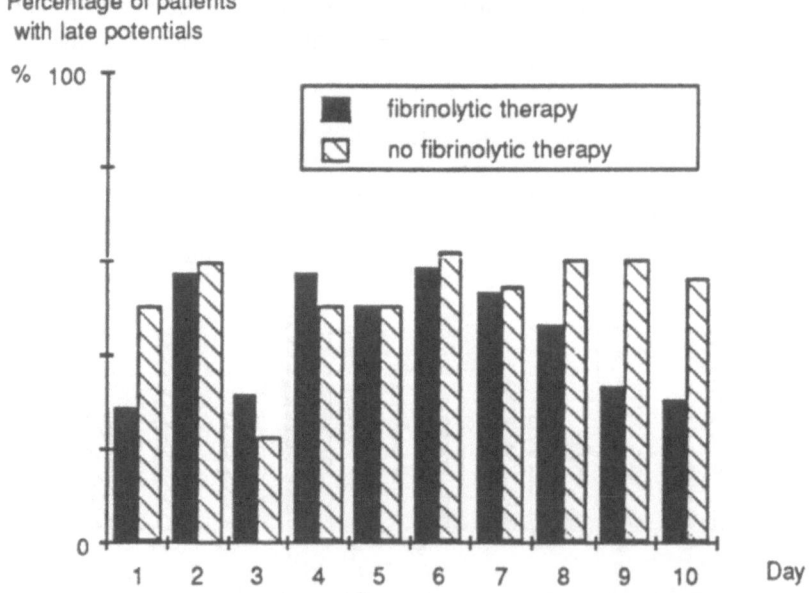

Figure 5. Incidence of late potentials in patients with and without fibrinolytic therapy. There was no statistically significant difference between the two groups (Fisher-exact-Test).

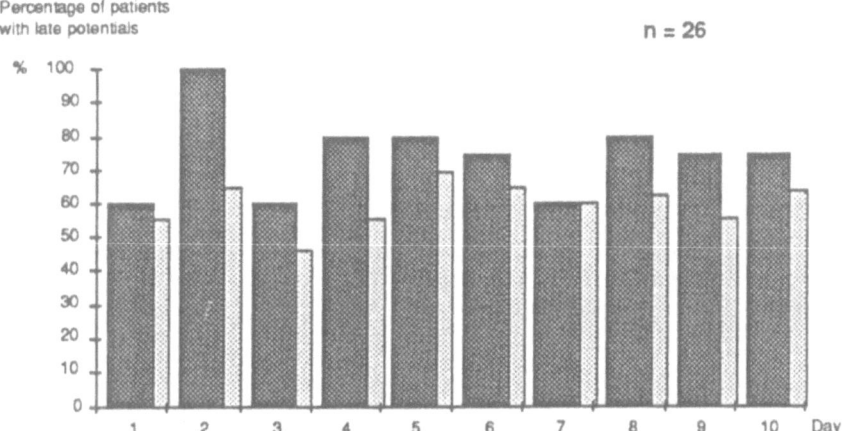

Figure 6. Incidence of late potentials in patients with left ventricular failure and pulmonary congestion ▇▇▇▇▇ in comparison to the incidence in the overall group ░░░░░ There was a significant difference ($p < 0.05$) between the two groups.

Conclusions

The incidence of late potentials in daily measurements during the first 10 days after acute myocardial infarction varied between 40% on the third day and 60% on the fifth day. There was no distinct tendency apparent over the course of the study. The site of the infarction was not related to the incidence of late potentials. Patients receiving a fibrinolytical therapy showed a lower incidence of late potentials than patients without. The difference, however, was not significant. The incidence of late potentials on the day of maximum levels of creatinine phosphokinase MB isoenzyme did not differ significantly from the incidence on the other days of the study. Patients whose acute infarction was complicated by left ventricular failure and pulmonary congestion, however, showed a significantly higher frequency of late potentials than patients without these complications.

16. High resolution electrocardiography. Basic and clinical aspects*

NABIL EL-SHERIF, MARK RESTIVO, WILLIAM CRAELIUS,
RAPHAEL HENKIN, GEORGE KELEN, JOHN M. FONTAINE,
SHANTHA N. URSELL & GIOIA TURITTO

State University of New York, Health Science Center and the Veterans Administration Medical Center, Brooklyn, New York, U.S.A.

Introduction

There are several low level electrocardiographic (ECG) potentials whose manifestations on the body surface are too small to be detected by routine measurement techniques. These include the potentials produced by the His-Purkinje system and by slow conduction in depressed ventricular myocardium (usually called late potentials). These potentials are small because the activation front is slow and fractionated or the mass of tissue undergoing depolarization is small or both. However, the measurement of the bioelectric potentials produced by these tissues is important for diagnostic purposes. Identification of the His-Purkinje potential can localize the site of atrio-ventricular conduction disorders, and the detection of late potentials may identify patients at high risk of malignant tachyarrhythmias. The problem in identifying these potentials is that the signal is smaller than the electric noise produced by various sources. Two different techniques have been utilized to improve signal-to-noise ratio: 1) temporal averaging (usually referred as to as signal averaging). This technique is applicable only to repetitive ECG signals and cannot detect moment by moment dynamic changes in the signals. 2) Low noise or high resolution ECG, which utilizes spatial averaging techniques, as well as other noise reducing measures, to record the His-Purkinje signal and late potentials on a beat-to-beat basis. The signal averaged technique has been utilized more often in the last few years and the averaged signal can be analyzed in either the time or frequency domain.

---

* Supported by National Institutes of Health Grants, HL 31341, HL 36680 and HC 65067 and by the Veterans Administration Medical Research Funds.

V. Hombach. H. H. Hilger and H. L. Kennedy (eds). Electrocardiography and Cardiac Drug Therapy. ISBN 978-94-010-6976-2
© 1989. Kluwer Academic Publishers, Dordrecht –

In this chapter we will review: A) System design and electrophysiologic instrumentation of the high resolution electrocardiogram; B) Experimental electrophysiologic substrate of late potentials; C) Clinical applications of the high resolution ECG; and D) New technical and physiologic advances.

System design and electrophysiologic instrumentation

The signal averaged ECG

Temporal averaging is a process whereby fixed intervals of a noisy signal are aligned temporally with respect to a reference point, and then summed. In the ideal case, N averages will reduce the noise by a factor of $1/SQR[N]$, while leaving the signal unaffected [1]. In practice, certain features of both noise and signal may limit the efficacy of signal averaging. The two conditions for optimal averaging are: a) the noise contaminant must be both random and stationary, and b) the signal of interest should be precisely synchronized to a stable reference time, or fiducial point.

A basic averaging system consists of: a) an ECG amplifier having high resolution and gain, b) high fidelity bandpass filters, c) a system for temporally aligning successive cardiac cycles, and d) a digital processor for the storage, averaging, and display of signals. Several such systems have been used, with designs ranging widely in complexity. Filter designs include analog bandpass circuits [2], linear digital filters [3], and bidirectional digital filters [4, 5]. Temporal alignment schemes range in complexity from simple R wave amplitude triggers [2] to QRS cross-correlation algorithms [6, 7]. Some alignment methods use the derivative of the QRS as the alignment signal [8, 9], while others use the wideband QRS [5]. Some QRS recognition algorithms, although not specifically designed for signal averaging, use an adaptive QRS threshold, whereby the waveforms from multiple beats specify threshold or contour limits, in order to optimize QRS detection [10–13].

To choose the optimal design for averaging, comparative performance characteristics are needed. Unfortunately, they are not available because standardized testing procedures for averaging systems do not exist. An obstacle to establishing standards has been the inability to directly measure the temporal misalignment. Because the waveshapes themselves are complex and vary from cycle to cycle, there are no a priori criteria by which to predict or quantify their alignment in time. Some attempts have been made to estimate alignment errors by modeling the QRS as a regular wave such as sine, and calculating the effects of amplitude variations and added noise

174

on a trigger system [14, 15], yet they offer no direct measure of alignment errors. A common method used to estimate alignment error is to measure a quantity called 'trigger jitter'. This is done by observing the range in temporal displacements of successive triggered QRS complexes on an oscilloscope screen. Reported values of jitter have ranged between 0.5 and 2 ms. Since the QRS shapes change in complex ways from beat to beat within that time resolution, the measurement of trigger jitter suffers from considerable arbitrariness. A more systematic method will be preferable. We have recently described a QRS detector system whereby temporal alignment accuracy and frequency response can be monitored during averaging and can be optimized for each patient [16]. The system shown in Figure 1 consists of two comparators, one based on amplitude, the other

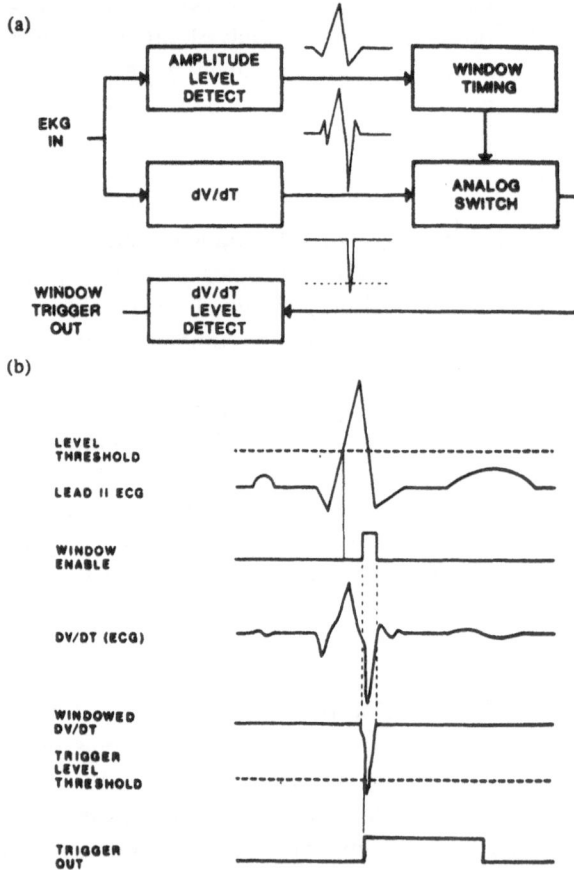

Figure 1. Design of QRS recognition system. (a) Schematic diagram. (b) Timing diagram (from Craelius et al. (1986) Criteria for optimal averaging of cardiac signals. IEEE Trans Biomed Eng BME-33:957, with permission).

based on slope within a specified interval. The ECG signal is high-pass filtered at a cutoff of 1 Hz to reduce baseline drift, and low-pass filtered at a cutoff of 500 Hz. The signal is fed into two circuits: a) an amplitude level detector, consisting of a comparator and b) a differentiator. The level detector triggers a timing circuit that sends a variable width pulse after a delay to an analog switch. The switch gates a selected portion of the differentiated signal and transmits this to a second comparator. If the slope is above the specified threshold, the final trigger pulse is generated. The final pulse is known as the 'window trigger', since it is based on a windowed portion of the QRS slope. It is used as the QRS alignment point for signal averaging, has a duration set just below the expected minimum ST interval of 300 ms, and is nonretriggerable. While all alignment systems are subject to some arbitrariness, one whose accuracy can be empirically measured and adjusted seems preferable. The window trigger system offers this advantage; it is not based on computed estimates and it can operate in real time. Moreover, the step response estimator of temporal misalignment can be readily incorporated into any alignment system, such as cross-correlation, in order to provide feedback on its accuracy.

The low noise beat-to-beat ECG

There are two major limitations for recording the His-Purkinje signals and late potentials by the signal averaging technique [17, 18]: a) it will not be able to detect dynamic (beat-to-beat) changes in the signal during sinus rhythm, and b) the signal averaged ECG can not be recorded during complex cardiac arrhythmias. We have recently designed two low noise ECG systems to record low amplitude His-Purkinje potentials and delayed depolarization potentials from the body surface on a beat-to-beat basis [17]. In one system, a bipolar electrode was utilized and the noise level was optimally reduced to 2 to 2.5 μv by a combination of noise-reduction techniques. In the second system, better noise reduction (1 to 1.5 μv) was achieved by utilizing spatial averaging from 16 pairs of electrodes and a specially designed volume conductor electrode. Other investigators have also reported on the use of a low noise, high resolution ECG for recording His-Purkinje potentials and/or late potentials [19–22]. In the spatial averaging technique, the potentials simultaneously recorded from multiple pairs of electrodes are averaged. The averaging reinforces the identical signals and attenuates uncorrelated potentials. Our recent observations suggest that electromyographic (EMG) potentials from skeletal muscle activity are the most significant source of noise [17, 23]. In spatial averaging, the optimal distance between pairs of surface electrodes is of crucial significance. If the interelectrode distance is small, EMG noise as well as the ECG signal from each pair would be correlated and spatial averaging would not enhance the signal-to-noise ratio. In a recent study from our laboratory, it was found that significant improvement in ECG to EMG noise ratio can be obtained by spacing electrode pairs 6 inches apart [23]. However, a somewhat closer interelectrode distance (2–4 inches) may be more practical, given the constraints of the number of electrodes that could be spatially averaged and, at the same time, maintain similar vectorial orientation of each electrode in reference to the ECG signal. In a recent study by Hombach et al. [21], an interelectrode distance of 15 mm, which seems to be less than optimal, was chosen.

In the low noise ECG system described by Flowers et al. [19] spatial averaging from multiple 'very closely spaced' electrodes was utilized. Further noise reduction was attempted by the use of a digital logic circuit that examines instantaneous polarity from each of the parallel input signals. The system would enhance signals with identical polarities and suppress those with non-identical polarities. Although this would reduce electrode and amplifier noise, it will not solve the problem of synchronous EMG potentials.

An improvement in ECG signal to EMG noise can be obtained by recording signals not from the precordial surface but a certain distance away from it with the help of a volume conductor electrode [17, 23]. When an electrode is placed directly on the chest surface, the potential recorded can be expressed by the solid angle model. It is directly proportional to the product of the potential difference of the activating biogenerator, the solid angle subtended by it, and a constant incorporating the conductivity of the medium. It is evident that if other variables do not alter and if the electrodes were to be moved distal to the chest surface with a conducting medium in between, the reduction in the solid angle of the cardiac generator would be less than for the EMG generator. This is because the ECG biogenerator is more distal to the skin surface than the EMG biogenerator. Hence, an improvement in the signal-to-noise ratio would occur even though both signals undergo attenuation. Recently, the concept of the volume conductor electrode was tested experimentally and the electrode was shown to result in significant reduction of EMG as compared to the ECG signal [23].

Experimental electrophysiologic substrate of late potentials

The origin of late potentials is believed to be myocardial zones with depressed electrophysiological properties which may provide the substrate

for reentrant excitation. Delayed activation potentials were initially described from the ischemic regions of the canine heart [24–27]. The relation
between delayed ventricular activation in ischemic myocardial zones and
ventricular arrhythmias based on a circus movement of excitation in the
post-infarction heart has been extensively investigated [28–31]. Several
investigators have shown that late potentials appear to correspond to
delayed and fragmented activation, which has been observed in epicardial
and endocardial electrograms recorded in animals [4, 32] and in patients
with ventricular tachyarrhythmias [33]. None of these studies, however,
correlated the presence of late potentials on the body surface recording
with ventricular activation maps of reentrant circuits. This was recently
investigated in a study from our laboratory utilizing the post-infarction
canine model of reentrant escitation [2]. In this model, reentrant circuits
commonly develop in the surviving ischemic epicardial layer overlying the
infarction and analysis of epicardial activation usually reflects the entire
reentrant circuit. Epicardial activation maps were constructed from 62
epicardial electrograms using a computerized multiplexer system. To assess
the relative contribution of electrically active regions to their detection on
the body surface, we constructed a synthesized root mean square (RMS)
composite electrogram. The composite was constructed by squaring the
individual epicardial electrograms, adding them, then taking the square
root of the sum. This eliminates the possibility of electrogram cancellation.
Body surface X, Y and Z leads were signal averaged, high pass filtered and
vector summed to record a signal averaged ECG. Late potentials in the
signal averaged ECG correlated in time with those in the 62 electrograms
and in the synthesized composite electrogram. Although the synthesized
composite electrogram showed late potentials that bridged the diastolic
interval, in the signal averaged ECG, 20 to 80 ms of the mid diastolic
interval sometimes failed to show late potentials. The late potentials-free
diastolic interval corresponded to very slow conduction of the reentrant
wavefront and to electrograms <0.1 mv. The results from one of the
experiments are shown in Figure 2. In this experiment a reentrant beat, V1
was consistently induced by a single premature stimulus, S2. A polar
projection of epicardial activation of the reentrant circuit is shown on the
right. Isochrones of activation are drawn at 20 ms intervals and the arcs of
functional conduction block are represented by the heavy solid lines. On
the left of Figure 2 is shown the XYZ vector sum of the signal averaged
ECG. Diastolic activity is seen following the S2 and preceding V1.
However, during a period of 70 ms in the mid diastolic interval, activity
was not present or was less than the noise level of the recording technique.
The mid diastolic interval corresponded in time to the slowly conducting
common reentrant wavefront as shown in the map to the right. On the

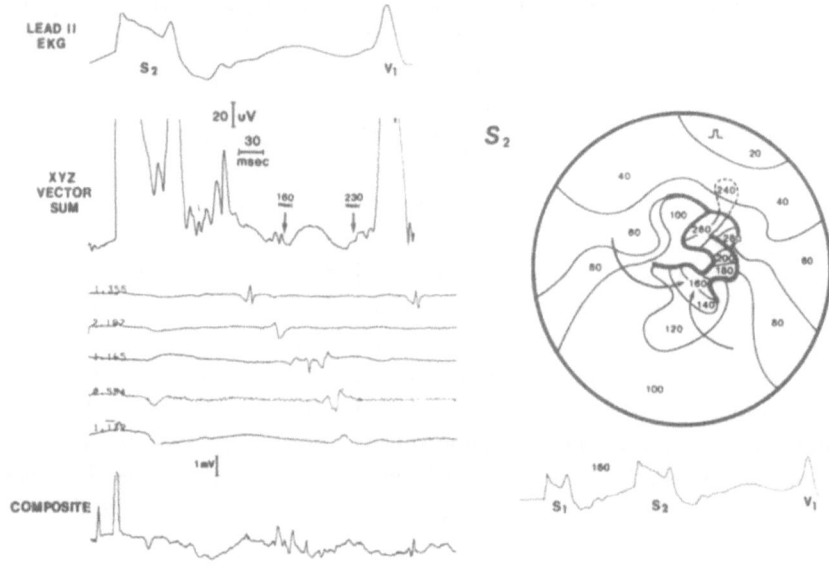

Figure 2. Recordings obtained from a 4-day-old canine post-infarction heart showing that the electrical activity of the slowly conducting part of the reentrant circuit could not be detected as mid diastolic potentials in the body surface signal averaged ECG. See text for details.

other hand, continuous diastolic activity was evident in the epicardial electrograms and in the composite electrogram. The selected epicardial electrograms shown in Figure 2 corresponded to the interval from 160 to 230 ms, where surface activity was not detected. The electrograms in this interval were recorded from a thin (1–2 mm) surviving epicardial layer overlying the core of the infarct. Some electrograms in this area were of reasonable amplitude (>1 mv), while others exhibited multiphasic electrotonic deflections, and others had low amplitude slow deflections (<0.1 mv). Those electrograms reflected very slow conduction through a narrow pathway surrounded by functionally blocked tissue. The small mass of active tissue which comprised the slowest part of the reentrant circuit was not reflected in the body surface recordings. Thus, our studies have shown that late potentials correlate with delayed epicardial activation in an area overlying the infarct. During reentrant activation, however, complete diastolic activity on the body surface may not be detected if the mass of electrically active cells is too small and/or if very slow conduction in part of the circuit generates low amplitude extracellular potentials.

Are regions of delayed activation during a basic rhythm the responsible arrhythmogenic substrate for reentry?

The relationship between myocardial zones showing conduction delay during sinus rhythm and spontaneous or induced reentrant rhythms is complex. Reentry requires a critical balance between the length of the zone of unidirectional block and the degree of conduction delay of the circulating wavefront [34]. The zones of unidirectional block are not represented in the signal averaged ECG and the degree of conduction delay necessary for reentry may bear little relationship to the degree of conduction delay during sinus rhythm. We have recently conducted a study in the 4-day-old canine post-infarction model of reentry to determine if regions of delayed activation during a basic rhythm (sinus rhythm or S1-S1 ventricular pacing) are the responsible arrhythmogenic substrate for reentry [35]. Reentrant rhythms were induced by programmed electrical stimulation. The signal averaged ECG during basic rhythm at a cycle length of 4000–500 ms detected late potentials, which corresponded temporally with the region of latest epicardial activation times. Subsequent signal averaging of reentrant circuits revealed that sites of late potentials during the basic rhythm were

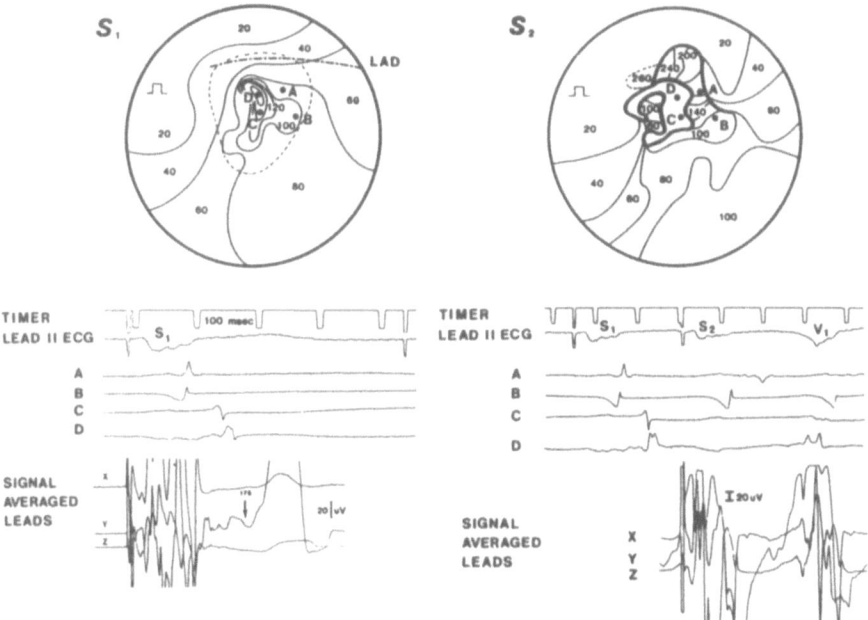

Figure 3. Recordings obtained from a 4-day-old canine post-infarction heart showing that regions responsible for late potentials during the basic rhythm were not part of the slow common reentrant pathway during reentrant activation. See text for details.

now always responsible for late potentials detected during reentrant activation. Examination of activation maps of these beats confirmed that the regions responsible for late potentials during a basic rhythm were not part of the final common reentrant pathway during reentrant activation. Regions of marked delay, Wenckebach or 2:1 conduction during the basic rhythm usually blocked during S2 and did not participate in the reentrant process. This is illustrated in Figure 3 obtained from one of the experiments. Shown from top to bottom are the epicardial activation map, surface ECG and selected epicardial electrograms and X, Y and Z leads of the signal averaged ECG. Recordings on the left were obtained during basic right ventricular pacing at an S1-S1 cycle of 400 ms. Recordings on the right were obtained during premature stimulation (S2) that initiated a reentrant beat (VI). During S1 stimulation the most delayed epicardial activation sites were in the center of the ischemic zone represented by epicardial electrograms C and D. These sites were reflected by late potentials in the signal averaged ECG. However, during reentrant activation induced by S2 stimulation, electrograms C and D showed conduction block and their sites did not participate in the reentrant circuit as shown in the activation map on the right. On the other hand, mid diastolic activity during reentry is represented by electrograms A and B. These sites contributed to the diastolic potentials during reentry but not to the late potentials during the basic rhythm.

Clinical applications of the high resolution ECG

Detection of His-Purkinje potential

The signal averaged ECG

The feasibility of recording His-Purkinje electrograms from the body surface by signal averaging techniques has been clearly established [36–43]. Although the technique for non-invasive recording of the His bundle electrogram has been in existence for several years, it has not enjoyed widespread application for two reasons: i) an invasive procedure is often necessary for other electrophysiologic measurements, and ii) because of technical problems. The quality of the non-invasive recording and the definite presence of the His bundle electrogram have often been questioned. Two problems have been prominent: i) it has been difficult to extract the small amplitude His bundle potential from the noise of the system. A signal-to-noise ratio of at least 2 to 3 is required to isolate the signal; ii) the terminal atrial activity often overlaps with the His bundle electrogram, making the two indistinguishable. Attempts to separate atrial from His bundle potentials by optimal bandpass filtering have not been successful [44]. Some investigators [45] have attempted to separate the atrial activity from the His bundle potential by prolonging the PR interval with the help of pharmaceutical agents. This procedure can give satisfactory recordings in some patients but it makes the technique more difficult to implement. One method that can increase the probability of recording His bundle activity is simultaneous signal averaging of multiple vectorial leads. In a study from our laboratory [46], we found that a reliable His bundle electrogram could be obtained with this technique in 18 to 30% more patients (depending on the vector) than when a single lead measurement was used. There are several advantages to this technique: i) it allows one to validate the His bundle potential in more than one lead. We found that no single lead was statistically superior and that any of the vectorial leads could display the maximal amplitude of the His bundle potential (Figure 4; ii) in some cases with atrial activity overlap, one lead showed an isoelectric terminal atrial vector that permitted recognition of the onset of the His potential. We consider it essential that at least a 10 ms isoelectric region be present between the atrial activity and the His deflection. The 10 ms interval was chosen primarily for ease of visual interpretation. This was the major reason that our overall success rate of 55% with three vectorial leads was less than that observed by some other investigators with

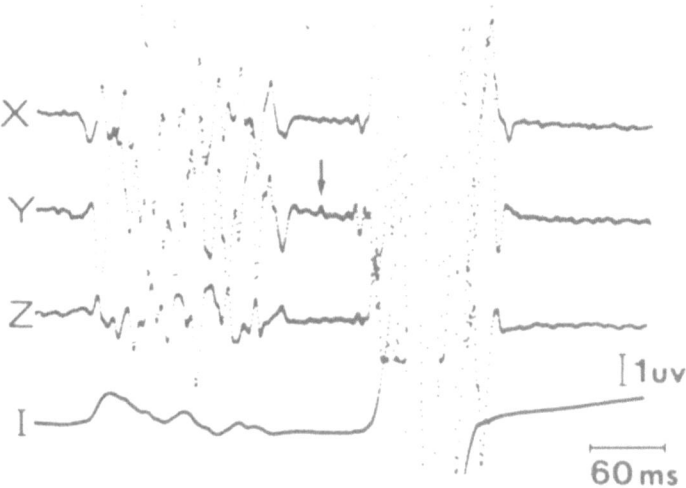

Figure 4. X, Y and Z leads recordings of the signal averaged ECG in a 50-year-old man. The His bundle potential is only evident in the Y lead (marked by arrow). A simultaneous low gain lead I electrocardiogram is also shown (from Mehra et al. (1982) Noninvasive His bundle electrogram: value of three vector lead recording. Am J Cardiol 49:344, with permission).

182

a single lead measurement [43 45]; iii) the likelihood of bundle branch potentials being considered as His bundle potentials is also reduced by recording from multiple leads. In some of our patients certain vector leads showed large bundle branch potentials and a diminutive His bundle electrogram. A multivectorial recording was essential to distinguish the earliest deflection, which was the His bundle potential.

The low noise beat-to-beat ECG

In a study from our laboratory [17], the low noise ECG identified the His bundle potential in 43% of patients compared with 71% recorded in the signal averaged ECG from the same patients. The HV intervals measured by the two techniques were remarkably similar [correlation coefficient $(r) = 0.97$, probability $(p) < 0.001$] (Figure 5). The lower yield of the low noise ECG was attributed to less optimal reduction of noise level with this technique compared to the signal averaged ECG. Higher success rate was reported by other investigators who utilized different noise-reducing techniques [19, 20]. The clinical advantage of identifying the His-Purkinje potential from a surface recording on a beat-to-beat basis is obvious particularly when compared with the signal averaged ECG. Only the low noise ECG is helpful in situations where there is a dynamic change of the temporal relation between the atrial and ventricular potentials [17, 20].

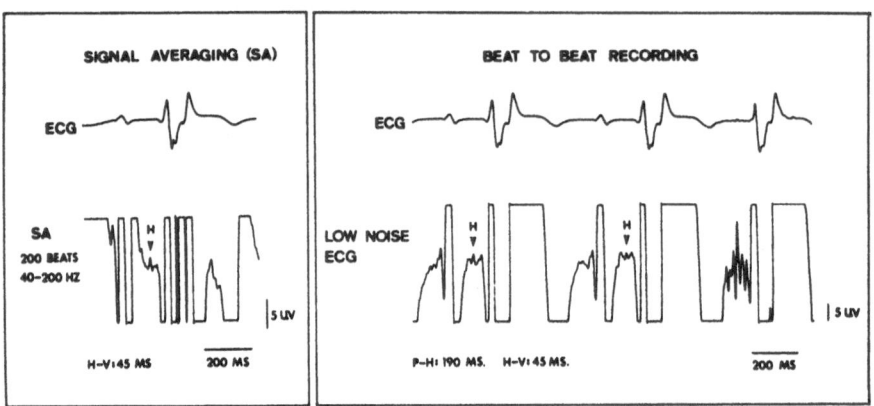

Figure 5. Recordings of the His bundle potential (H) by both the signal averaged ECG (left panel) and the low noise beat-to-beat ECG (right panel) in a 76-year-old man. A discrete and remarkably similar H potential with an HV interval of 45 ms is seen in both recordings. Of the three consecutive beats in the low noise ECG, the third is a supraventricular premature beat. The preventricular segment of this beat is obscured by potentials originating from an ectopic P wave with a short PR interval (From El-Sherif et al. (1983) Appraisal of a low noise electrocardiogram. J. Am Coll Cardiol 1:456, with permission).

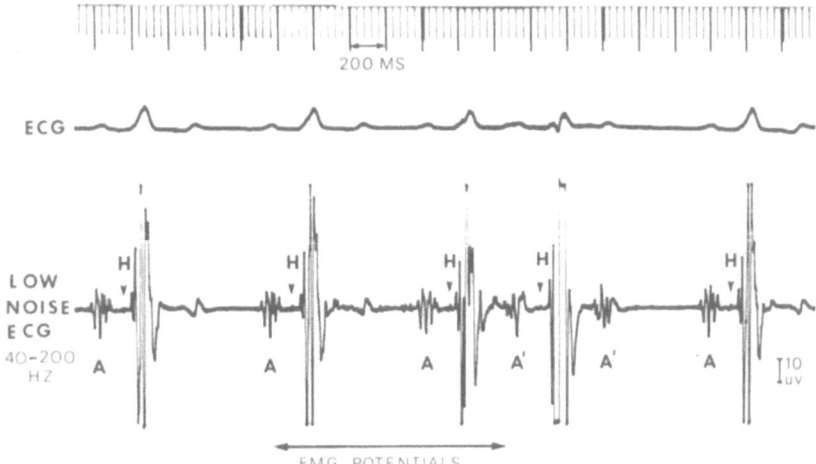

Figure 6. Value of the low noise ECG for the diagnosis of complex cardiac arrhythmias. Recordings obtained from a 63-year-old man. The standard ECG lead (top) shows sinus rhythm, first degree AV block, left bundle branch block and a single premature beat with a QRS configuration slightly different from that of the sinus beat. The low noise ECG (bottom) shows a distinct His bundle potential (H) with an AH and AV intervals of 180 and 55 ms, respectively, reflecting AV nodal conduction delay. The recording also reveals the presence of two atrial premature beats with the first beat showing further prolongation of the AH interval and the second blocking at the level of the AV node. Note the periodic increase of electromyographic (EMG) potentials associated with respiration (from El-Sherif et al. (1983) Appraisal of low noise electrocardiogram. J Am Coll Cardiol 1:456, with permission).

This encompasses a wide spectrum of clinically relevant disorders of the cardiac rhythm that include all examples of second and third degree AV block, AV dissociation, atrial and ventricular premature depolarizations and tachyarrhythmias (Figure 6).

Detection of late potentials

The signal averaged ECG

Late potentials in patients with spontaneous or induced ventricular tachyarr-hythmias. Several investigators have shown correlation of late potentials with the occurrence of sustained ventricular tachycardia especially in the post-infarction period. The incidence of late potentials in patients with recurrent sustained ventricular tachycardia (VT) varies from 66% to 90% [47–49]. Late potentials may also be an indication of increased vulnerability in patients without previously documented spontaneous ventricular tachy-arrhythmias. The predictive value of late potentials and programmed electrical stimulation was assessed prospectively in 379 patients without a history of sustained VT, dizziness or syncope [50]. No correlation was found between the two techniques and the occurrence of sudden cardiac death. However, the combined use of signal averaged ECG and program-med stimulation helped to identify subgroups at markedly different risk of developing spontaneous symptomatic VT. The highest predictive value for subsequent sustained VT was reached by a combination of late potentials of 40-ms duration or more, the induction of monomorphic sustained VT at rates below 270 beats/min, and an interval after myocardial infarction less than 6 weeks. We have recently conducted a prospective study to evaluate the value of several clinical variables, left ventricular function indices, Holter ECG characteristics, and the signal averaged ECG in predicting the inducibility of sustained ventricular tachyarrhythmias in 100 patients with spontaneous non-sustained ventricular tachycardia [51]. The patients were divided into three groups based on the results of programmed stimulation: Group I, 21 patients with induced sustained monomorphic VT, Group II, 12 patients with induced ventricular fibrillation, and Group III, 67 patients with no induced sustained ventricular tachyarrhythmias. The following variables were significantly more common in Group I compared to Group III: history of syncope/presyncope, left ventricular ejection fraction <0.40, and the presence of late potentials in the signal averaged ECG. On the other hand, no significant difference was found between Groups II and III except for age. The sensitivity, specificity and predictive accuracy of late potentials were 62%, 90% and 83%, respectively (Figure 7). The predic-tive accuracy of late potentials was not significantly different in patients with coronary artery disease or non ischemic dilated cardiomyopathy, nor in patients with short or long runs of spontaneous non-sustained VT. Using stepwise discriminant function analysis, no combination between late potentials, ejection fraction and history of syncope/presyncope provided an improvement in predicting the induction of sustained monomorphic VT, in comparison with late potentials alone. No combination of variables predic-ted the induction of ventricular fibrillation. Our study shows that the signal averaged ECG represents the most accurate single non-invasive screening test to predict the induction of sustained monomorphic VT. The failure to predict the induction of ventricular fibrillation may reflect the lack of clinical significance of this response to programmed stimulation in patients with non-sustained VT.

Incidence and prognostic significance of late potentials in the post-infarction patients. The incidence and prognostic significance of late potentials in the

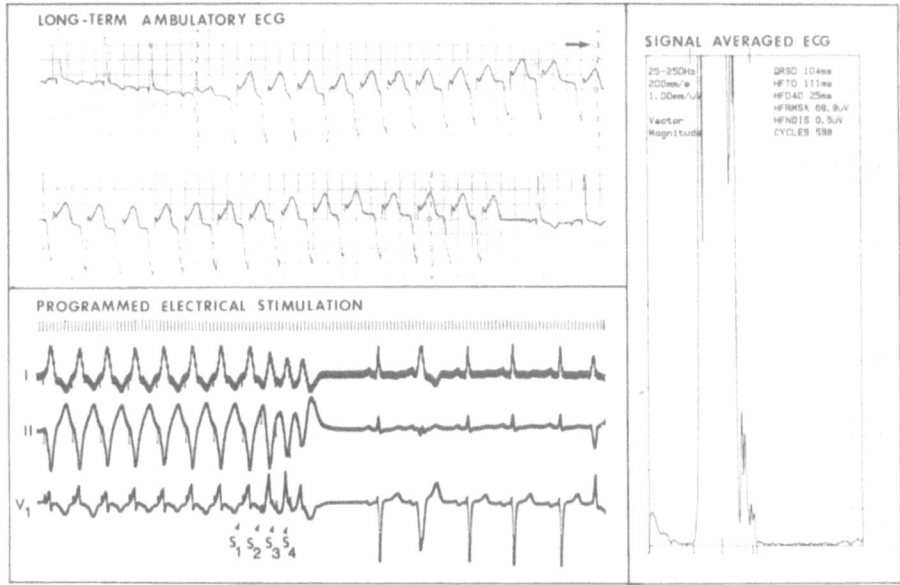

Figure 7. Recordings of ambulatory ECG, programmed electrical stimulation and the signal averaged ECG from a 41-year-old man with non-ischemic delated cardiomyopathy. The patient had no history of syncope/presyncope. Ejection fraction by radionuclide ventriculography was 16%. A 24-hour ambulatory ECG showed frequent ventricular premature complexes (average 240/hour) and 6 runs of non-sustained ventricular tachycardia. The longest run lasted for 11.4 seconds and had an average rate of 134 beats/min (shown in the figure). The signal averaged ECG was normal and there was no inducible arrhythmia on programmed stimulation.

post-infarction period vary widely in different studies. A low incidence of 16% was reported by Kertes et al. in a group of 43 patients when the recording was obtained in the immediate post-infarction period [52]. Late potentials were defined as RMS low amplitude signals of $<10 \ \mu v$ of the unfiltered signal averaged QRS. The signal averaged ECG was recorded before the onset of ventricular fibrillation in 7 patients and in only one did the record show late potentials. In a study from our laboratory [53] the signal averaged ECG was recorded in 50 patients between 1 and 10 days post-infarction. The duration of low amplitude signals of $<40 \ \mu v$ (LAS40) was >42 ms in 44% of the patients, the RMS voltage in the terminal 40 ms of the QRS (RMS40) was $<20 \ \mu v$ in 42% and the total duration of the averaged QRS was >120 ms in 42%. In a more recent study [54] the incidence of abnormalities on the signal averaged ECG was 31% in a group of 70 patients studied in the first two months post-infarction. This was based on the presence of RMS40 $<25 \ \mu v$ and/or a total averaged QRS duration >120 ms. In a study by Breithardt et al. [55] the incidence of late potentials was 50.6% in a group of 160 patients. The signal averaged ECG was obtained between 7 and 109 days (median: 25.5 days) after infarction. Late potentials were identified visually as low amplitude signals at the end of the averaged QRS. Late potentials of <20-ms duration were observed in 20.6% of the patients whereas late potentials of >20-ms duration were present in 30% of the patients. In the latter group late potentials were more frequent in patients with inferior infarction (38.6%) than in those with anterior infarction (17.9%). Follow-up (mean + standard deviation, 7.7 + 3.2 months) showed the recording of late potentials was able to predict the subsequent occurrence of symptomatic sustained VT after discharge from hospital. These data have recently been extended to a total of 511 patients in whom follow-up was greater than 6 months [56]. The prevalence of sudden cardiac death was greater in patients with late potentials than in those without them. The rate of sudden death (<24 hours) after one year was 0.95% in patients without and 3.1% in patients with late potentials ($p < 0.01$). However, if only cases dying within one hour were considered, the difference was no longer significant. On the other hand, the signal averaged ECG proved to be more predictive of subsequent occurrence of sustained VT with a sensitivity of 78.6% and a specificity of 63.3%. In a study by Denniss et al. [57], 26% of 307 patients had an abnormal signal averaged ECG defined as a total duration of the signal averaged unfiltered QRS of >140 ms. Patients were also subjected to programmed stimulation 7–28 days post-infarction. There was a significant correlation ($p < 0.01$) between the presence of delayed potentials and the ability to induce VT but not ventricular fibrillation. The study found that in survivors of recent infarction who have not had spontaneous ventricular tachyarrhythmias, inducible VT, (but not inducible ventricular fibrillation) at programmed stimulation predicts a significant risk of sudden death and/or arrhythmic events. A similar risk was found for patients with delayed potentials in the signal averaged ECG. However, there was incomplete correspondence between the two tests with respect to correct identification of patients who suffered cardiac events during follow-up. Multiple logistic regression analysis showed that inducible VT and delayed potentials were not independent predictors of either mortality or primary arrhythmic events. By contrast, anterior infarction was an independent predictor of mortality ($p < 0.01$) while pulmonary congestion on the chest X-ray was the only variable tested that was an independent predictor of spontaneous ventricular tachyarrhythmias ($p < 0.02$). The risk of developing spontaneous VT and/or sudden death over the following year was prospectively assessed by Kuchar et al. [58] in 165 patients who survived acute myocardial infarction. The signal averaged ECG was performed before hospital discharge (10.5 + 6.1 days after initial presentation, range 7 to 40 days). An abnormal signal averaged ECG was defined as the presence of RMS40 <20 μv and/or a total filtered QRS duration >120 ms utilizing a high bandpass frequency of 40 Hz. The incidence of abnormal signal averaged ECG was 41%. Abnormalities on signal averaged ECG were more common in inferior infarction (56%) than in anterior infarction (35%) and non-Q wave infarction (29%). The sensitivity of the signal averaged ECG as a predictor of arrhythmic events was 92% with a specificity of 62%. Multivariate logistic regression determined that abnormal signal averaged ECG and left ventricular ejection fraction <0.40 provided independent information. However, evidence of complex ventricular ectopy during Holter monitoring was not found to be significant in the multivariate model.

Differences in the reported incidence and prognostic significance of abnormal signal averaged ECG in the post-infarction period can be explained by: 1) differences in the recording technique and in the definition of an abnormal recording; 2) the time of the recording in the post-infarction period; and 3) the difference in the incidence of late potentials between anterior and inferior myocardial infarction. At present, general guidelines could be suggested regarding optimal techniques for the recording of the time domain signal averaged ECG. The use of a bidirectional filter [59], an iterative cross-correlation procedure to optimize QRS alignment and a computer algorithm to identify abnormal indices is usually recommended. There is, however, some controversy regarding the use of high bandpass filters. Some investigators analyzed unfiltered averaged signals [52, 57], while others found that high bandpass filtering is necessary to reject the low frequency activity present in the ST-T segment. The use of a high bandpass filter can significantly influence the numeric criteria that have been suggested for analysis of the signal averaged QRS. These include the root mean square voltage of the terminal (usually 40 ms) signals of the QRS, the duration of signals of less than a certain amplitude (usually 40 μv), and the total duration of the averaged QRS. In a study by Simson et al. [59] applying a 25-Hz high bandpass filter, 92% and 72% of patients with VT after myocardial infarction could be correctly identified based on a low amplitude signal in the last 40 ms of the QRS <25 μv and QRS duration >120 ms, respectively. On the other hand, Denes et al. [60] suggested that a high bandpass filter of 40 Hz could better distinguish between normal subjects and patients with VT based on an abnormal low amplitude signal in the last 40 ms of the averaged QRS <20 μv. The importance of the time of recording of the signal averaged ECG in the post-infarction period was recently emphasized in a study from our laboratory [54]. Serial signal averaged ECGs were obtained 0–5 days, 6–30 days and 31–60 days post-infarction in 70 patients with acute myocardial in-

188

farction. The study has shown that abnormal recordings appear early (within the first five days after infarction) in 45% of the cases and late (between 6 and 30 days after infarction) in the remaining 55%. The recording returned to normal in 50% of the patients within 60 days of infarction (Figure 8). Some studies have documented a similar trend towards a decreased incidence of late potentials in the late phases of myocardial infarction [58]. The dynamic nature of abnormalities in the signal averaged ECG illustrates the limitations of investigations based on a single recording in the post-infarction period. Our study suggests that in order to achieve maximal sensitivity, the optimal time for signal averaging should be between two and four weeks post-infarction. However, the prognostic significance of transient versus more lasting abnormalities in the signal averaged ECG has yet to be established.

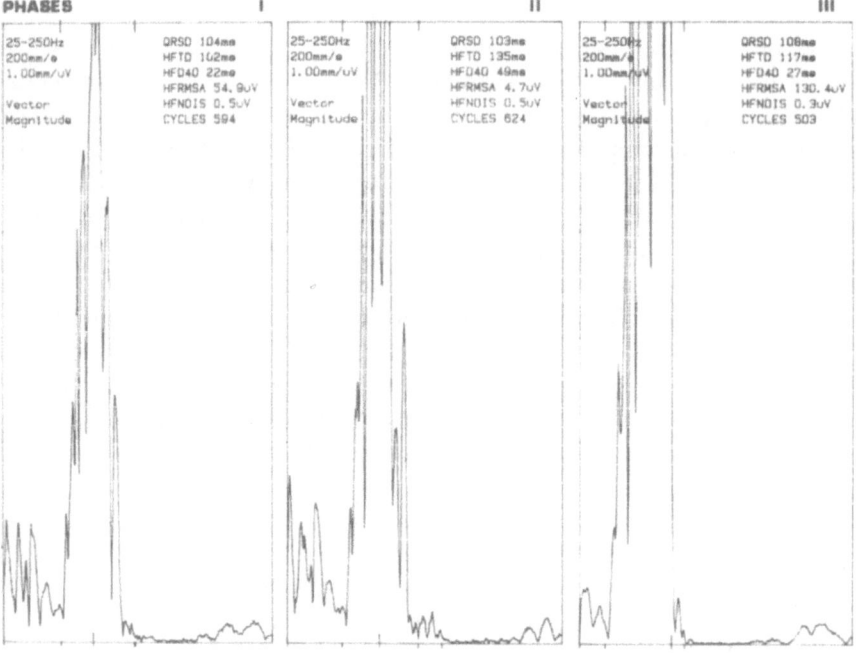

Figure 8. Time course of the signal averaged ECG in a patient with acute anterior wall myocardial infarction. The vector magnitude recording of the filtered QRS complex is shown. The three recordings from left to right were obtained 4, 9 and 35 days post-infarction, respectively. The abnormalities in the signal averaged ECG were first observed in the record obtained 9 days post-infarction as RMS40 of 4.7 uv and total duration of the filtered QRS at 135 ms. The record normalized by the 35th day post-infarction.

Comparison of time and frequency domain analysis of late potentials in the signal averaged ECG. In most studies, late potentials have been identified in the time domain by analysis of the highly amplified terminal QRS complex after signal averaging and usually high pass filtering and vector summation. It has recently been suggested that an alternative and perhaps more clinically sensitive and/or specific way to detect abnormal high frequency activity in the terminal QRS and ST segment is to perform frequency analysis using the Fast-Fourier transform (FFT) technique on the appropriate visually identified segment of the signal averaged ECG [61–63]. Late potentials in the time domain should correspond to disproportionately high levels of power in the frequency spectrum above 20 Hz [61, 62]. Increased accuracy of detection of patients prone to sustained VT has been suggested [61–63].

Using a microcomputer based system capable of performing time and frequency domain analyses on the same set of acquired data and signal averaged raw data, we conducted a study to correlate late potentials revealed by the conventional time domain technique with the results of FFT analysis performed according to previously reported techniques [64]. Data from 10 patients who satisfied the criteria for late potentials in the time domain signal averaged ECG were analyzed. All patients had spontaneous and/or inducible VT. Data from 10 healthy normal subjects were also analyzed. The study found that it is difficult to distinguish patients with spontaneous and/or inducible VT (and late potentials in the time domain recording) from normals (without late potentials) on the basis of the proportion of high frequency content in the FFT of the terminal QRS and ST segment utilizing previously reported techniques. A major difficulty was the inability to reproducibly select the same length and position of the QRS-ST segment subjected to FFT analysis. A very small change in the analyzed segment length of the order of 10 ms changed the computed FFT parameters by several hundreds percent, certainly sufficient to cross any boundary of normalcy.

Figures 9 and 10 illustrate the time and frequency domain analyses of the signal averaged electrogram from a 57-year-old man with an old anterior wall myocardial infarction, episodes of spontaneous non-sustained VT and inducible sustained monomorphic VT on programmed stimulation. The lower plot in Figure 9 shows the three averaged orthogonal leads while the upper plot illustrates the time domain vector magnitude calculated by taking the square root of the sum of the rectified three leads. Late potentials were present based on a RMS40 of 16.7 μv and a LAS40 of 66.0 ms. Figure 10 illustrates two examples of frequency domain analysis, calculated from the three averaged orthogonal leads shown in Figure 9. The left panel in Figure 10 illustrates the analyzed FFT plots for segment 1

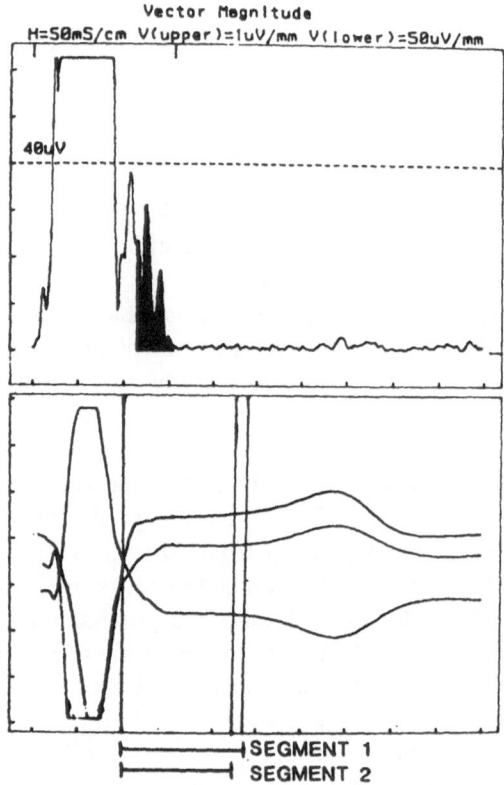

```
QRS Duratlon = 154.5 mS
RMS-40 = 16.7 uV    LAS-40 = 66.0 mS

Nolse (vector) = 0.9 uV


          Vector Magnitude
H=50mS/cm V(upper)=1uV/mm V(lower)=50uV/mm
```

40uV

├────────────┤ SEGMENT 1
├────────────┤ SEGMENT 2

Figure 9. The signal averaged ECG in the time domain mode from a 57-year-old man with old anterior wall myocardial infarction and recurrent ventricular tachycardia. The X, Y and Z leads are shown on the bottom and the vector magnitude on the top. Note the presence of late potentials. See text for details.

(the segment comprised the last 40 ms of the QRS and the ST segment up to what was considered to be the onset of the T wave). The length of this segment was 139.5 ms and the averaged area ratio 1 (13.61) suggests that the patient does not have significant frequency components in the 20–50 Hz range. In contrast, when averaged area ratio 1 was computed for a slightly shorter segment length of 129.0 (segment 2, obtained by moving the cursor used to define the onset of the T wave to the left) it was greater than that calculated for segment 1 (67.00 versus 13.61 respectively). This exceeded the criterion of significance for area ratio 1 of >20 [62,63].

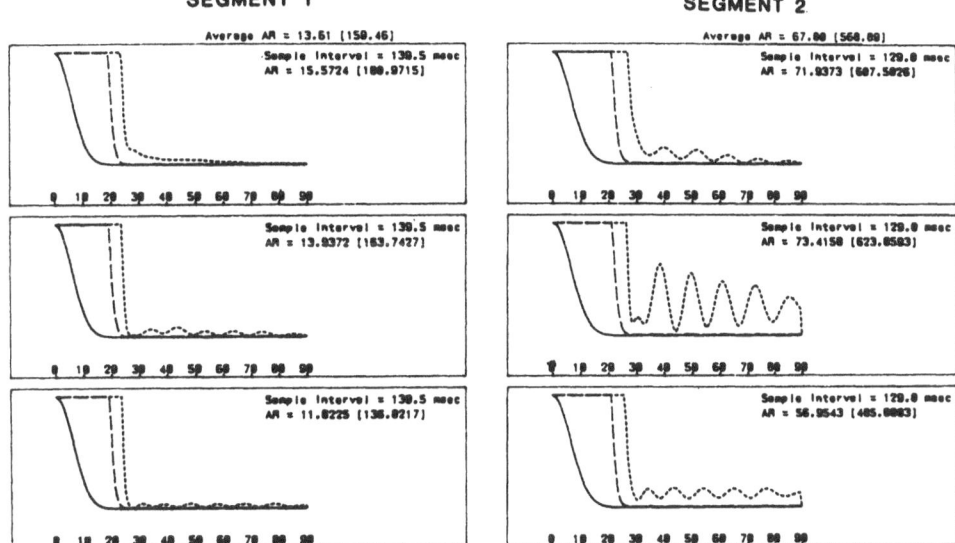

Figure 10. The Fast-Fourier Transform (FFT) analysis from the same patient shown in Figure 9. The FFT plot of segments 1 and 2 as outlined in Figure 9 are shown on the left and right panels, respectively. The calculated area ratios for the two segments are markedly different. See text for details.

Values for area ratio 2 were also calculated (shown in brackets in Figure 10) and these too showed a significant increase as the segment was shortened. Figure 11 illustrates the changes in computed area ratio 1 from the same patient when the analyzed segment was shortened in 10 steps of 1.5 ms each. Position 0 on the abscissa corresponds to the longest segment of 139.5 ms as shown in Figure 9, while position 13.5 reflects the shortest segment of 126.0 ms. The right border of each segment remained fixed and demarcated the terminal 40 ms of the QRS complex as shown in Figure 9. The graph illustrates that decreasing the length of the analyzed segment resulted in a consistent increase in area ratio 1, reflecting an increased proportion of high frequency components in the analyzed segment. A decrease in segment length of 3 ms was enough to change area ratio 1 from less than to more than 20, the suggested index of significance [62, 63] (i.e. from false negative to true positive). Our study suggests that while frequency domain analysis of ECG signals remains an attractive possibility, to be clinically useful a technique using frequency analysis should yield reproducible results that are independent of arbitrary factors such as precise length and position of analyzed signal sample. At present, in contrast to time domain analysis, frequency domain analysis techniques are not developed enough to warrant large scale clinical trials.

192

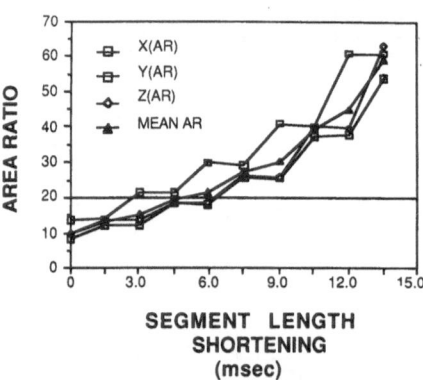

Figure 11. Diagrammatic illustration of the area ratio from the same patient shown in Figures 9 and 10 calculated for 10 different segments. Note that decreasing the length of the analyzed segment resulted in a consistent increase in the calculated area ratios. See text for details.

The low noise beat-to-beat ECG

In a study from our laboratory [65], we analyzed the low noise ECG for the presence of late potentials in 18 normal volunteers and in 20 patients with various disorders of cardiac rhythm. None of the patients had had myocardial infarction in the past year. Late potentials were recorded in only two patients (7%). On the other hand, late potentials in the low noise ECG were recorded in 15 of 21 patients within the first three weeks following acute myocardial infarction (71%). Twelve of the 15 patients had episodes of VT and/or ventricular fibrillation either spontaneously or during programmed stimulation. Only one of the remaining six patients who had no late potentials had spontaneous episodes of VT. The late potentials varied in amplitude between 2 and 25 μv and were continuous with high amplitude, high frequency components in the late QRS complex. The late potentials extended up to 280 ms from the onset of the QRS complex (20 to 190 ms from the end of the QRS complex; the latter was approximately defined from normal standard leads I, aVF and V1 that were recorded simultaneously with the low noise ECG). The late potentials remained constant in successive sinus beats in nine patients, probably reflecting a 1:1 conduction pattern in ischemic myocardium. In six patients, the late potentials varied in configuration and timing in successive sinus beats, probably reflecting a Wenckebach conduction pattern. In such patients the low noise ECG was usually superior to the signal averaged recording. In four patients, the late potentials were recorded during spontaneous ventricular premature beats. In two patients, late potentials were reproducible only in

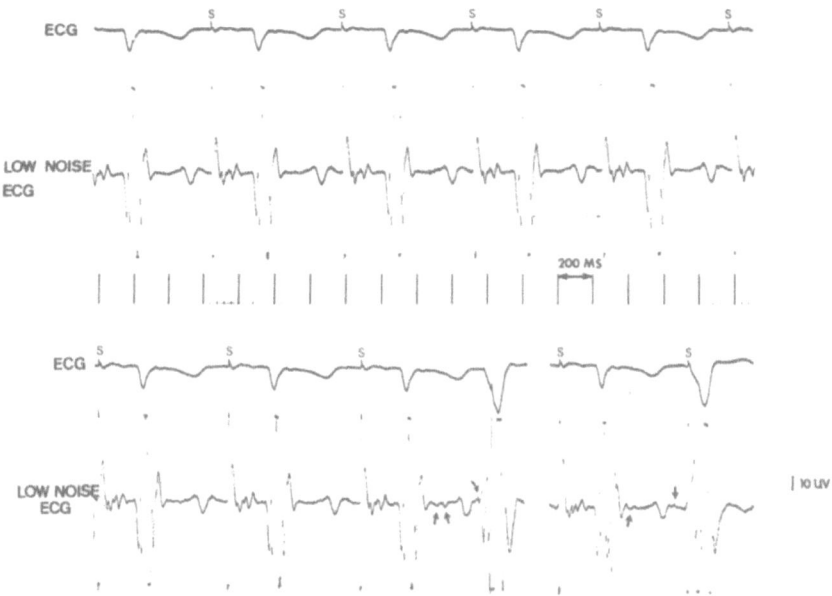

Figure 12. A low noise ECG recording from a patient 3 weeks post-infarction showing an atrial paced rhythm and spontaneous ventricular premature complexes (VPCs). No late potentials were seen during the atrial paced beats. However, late potentials were consistently seen in the diastolic interval preceding spontaneous VPCs both in the early and late parts of the ST-T segments (arrows, lower panel). Note that the diastolic potentials are unrelated to the coupling interval of the VPCs (from El-Sherif et al. (1983) Appraisal of a low noise electrocardiogram J Am Coll Cardiol 1:456, with permission).

Table 1. Low noise ECG in normals and post-infarction patients

---

  I. Control Group: 28 patients, no MI[2] in last year, no
       LP[1] in 2 (7%)   spontaneous VT[4]
 II. Post-infarction Group: 21 patients, MI[2] within 3 weeks
       LP[1] in 15 (71%)
     A) spontaneous or   induced VT[4]/VF[3]: 13 patients
     B) no spontaneous   VT[4]/VF[3]: 8 patients

Positive predictive value: 80%
Negative predictive value: 83%
Total predictive value: 81%

---

[1] LP–late potentials; [2]MI–myocardial infarction; [3]VF–ventricular fibrillation; [4]VT–ventricular tachycardia.

the ST segment preceding a ventricular premature beat (Figure 12). Multiform ventricular premature complexes recorded in two other patients did not appear to be related to the late potentials. A low noise ECG was not recorded during VT in any of the patients. The results are summarized in Table 1 and show a positive predictive value of 80%, a negative predictive value of 83% and a total predictive value of 81%.

Comparison of late potentials in the low noise ECG and the signal averaged ECG

We compared the incidence of late potentials in the low noise ECG and the signal averaged ECG in 20 patients [65] (Table 2). The signal averaged ECG was recorded in nine patients in whom a low noise ECG did not reveal late potentials. In two patients, late potentials, 2–5 μv in amplitude and 20–40 ms in duration, were recorded. On the other hand, in 11 patients in whom a low noise ECG revealed late potentials, a signal averaged ECG showed late potentials of similar duration in eight patients but failed to show consistent late potentials in three. In two of these three patients, the late potentials in the low noise ECG varied from beat-to-beat. No signal averaged ECG was recorded when late potentials and spontaneous ventricular arrhythmias in the low noise ECG were present. In three patients, late potentials in both the low noise ECG and signal averaged ECG were correlated with localized delayed potentials recorded from endocardial catheter electrodes. This is illustrated in Figures 13 and 14 obtained from a 54-year-old patient 7 days following an inferior wall infarction. Figure 13 shows the signal averaged ECG on top and the low noise ECG on bottom. Late diastolic potentials of 80 ms duration (measured from the end of QRS) were recorded in both the unfiltered and filtered low noise ECG. On the other hand, in the signal averaged ECG, only the V lead showed late potentials of 80 ms duration corresponding to the ones in the low noise ECG. Both the X and Z leads showed delayed potentials of only 40 ms duration. Figure 14 illustrates electrode catheter recordings from proximal

Table 2. Comparison of low noise ECG and signal averaged ECG (20 patients)

	Low noise ECG	Signal averaged ECG
Group A(LP[1])	11	8
Group B (no LP[1])	9	7*

* Two patients had LP 2–5 μv in amplitude and 20–40 ms in duration; [1]LP–late potentials.

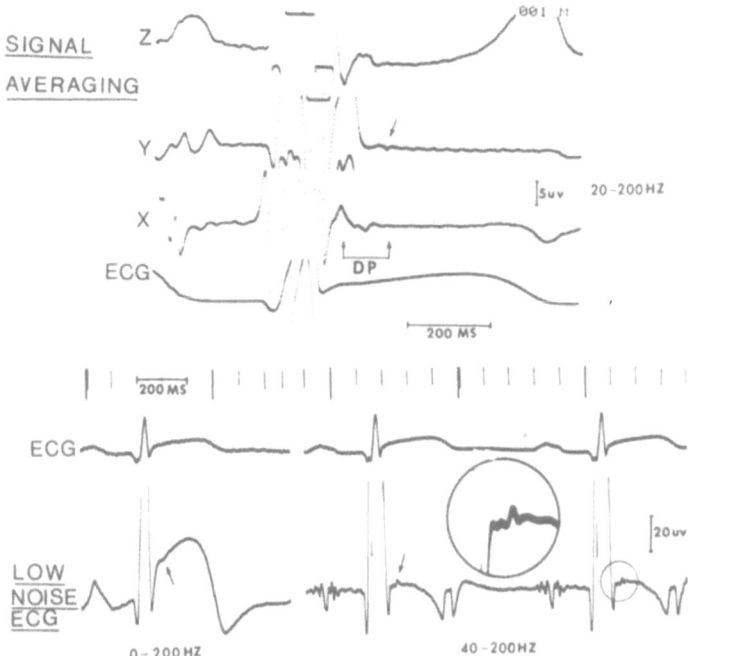

Figure 13. Comparison of the signal averaged ECG (top) and the low noise ECG (bottom) in a patient one week post-inferior wall myocardial infarction (see text for details). DP, delayed potentials (from El-Sherif et al. (1985) Late potentials and arrhythmogenesis. PACE 8:440. with permission).

and distal right septal myocardium from the same patient obtained during an electrophysiologic study. The distal septal electrogram showed the presence of a late potential. The occurrence of a spontaneous ventricular premature beat at a short coupling interval (labeled X) resulted in marked fractionation of the late potentials (labeled DP). The figure illustrates a tachycardia-dependent lengthening of the duration of late diastolic potentials which is consistent with the known response of conduction in ischemic myocardial zones [27].

In a larger series of patients, Hombach et al. compared the recording of late potentials from body surface using the signal averaged ECG and the low noise beat-to-beat technique and reported similar results [22]. Concordant results were found in 39 of 53 patients (late potentials were retrieved by both techniques in 24 or 53 patients and no late potentials were recorded by both techniques in 15 of 53 patients). On the other hand, discordant results were found in 14 of 53 patients (late potentials were recorded by the beat-to-beat technique but not in the signal averaged ECG in 12 patients while the opposite was true in two patients). Dynamic changes of late potentials were only detectable by the beat-to-beat technique.

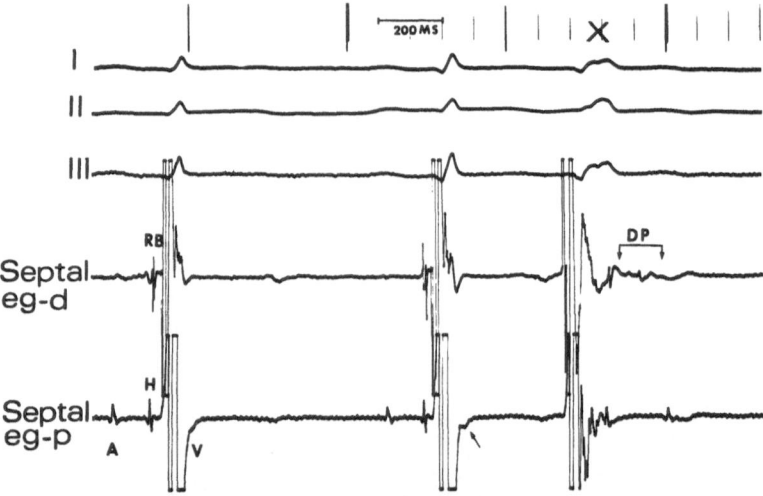

Figure 14. Electrode catheter recordings of proximal and distal septal electrograms (septal eg-p and Septal eg-d, respectively) from the same patient as in Figure 13. The arrows point to a late potential during sinus rhythm. X is a spontaneous ventricular premature complex that resulted in tachycardia-dependent fractionation of the late diastolic potential (DP). (From El-Sherif et al. (1985) Late potentials and arrhythmogenesis. PACE 8:440, with permission).

Our data as well as those of Hombach et al. suggest that the beat-to-beat, low noise ECG may provide complimentary data to the signal averaged ECG in some patients, particularly when there is a beat-to-beat variation of the signal and/or in the presence of spontaneous ventricular arrhythmias. However, there are current limitations of the technique of low noise ECG. There is an obvious lack of standardization between different laboratories regarding equipment design, methods of recording and analysis of the low noise ECG. In spite of these limitations, recording of late potentials on a beat-to-beat basis has the exciting potential of directly identifying malignant 'reentrant' versus benign 'focal' ventricular rhythms.

D. New technical and physiologic advances

Signal averaging of Holter ECG recordings

It is possible that dynamic changes in late potentials can occur prior to the onset of spontaneous tachyarrhythmias that may not be present otherwise during arrhythmia-free periods. We have recently described a technique for signal averaging of high gain Holter ECG recordings [66]. In a preliminary study [67] we performed signal averaging on multiple 1000 beat aliquots acquired from 24 hour Holter tapes of 7 patients with sustained or non-sustained VT. Between 4 and 11 aliquots each of about 15 minutes, spanning 24 hours overall were examined from each subject tape. The mean and standard deviation (SD) of the RMS40, LAS40 and total QRS duration were measured for each subject, with RMS40 $<25~\mu v$ and LAS40 >38 ms considered abnormal. All 5 subjects with late potentials also had late potentials on each Holter aliquot examined, with very similar and constant morphology reflected in the low scatter of late potential parameters within each subject data set. However, in two patients without late potentials on real time signal averaged ECG, late potentials were seen in some but not all of the Holter aliquots, such that real time signal averaging performed at various times during the day would have yielded conflicting results as to late potentials presence. Although in those two patients we could not correlate the appearance of late potentials with the occurrence of episodes of non-sustained VT on the Holter tape, it is possible that in a large scale study a correlation between dynamic changes of late potentials and spontaneous ventricular tachyarrhythmias could be established.

Analysis of periodicity of late potentials

Our electrophysiologic observations in the post-infarction canine heart suggest that there is a close association between myocardial zones showing a Wenckebach conduction pattern and the chance for development of spontaneous reentry. The presence of areas of 2:1 block also may prove to be a strong marker for spontaneous reentry. The rationale is as follows: since conduction in ischemic myocardium is characteristically tachycardia-dependent [27], it is expected that zones showing a 2:1 pattern usually would revert to a Wenckebach conduction pattern and then a 1:1 delayed conduction pattern on slowing of the heart rate. Thus a body surface recording that would be able to discern the presence of myocardial zones showing 2:1 or Wenckebach periodicity may prove to represent a better electrophysiologic marker for the propensity to develop reentrant arrhythmias as contrasted to a recording that reflects primarily areas of conduction delays in a 1:1 pattern. A signal averaged ECG will not be able to detect periodicity of late potentials since the periodic absence of signals simply reduces the averaged signal. A low noise ECG can potentially record dynamic beat-to-beat changes of late potentials. However, because of the very low amplitude of these potentials in relation to noise, a high degree of resolution of signal-to-noise ratio is required. We have investigated a novel approach to detect periodicity of late potentials using FFT techniques [68]. In the frequency domain, patterns that occur with any regularity, whether their period is the basic heart rate or some fraction of

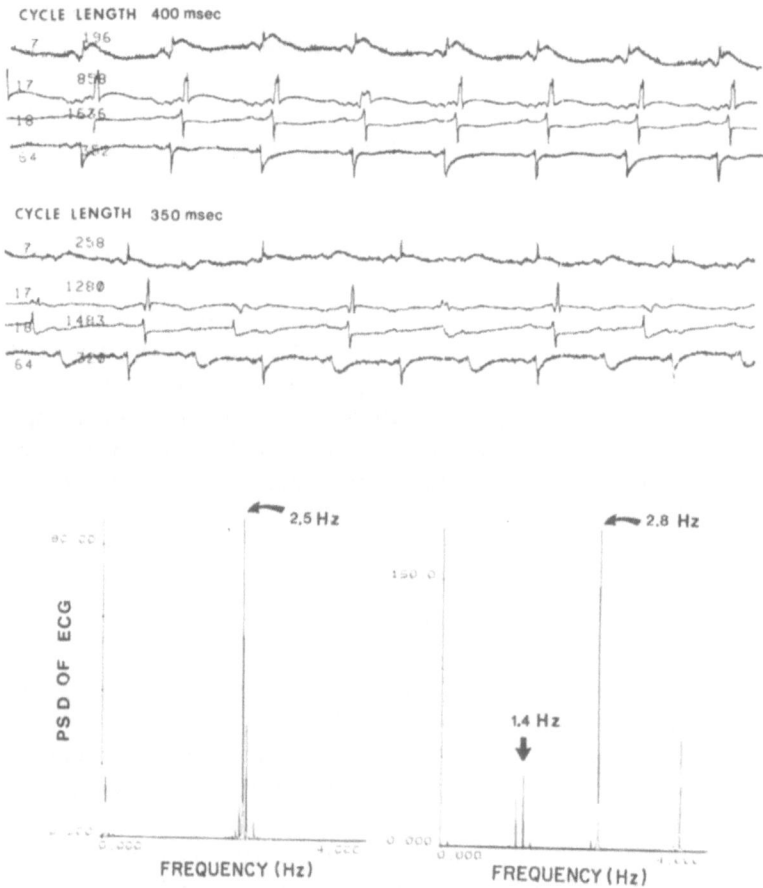

Figure 15. Time and spectral analyses of the ECG signals from a 4-day-old post-infarction canine heart. A tachycardia-dependent 2:1 conduction block in some of the epicardial electrograms obtained from the ischemic epicardial zone was associated with the appearance of a subharmonic at 1.4 Hz in the spectral recording. See text for details. (From Craelius et al. (1986) Rhythm analysis of arterial blood pressure. IEEE Trans Biomed Eng BME-33:1166, with permission).

the heart rate can be detected as sub-harmonics. An example of the Fourier analysis of the ECG is shown in Figure 15. The top record shows selected bipolar electrograms recorded from the epicardial surface of a 4-day-old post-infarction canine heart. The recording at a cardiac cycle length of 400 ms shows a 1:1 conduction pattern. When the cycle length was shortened to 350 ms, 2:1 conduction block developed in the ischemic epicardial zone resulting in alternation of the electrogram configuration. The bottom of the Figure shows the power spectral densities of the surface

ECG lead recorded from the post-infarction dog whose epicardial recordings are shown on top. The record on the left shows the spectrum of the ECG recorded during a 5-minute period at a constant cycle length of 400 ms. The spectrum has a single peak at a frequency of 2.5 Hz, as expected if a 1:1 activation pattern occurred every 400 ms. In the record on the right, the cardiac cycle length was decreased to 350 ms. A major peak occurred at 2.8 Hz corresponding to the cardiac cycle length. However, a second peak became evident at 1.48 Hz, one half of the basic cycle length. This subharmonic is evidence for an event occurring with 2:1 periodicity induced by shortening the cardiac cycle length, most probably 2:1 conduction block in one or more ischemic epicardial zones. Further experimental and clinical studies will be required to investigate the feasibility of detecting periodicity of late potentials from spectral analysis of the ECG and its predictive value as a marker of reentrant ventricular arrhythmias.

Conclusions

In the last 15 years, a number of techniques for obtaining a high resolution ECG were investigated and were shown to be able to detect His-Purkinje and late potentials from body surface recordings. Although the retrieval rate is currently limited, the recording of the His-Purkinje potential particularly on a beat-to-beat basis can provide valuable clinical information. On the other hand, late potentials are proving to be a valuable marker for the propensity to develop serious 'reentrant' ventricular arrhythmias, particularly in the post-infarction period. The high resolution ECG owes a large part of its appeal to its being a relatively simple non-invasive test. However, there is an urgent need for the meeting of mind among investigators interested in this technique to establish standardized criteria for equipment design, methods of recording and analysis of the ECG signal in order to foster a better climate for the exchange of clinical data. Further, more basic studies are needed to understand the electrophysiologic substrate of late potentials and large scale multicenter clinical studies are required to provide a definitive evaluation of their prognostic significance.

References

1. Ros HH, Koeleman ASM, Van der Akker TJ (1981) The technique of signal averaging and its practical application in the separation of atrial and His-Purkinje activity. In: Hombach V, Hilger HH (eds) Signal averaging technique in clinical cardiology. New York: Schattauer Verlag, pp 3–14

2. Restivo M, El-Sherif N, Kelen GJ, Henkin R, Craelius W, Gough WB (1985) Correlation of late potentials on the body surface and ventricular activation maps of reentrant circuits in the post-infarction dog heart. Circulation Abstr 72:Suppl. III-11.

3. Abboud S, Belhassen B, Laniado S, Sadeh D (1983) Non-invasive recording of late ventricular activity using an advanced method in patients with a damaged mass of ventricular tissue. J. Electrocardiol 16:245.

4. Simson MB, Euler D, Michelson EL, Falcone RA, Spear JF, Moore EN (1981) Detection of delayed ventricular activation on the body surface in dogs. Am J Physiol 24:H363

5. Berbari E, Collins S, Salu Y, Arzbaecher R (1983) Orthogonal surface lead recordings of His-Purkinje activity: comparison of actual and simulated waveforms. IEEE Trans Biomed Eng BME-30:160

6. Abboud S, Sadeh D (1982) The waveforms' alignment procedure in the averaging process for external recording of the His bundle activity. Comput Biomed Res 15:212

7. Wolf HK, MacInnis PJ, Stock S, Helppi RK, Rautaharju PM (1972) Computer analysis of rest and exercise electrocardiograms. Comput Biomed Res 5:329

8. Wajszczuk WJ, Moskowitz MS, Bauld T, Dabos P, Weiss R, Rubenfire M (1978) Non-inverse external recording of cardiac conduction system (His bundle) activity. Med Instrum 12:282

9. Brandon CW, Brody DA (1970) A hardware trigger for temporal indexing of the electrocardiographic signal. Comput Biomed Res 3:47

10. Goovaerts HG, Ros HH, Van Der Akker TJ, Schneider H (1976) A digital QRS detector based on the principle of contour limiting. IEEE Trans Biomed Eng BME-23:154

11. Borjesson PO, Pahlm O, Sornmo L, Nygards ME (1982) Adaptive QRS detection based on maximum a posteriori estimation. IEEE Trans Biomed Eng BME-29:341

12. Thakor NV, Webster JG, Tompkins WJ (1983) Optimal QRS detector. Med Biol Eng Comput 21:343

13. Tremblay G, LeBlanc AR (1985) Near-optimal signal preprocessor for positive cardiac arrhythmia identification. IEEE Trans Biomed Eng BME-32:141

14. Uijen GJH, deWeerd JPC, Vendrik AJH (1979) Accuracy of QRS detection in relation to the analysis of high-frequency components in the electrocardiogram. Med Biol Eng Comput 17:492

15. Fraden J, Neuman MR (1980) QRS wave detection. Med Biol Eng Comput 18:125

16. Craelius W, Restivo M, Assadi MA, El-Sherif N (1986) Criteria for optimal averaging of cardiac signals. IEEE Trans Biomed Eng BME-33:957

17. El-Sherif N, Mehra R, Gomes JAC, Kelen G (1983) Appraisal of a low noise electrocardiogram. J Am Coll Cardiol 1:456

18. El-Sherif N (1984) The low noise (high resolution) electrocardiogram. Int J Cardiol 6:185

19. Flowers NC, Shvartsman V, Kennelly BM, Sohi GS, Horan LG (1981) Surface recordings of His-Purkinje activity on an every beat basis without digital averaging. Circulation 63:948

20. Flowers NC, Shvartsman V, Horan LG et al (1983) Analysis of PR subintervals in normal subjects and early studies in patients with abnormalities of the conduction system using surface His bundle recordings. J Am Coll Cardiol 2:939

21. Hombach V, Kebbel U, Hopp H-W, Winter V, Hirche, H (1984) Non-invasive beat-to-beat registration of ventricular late potentials using high resolution electrocardiography. Int J Cardiol 6:167

22. Hombach V, Hopp H-W, Kebbel U, Treis I, Osterpey A, Eggeling T, Winter U, Hirche H, Hilger HH (1986) Recovery of ventricular late potentials from body surface using the signal averaging and high resolution ECG techniques. Clin Cardiol 9:361

23. Mehra R, Restivo M, El-Sherif N (1983) Electromyographic noise reduction for high

resolution electrocardiography. In: IEEE Frontiers of Engineering and Computing in Health Care. New York:IEEE, p 298

24. Waldo AL, Kaiser GA (1973) A study of ventricular arrhythmias associated with myocardial infarction in the canine heart. Circulation 47:1222

25. Boineau JP, Cox JL (1973) Slow ventricular activation in acute myocardial infraction in the canine heart. A source of reentrant premature ventricular contractions. Circulation 48:702

26. El-Sherif N, Scherlag BJ, Lazzara R (1975) Electrode catheter recordings during malignant ventricular arrhythmias following experimental acute myocardial ischemia. Circulation 51:1003

27. El-Sherif N, Scherlag BJ, Lazzara R, Hope RR (1977) Reentrant ventricular arrhythmias in the late myocardial infarction period. I. Conduction characteristics in the infarction zone. Circulation 55:586

28. Janse MJ, VanCapelle FJL, Morsink M, Kleber AG, Wilms-Schopmaan F, Cardinal R, D'Alnoncourt CN, Durrer D (1980) Flow of "injury" current and patterns of excitation during early ventricular arrhythmias in acute regional myocardial ischemia in isolated porcine and canine hearts. Circ Res 47:151

29. El-Sherif N, Smith RA, Evans K (1981) Ventricular arrhythmias in the late myocardial infarction period in the dog. 8. Epicardial mapping of reentrant circuits. Circ Res 49:255

30. Mehra R, Zeiler RH, Gough WB, EL-Sherif N (1983) Reentrant ventricular arrhythmias in the late myocardial infarction period 9. Electrophysiologic-anatomical correlation of reentrant circuits. Circulation 67:11

31. El-Sherif N, Mehra R, Gough WB, Zeiler RH (1983) Reentrant ventricular arrhythmias in the late myocardial infarction period. Interruption of reentrant circuits by cryothermal techniques. Circulation 68:644

32. Berbari EJ, Scherlag BJ, Hope RR, Lazzara R (1978) Recording from the body surface of arrhythmogenic ventricular activity during the S-T segment. Am J Cardiol 41:697

33. Simson MB, Untereker WJ, Spielman SR, Horowitz LN, Marcus NH, Falcone KA, Harken AH, Josephson ME (1983) The relationship between late potentials on the body surface and directly recorded fragmented electrograms in patients with ventricular tachycardia. Am J Cardiol 51:105

34. Gough WB, Mehra R, Restivo M, Zeiler RH, El-Sherif N (1985) Reentrant ventricular arrhythmias in the late myocardial infarction period in the dog. 13. Correlation of activation and refractory maps. Circ Res 57:432

35. Restivo M, Henkin R, Craelius W, El-Sherif N (1986) Are regions of delayed activation during a basic rhythm the responsible arrhythmogenic substrate for reentry (abstr.)? J Am Coll Cardiol 7:85A

36. Berbari EJ, Lazzara R, Samet P, Scherlag BJ (1973) Noninvasive technique for detection of electrical activity during the P-R segment. Circulation 48:1005

37. Flowers NC, Hand RC, Orander PC, Miller CB, Walden MO, Horan LG (1974) Surface recording of electrical activity from the region of the bundle of His. Am J Cardiol 33:384

38. Stopczyk MJ, Kopec J, Zochowski RJ, Pleniak M (1973) Surface recording of electrical heart activity during the P-R segment in man by computer averaging technique. Int Res Com Sys 11:73

39. Hishimoto Y, Sawayama T (1975) Noninvasive recording of His bundle potential in man. Br Heart J 37:635

40. Furness A, Sharratt GP, Carson P (1975) The feasibility of detecting His bundle activity from the body surface. Cardiovsc Res 9:390

41. Berbari EJ, Scherlag BJ, El-Sherif N, Befeler B, Aranda JM, Lazzara R (1976) The His-Purkinje electrocardiogram in man. Circulation 54:219

202

42. Vincent R, Stroud NP, Jenner R, English MJ, Woollons DJ, Chamberlain DA (1978) Noninvasive recording of electrical activity in the PR segment in man. Br Heart J 40:124

43. Wajszczuk WJ, Stopczyk MJ, Moskowitz MS, Zochowski RJ, Bauld T, Dabos PL, Rubenfire M (1978) Noninvasive recording of His-Purkinje activity in man by QRS-triggered signal averaging. Circulation 58:95

44. Berbari EJ, Lazzara R, Scherlag BJ (1979) The effects of filtering the His-Purkinje system electrocardiogram. IEEE Trans Biomed Eng 2:82

45. McKenna WJ, Rowland E, Mortara D, Dawson RE, Krikler DM (1979) Noninvasive recording of the His bundle electrogram (abstr.). Proc VIth World Symposium on Cardiac Pacing. PACE 2:1978

46. Mehra R, Kelen GJ, Zeiler RH, Zephiran D, Fried P, Gomes JAC, El-Sherif N (1982) Noninvasive His bundle electrogram: value of three vector lead recordings. Am J Cardiol 49:344

47. Kanovsky MS, Falcone RA, Dresden CA, Josephson ME, Simson MB (1984) Identification of patients with ventricular tachycardia after myocardial infarction: signal-averaged electrocardiogram, Holter monitoring, and cardiac catheterization. Circulation 70:264

48. Denes P, Uretz E, Santarelli P (1984) Determinants of arrhythmogenic ventricular activity detected on the body surface QRS in patients with coronary artery disease. Am J Cardiol 53:1519

49. Buckingham TA, Ghosh S, Howan SM, Thessen CC, Redd RM, Stevens LL, Chaitman BR, Kennedy HL (1987) Independent value of signal-averaged electrocardiography and left ventricular function in identifying patients with sustained ventricular tachycardia and coronary artery disease. Am J Cardiol 59:568

50. Breithardt G, Borggrefe M, Haerten K (1986) Ventricular late potentials and inducible ventricular tachyarrhythmias as a marker for ventricular tachycardia after myocardial infarction. Eur Heart J 7(Suppl A):127

51. Turitto G, Fontaine J, Macina G, Caref E, Ursell S, Stavens C, El-Sherif N et al. (1987) Signal averaged ECG predicts the inducibility of sustained ventricular tachycardia in patients with spontaneous non-sustained tachycardia (abstr.). J. Am Coll Cardiol 9:151A

52. Kertes PJ, Glabus M, Murray A, Julian DG, Campbell RWF (1984) Delayed ventricular depolarization: correlation with ventricular activation and relevance to ventricular fibrillation in acute myocardial infarction. Eur Heart J 5:974

53. Gomes JA, Mehra R, Barreca P, El-Sherif N, Hariman R, Holtzman R (1985) Quantitative analysis of the high-frequency components of the signal-averaged QRS complex in patients with acute myocardial infarction: a prospective study. Circulation 72:105.

54. Turitto G, Macine G, Caref E, Mittleman R, Henkins R, El-Sherif N (1886) Lack of correlation between Holter recording and signal averaged electrocardiogram in the post-infarction period (abstr.). Circulation 74(Suppl 2):II-402

55. Breithardt G, Schwarzmayer J, Borggrefe M, Haerten J, Seipel L (1983) Prognostic significance of late ventricular potentials after acute myocardial infarction. Eur Heart J 4:487

56. Breithardt G, Borggrefe M (1986) Pathophysiological mechanisms and clinical significance of ventricular late potentials. Eur Heart J 7:364

57. Denniss AR, Richards DA, Cody DV, Russell PA, Young AA, Cooper MJ, Ross DL, Uther JB (1986) Prognostic significance of ventricular tachycardia and fibrillation induced at programmed stimulation and delayed potentials detected on the signal-averaged electrocardiogram of survivors of acute myocardial infarction. Circulation 74:731

58. Kuchar DL, Thorburn CW, Sammel NL (1986) Late potentials detected after myocardial infarction: natural history and prognostic significance. Circulation 74:1280

59. Simson MB (1981) Use of signals in the terminal QRS complex to identify patients with ventricular tachycardia after myocardial infarction. Circulation 64:235

60. Denes P, Santarelli P, Hauser RG, Uretz EF (1983) Quantitative analysis of the high frequency components of the terminal portion of the body surface QRS in normal subjects and in patients with ventricular tachycardia. Circulation 67:1129

61. Cain ME, Ambos HD, Witkowski FX, Sobel BE (1984) Fast-Fourier transform analysis of signal-averaged electrocardiograms for identification of patients prone to sustained ventricular tachycardia. Circulation 69:711

62. Cain ME, Ambos HD, Markham J, Fischer AE, Sobel BE (1985) Quantification of differences in frequency content of signal-averaged electrocardiogram between patients with and without sustained ventricular tachycardia. Am J Cardiol 55:1500

63. Lindsay BD, Ambos HD, Schechtman KB, Cain ME (1986) Improved selection of patients for programmed ventricular stimulation by frequency analysis of signal-averaged electrocardiograms. Circulation 73:675

64. Henkin R, Kelen G, El-Sherif N (1986) Correlation between late potentials and frequency (FFT) analysis of signal averaged ECG—importance of analyzed segment duration (abstr.). Circulation 74(Suppl II):II-781

65. El-Sherif N, Gomes JAC, Restivo M, Mehra R (1985) Late potentials and arrhythmogenesis. PACE 8:440

66. Kelen GJ, Henkin R, Restivo M, Zeiler RH, Caref EB, El-Sherif N (1986) Signal averaging of high gain Holter EKG recordings. Validation of a new technique for detection of after potentials (abstr.). J Am Coll Cardiol 7:104A

67. Kelen GJ, Henkin R, Howard M, Ferraro C, El-Sherif N (1987) Serial signal averages from Holter tapes may reveal intermittent or changing late potentials (abstr.). PACE: (in press)

68. Craelius W, Chen VKH, Restivo M, El-Sherif N (1986) Rhythm analysis of arterial blood pressure. IEEE Trans Biomed Eng BME-33:1166

17. Clinical and prognostic significance of ventricular late potentials – Experience with the averaging technique

GÜNTER BREITHARDT, MARTIN BORGGREFE,
ANDREA PODCZECK, KLAUS HAERTEN,
& ANTONIO MARTINEZ-RUBIO*

Hospital of the University of Düsseldorf, Department of Cardiology, Pneumology and Angiology, University of Düsseldorf, Düsseldorf, F.R.G.

Key words: ventricular late potentials, sustained ventricular tachycardia, sudden cardiac death, prognosis after myocardial infarction

Introduction

In experimental studies, delayed fractionated electrical activity has been detected during diastole in regions of experimental myocardial infarction [1–4]. These potentials are characterized by multiple low-amplitude spikes that are sometimes separated by isoelectric intervals. It has been suggested that the presence of such electrograms during sinus rhythm indicates sites for potential reentrant circuits. The pathophysiological mechanisms leading to late potentials have been discussed extensively in a recent review article [5].

Delayed and fractionated potentials have been observed during intra-operative epicardial and endocardial mapping [6–9] and endocardial catheter mapping in patients with ventricular tachycardia [10, 11]. Since the pioneering work by Berbari et al. [12] and Fontaine et al. [7], it has become possible to record ventricular late potentials non-invasively using appropriate recording and filtering techniques (Figure 1). Since then, a great number of clinical studies, mostly in patients with documented ventricular tachycardia have been published using the signal-averaging technique in the time-domain [7, 12–19] as well as in the frequency-domain [20–22]. In addition, some studies have been concerned with the high-resolution ECG which attempts a beat-to-beat recording of late potentials (see this book).

---

* Supported by a grant from the C.I.R.I.T. (Comissio Interdepartamental per la recerca i l'innovació tecnològica), Generalitat de Catalunya, Spain.

V. Hombach, H. H. Hilger and H. L. Kennedy (eds), Electrocardiography and Cardiac Drug Therapy. ISBN 978-94-010-6976-2

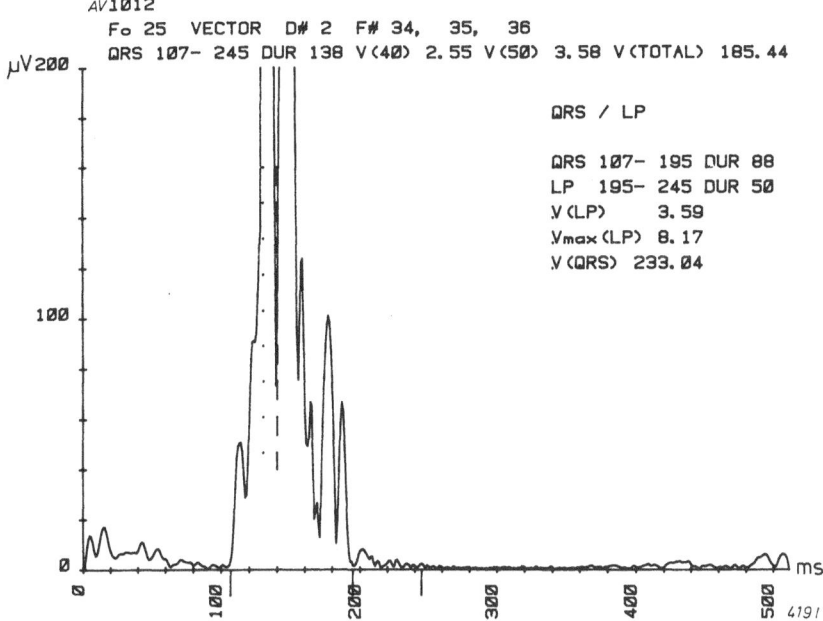

Figure 1. Signal-averaged and filtered recording of leads *X*, *Y*, *Z* (vector magnitude) using the software developed by M. Simson in a patient with ventricular tachycardia. QRS duration (DUR) in the highly amplified and filtered recording was 138 ms. The programme automatically identified the end of the total QRS-complex at 245 ms on the *x*-axis. The amplitude in the terminal 40 ms was low (V(40) = 2.55 μV). The onset of low-amplitude activity was automatically identified at 195 ms by the automatic recognition programme [27].

The purpose of this chapter is to review the presently available clinical studies using the signal-averaging technique in the time-domain in patients with documented ventricular tachycardia as well as the potential role of late potentials for identification of patients at risk of ventricular tachyarrhythmias after myocardial infarction.

Methodological aspects

With conventional methods of ECG recording, late potentials cannot be recovered from the body surface except in very rare cases [23–24]. However, using high-gain amplification and computer averaging techniques, these signals were first recorded in the experimental animal [12] and in patients with idiopathic ventricular tachycardia [7]. Because of the low amplitude of these signals in relation to the electrical noise produced by various sources [25], averaging of many identical beats is used to eliminate the remaining random noise. Thus, one of the requirements of the signal-averaging technique is that only identical beats are averaged. Premature ventricular beats have to be excluded either by rejecting all beats of a given prematurity [14] or more specifically by passing all ECG signals through a template recognition programme to reject ectopic beats and grossly noisy signals [18].

In how far the assumption that all beats of similar QRS morphology are identical with respect to the presence and timing of low-amplitude signals is correct, has been a matter of recent debate (see the chapter by Hombach). Beat-to-beat variation of the timing of ventricular late potentials may cause progressive attenuation of the low-amplitude tail of the highly amplified QRS complex. This may thus lead to cancellation of at least part or all of the signal to be recovered during the averaging process. Furthermore, another prerequisite for applying the signal-averaging process is stable triggering of the signal. In case of significant jitter of the triggering point, major parts of the high-frequency signal may be attenuated.

At the present time, no definite information is available in large groups of patients on how frequently attenuation or cancellation of ventricular late potentials occurs during the averaging process. Signal-averaging in the time-domain thus may have the limitation that it may loose information during the averaging process. From the practical point of view, its major advantage is that it does not require an especially shielded surrounding as is the case for high-resolution beat-to-beat recordings.

In our department, we have been operating with two different systems for signal-averaging. The first system was designed in 1978/79 [14, 26]. It used visual analysis of four separate precordial leads. In contrast, since 1982/83, we have additionally been using the signal-averaging system developed by M. Simson [18]. In addition to evaluating the root-mean-square (RMS) voltage in the last 40 ms of the terminal QRS-complex, we additionally devised a new algorithm for automatic detection of late potentials [27].

Incidence of late potentials in patients with documented ventricular tachycardia

In patients with previously documented sustained monomorphic ventricular tachycardia and/or fibrillation, ventricular late potentials (Figure 1) can be found in a high proportion of cases [14–19, 26–32]. Late potentials were found in 45 of 63 patients (71%) with documented ventricular tachycardia/fibrillation [28]. If only patients with coronary artery disease were considered, the proportion of patients with late potentials increased to 37 of

47 patients (79%). The voltage in the last 40 ms of the filtered QRS-complex was found to discriminate well between patients with and without ventricular tachycardia [18]. The root-mean-square voltage in the last 40 ms was $15 \pm 14.4 \ \mu V$ in patients with ventricular tachycardia but it was significantly greater in patients without $(74 \pm 77.7 \ \mu V; \ p < 0.0001)$. A threshold of 25 μV was suggested to discriminate between patients with and without ventricular tachycardia [18]. The QRS-duration was longer in patients with ventricular tachycardia (139 ± 26 versus 95 ± 10 ms; $p <$ 0.0001). Similarly, Freedman et al. [30] detected late potentials in 33 of 53 patients (62%) with ventricular tachycardia. Kanovsky et al. [32] studied 174 patients after myocardial infarction, 98 of whom had recurrent sustained ventricular tachycardia. By multivariate logistic regression analysis, the signal-averaged ECG, peak premature ventricular contractions > 100/h, and the presence of a left-ventricular aneurysm were found to be independently significant. Patients with congestive cardiomyopathy and a history of ventricular tachycardia were reported to have a significantly

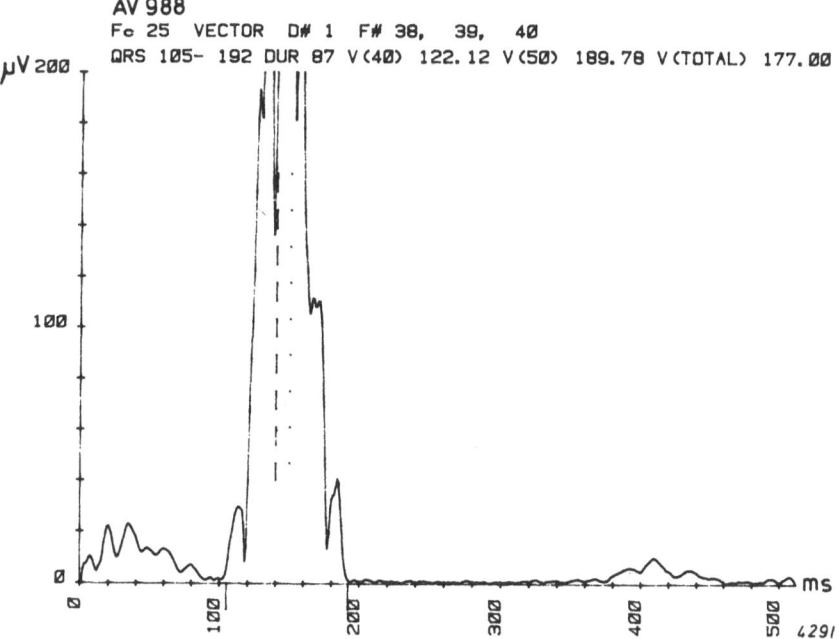

Figure 2. Signal-averaged and filtered recording of leads X, Y, Z (vector magnitude) using the software developed by M. Simson in a patient without a history of ventricular tachycardia and without structural heart disease. There is no low-amplitude activity at the end of the high-amplitude portion of the QRS-complex. The voltage in the last 40 ms of QRS was $122.12 \mu V$.

greater incidence of late potentials and a longer QRS-duration than those without ventricular tachycardia [33]. By use of Fourier analysis, it has been shown that patients with ventricular tachycardia have a higher frequency content in their terminal QRS-complex compared to normals [20, 22].

In contrast, electrical activity suggestive of slow-ventricular activation is almost never detected in subjects with normal left-ventricular function (Figure 2) [15, 16, 18, 28, 29, 33–36]. The signal-averaged ECG proved to be very specific as it did not detect delayed ventricular activity in patients in whom there was no delayed activity during epicardial intraoperative mapping [37]. However, it may miss delayed activity on the body surface in patients in whom it can be demonstrated by endocardial mapping.

Incidence of late potentials in patients without a history of ventricular tachyarrythmias

The major impact for the use of signal-averaging is, however, not so much in the field of retrospective analysis of patients with documented sustained ventricular tachycardia but in the application of signal-averaging for predicting prognosis especially after recent myocardial infarction. Thus, one of the major recent applications of signal-averaging for detection of late potentials has been the prospective study of patients with coronary artery disease who have no history of sustained ventricular tachyarrhythmias.

Previous work from our group has shown that ventricular late potentials cannot only be detected in patients with previously documented ventricular tachycardia but also in asymptomatic patients [28]. None of these patients had a history of ventricular tachycardia or fibrillation outside acute myocardial infarction. Late potentials could be detected in 49 of 146 patients (37.6%). These data indicate that in many of these patients, most of them having coronary artery disease with previous myocardial infarction, there probably is a substrate for reentrant arrhythmias which, however, has not yet manifested itself. Obviously, some trigger factor is needed to initiate ventricular tachycardia or fibrillation. These results have subsequently been confirmed by others [29, 32, 36].

The anatomic substrate for the occurrence of ventricular late potentials in these patients obviously is the appearance of interstitial fibrosis forming insulating boundaries between muscle bundles in the border zone of myocardial infarction [38]. The individual components of fragmented electrograms most probably represent asynchronous electrical activity in each of the separate bundles of surviving muscle under the electrode. The intrinsic asymmetry of cardiac activation due to fibre orientation may be accentuated by infarction and may predispose to reentry [38, 39]. The slow activation might result from conduction over circuitous pathways caused by the separation and distortion of the myocardial fibre bundles. The low amplitude of the electrograms from the border zone of myocardial infarction probably results from the paucity of surviving muscle fibres under the electrode because of the large amount of connective tissue, and not from depression of the action potentials [38]. The anatomic substrate for reentry seems to be present in regions where fragmented electrograms can be recorded which, thus, indicate slow inhomogeneous conduction. However, fragmented electrograms are probably found wherever myocardial fibres are separated by connective tissue, even if reentry does not occur in the region. This has recently shown by Kienzle et al. [40] who concluded that these electrograms may be associated with, but are not specific for sites of origin of ventricular tachycardia. The time course with which late potentials appear during acute myocardial infarction has only been studied in small groups of patients. Kertes et al. [29] found late potentials in 16% of patients with myocardial infarction without ventricular fibrillation. They were more common in inferior myocardial infarction (32%) than in other sites of infarction (4%). In 5 of 6 patients where late potentials were present on the admission averaged ECG, they had either disappeared or prominently reduced in duration on the second averaged ECG. In another study of patients with recent myocardial infarction [41], the prevalence of late potentials was much greater in patients with inferior wall infarction (63%) than in patients with anterior wall infarction (35%). One possible explanation for this difference might be that various left ventricular sites are activated at different times [42]. Since the infero-postero-basal areas of the left ventricle are activated late, an electrogram of a given duration from this site may clearly extend beyond the QRS-complex. However, an electrogram of long duration that may even be longer than one from the inferior wall may not extend beyond the QRS and may still be hidden within it if it originates from the anterior wall and thus begins early in the QRS-complex [42, 43].

Since late potentials were not only found in patients with but also without previously documented ventricular tachycardia, their presence proved neither highly sensitive nor specific for patients with clinically evident ventricular tachyarrhythmias. Additionally, there was a large overlap in the duration of late potentials among patients with ventricular tachycardia or fibrillation and patients without a history of these arrhythmias. The longer duration of late potentials in patients with ventricular tachycardia may indicate that in these cases, regional activation was more fragmented and possibly slower than in those without previously documented ventricular tachycardia.

Several reasons may be responsible for the fact that late potentials cannot be detected in all patients with documented ventricular tachycardia and/or fibrillation. This includes unstable triggering, too low amplitudes of the signals, too short signals occurring immediately at the end of the QRS-complex when filter ringing might occur, and, lastly, other mechanisms responsible for the genesis of ventricular tachycardia than reentry such as triggered automaticity [44, 45].

Prognostic significance of late potentials

During recent years, several studies have addressed the problem of the prognostic value of ventricular late potentials [46–50] including our own studies [41, 51].

Denniss et al. [46] studied 110 patients 7 to 28 days after acute myocardial infarction. The median day of study was 11. Follow-up of these patients ranged between 2 to 12 months (mean: 5 months). There was a significant difference in the subsequent occurrence of symptomatic sustained ventricular tachycardia during follow-up in patients without late potentials (1.1%) compared to those with late potentials (17.4%). The incidence of sudden cardiac death was not reported in the study. Kacet et al. [47] studied a population of 104 patients that were followed for 8.5 ± 4 months. The incidence of subsequent symptomatic sustained ventricular tachycardia in patients without late potentials was 4.5% compared to 28.9% in patients with late potentials. None of the patients without late potentials died suddenly compared to 13% of patients with late potentials. In another study, Kuchar et al. [48] reported the results of follow-up (3 to 12 months) of 123 patients that were studied 10 days (mean) after acute myocardial infarction. The incidence of major arrhythmic complications such as sudden death or symptomatic sustained ventricular tachycardia was only 1.4% in patients without late potentials compared to 20.5% in patients with late potentials. In a study by Höpp et al. [49], 50 patients were studied in the early post-infarction period. These patients were followed for 24 ± 5 months. 12 of 30 patients who had late potentials (37%) died suddenly. On the contrary, none of the 20 patients without late potentials died suddenly. The same authors studied another group of 200 patients with chronic, stable coronary artery disease [49]. Mean follow-up 20 ± 5 months. 108 of 200 patients had ventricular late potentials. 15 of these patients (13.9%) died suddenly compared to 4 of 92 patients (4.3%) without late potentials ($p < 0.001$). Von Leitner et al. [50] followed 518 patients who took part in a rehabilitation program after myocardial infarction. These patients were studied between 6–8 weeks after onset of infarction. During a mean follow-up period of 10 months, cardiac mortality was 1.5% in patients without late potentials compared to 7.3% in patients with ventricular late potentials. Sudden cardiac death occured in 0.9% of patients without late potentials compared to 3.6% of patients with late potentials. In none of these patients, symptomatic sustained ventricular tachycardia was reported.

Our own experience is based on two prospective studies. First, a prospective trial was initiated at Düsseldorf University in 1980 that used the methodology for recording of signal-averaged ECG's that was developed in our department between 1978 and 1979. This system was primarily based on a hard-wired signal-averager [14, 28, 41, 51, 52] which has also been used by other groups [34, 53, 54]. The second study was started in January 1983. It was extensively supported by the Federal Minister for Research and Technology (Bundesministerium für Forschung und Technologie, Bonn, Germany, F.R.). This study included male patients after recent Q-wave myocardial infarction. Signal-averaging was performed using the software programme by M. Simson [18], which includes bidirectional filtering and automated analysis of signal-averaged ECG's. This multicenter non-interventional study has been called the PILP-Study (Post-Infarction Late Potential-study). It has recently been completed after inclusion of almost 800 patients. Data analysis has not yet been completed.

In our first study which now includes 628 patients, only patients without a history of sustained ventricular tachycardia or fibrillation outside the acute phase of myocardial infarction, without a history of syncope, and without complete bundle branch block were included. The patients were selected if they either had survived recent myocardial infarction or if they were referred to our department because of a clinical indication for coronary angiography to establish or exclude the presence of coronary artery disease. In the first group, only patients with acute myocardial infarction were included that were admitted to the hospital on a primary referral basis. Thus, patients referred from other hospitals because of major complications of myocardial infarction were not included. Signal-averaging was done as previously described [14, 52]. Mean age of these patients was 54 ± 7.6 years. 469 patients had a history of previous myocardial infarction. 258 patients were included within the first 4 weeks after myocardial infarction, another 52 patients within the second month, whereas the remaining 259 patients were studied after more than two months after their myocardial infarction.

Mean follow-up duration was 39 ± 15.0 months. At the end of follow-up, 21 patients (3.3%) had died suddenly within one hour, mostly occurring either instantaneously or during sleep whereas another 3 patients (0.5%) died within one to 24 hours. There were another 14 cardiac deaths mostly due to reinfarction and myocardial failure. In addition, there were 14 patients (2.2%) who had survived an episode of symptomatic spontaneous sustained ventricular tachycardia that required some type of emergency intervention. Thus, in a total of 35 patients, a major arrhythmic event occurred during follow-up. The risk of major arrhythmic complications was 2.8 times greater in patients with late potentials of less than 40 ms duration compared to those without, and 9.3 times greater in those with a duration of 40 ms or more. The chance of sudden cardiac death within one hour was 3.3 and 5.4 times greater, respectively, whereas the chance for symptomatic sustained ventricular tachycardia was 2.0 and 17.4 times greater, respectively, depending on the duration of late potentials (less than 40 ms or greater). The chance of major arrhythmic complications such as sudden cardiac death or sustained symptomatic ventricular tachycardia was greatest in those patients who were studied within the first 4 to 8 weeks after their qualifying myocardial infarction.

Conclusions and clinical implications

Based on these presently available prospective studies, the presence of ventricular late potentials obviously heralds an increased risk for subsequent occurrence of sudden cardiac death or symptomatic sustained ventricular tachycardia. This mainly applies to patients who are studied after recent myocardial infarction [46–49] whereas patients who are included later and/or who are considered to be eligible for a cardiac rehabilitation programme [50], obviously have a much lower incidence of arrhythmic events. Thus, the predictive value of the presence of ventricular late potentials largely depends on under which clinical circumstances they can be detected. Patients who have survived for a long period after their myocardial infarction have a much lower risk of subsequent development of sudden cardiac death or symptomatic sustained ventricular tachycardia. This is obviously based on a selection process as patients at greater risk might have died in the meanwhile. In addition, our results show that the duration of late potentials might be of prognostic significance. The chance for development of an arrhythmic event, mainly symptomatic sustained ventricular tachycardia, is proportional to the duration of the late potentials.

With regard to the complex mechanisms that may lead to sudden cardiac death, it cannot be expected that any single method will be able to predict the occurrence of sudden cardiac death with 100% sensitivity. Sudden cardiac death may be due to chronic electrophysiological abnormalities as a consequence of regional slow conduction in the border zone of a previous myocardial infarction which is conventionally considered to be the electrophysiological substrate for ventricular late potentials.

The presence of regional slow conduction is mostly not sufficient for the spontaneous occurrence of ventricular tachyarrhythmias. Instead, some trigger factor such as spontaneous ventricular ectopic beats are necessary to alter the electrophysiological milieu in a way that tachycardia originates. However, most spontaneous ventricular arrhythmias detected during long-term ECG-recording are not harmful to the patient as they obviously do not induce ventricular tachycardia. Instead, some change in, for instance, the coupling interval or the sequence of ectopic beats, including the occurrence of short runs, may alter the electrophysiological milieu in a way that the prerequisites for reentry are met. Such transient occurrence of complex ventricular arrhythmias acting as trigger factor might also be induced by short, regional episodes of ischaemia induced by embolisation of platelet aggregates into the peripheral coronary system [55].

Another mechanism that may lead to sudden cardiac death is the occurrence of more extensive ischaemia due to reinfarction. There is no doubt that this may also lead to ventricular fibrillation and, thus, sudden cardiac death. Such a type of event, of course, cannot be predicted on the presence of preexisting indicators of regional slow conduction such as late potentials. However, it has been shown that preexisting myocardial damage increases the chance of ventricular fibrillation if regional ischaemia occurs at a site remote from that of preexisting cardiac damage [56].

Thus, it seems unjustified to expect any single method to be able to identify the individual patient at risk of sustained ventricular tachycardia and/or sudden death. Instead, a combination of various parameters including late potentials, spontaneous ventricular arrhythmias during long-term ECG-recording, extent of myocardial contractile disturbance (ejection fraction), and estimates of central nervous activity [57–58] might serve for further risk stratification in patients after recent myocardial infarction.

References

1. El-Sherif N, Scherlag BJ, Lazzara R, Hope RR (1977) Reentrant ventricular arrhythmias in the late myocardial infarction period. I. Conduction characteristics in the infarction zone. Circulation 55:686–702
2. El-Sherif N, Scherlag BJ, Lazzara R, Hope RR (1977) Reentrant ventricular arrhythmias in the late myocardial infarction period. II. Patterns of initiation and termination of reentry. Circulation 55:702–719
3. El-Sherif N, Lazzara R, Hope RR, Scherlag BJ (1977) Reentrant arrhythmias in the late myocardial infarction period. III. Manifest and concealed extrasystolic grouping. Circulation 56:225–234
4. Durrer D, Formaijne P, Van Dam R, Buller J, Van Lier A, Meyler F (1961) Electrogram in normal and some abnormal conditions. Am Heart J 61:303

5. Breithardt G, Borggrefe M (1986) Pathophysiological mechanisms and clinical significance of ventricular late potentials. Eur heart J 7:364–385
6. Fontaine G, Guiraudon G, Frank R (1978) Intramyocardial conduction defects in patients prone to ventricular tachycardia. III in: Sandoe E, Julian DG, Bell JW (eds) Management of ventricular tachycardia—role of mexiletine. Amsterdam: Excerpta Medica, pp 67–9
7. Fontaine G, Frank R, Gallais-Hamonno F, Allali I, Phan-Thuc H, Grosgogeat Y (1978) Electrocardiographie des potentiels tardifs du syndrome de post-excitation. Arch Mal Cœur 71:854–864
8. Klein H, Karp RB, Kouchoukos NT, Zorn GL, James TN, Waldo AL (1982) Intraoperative electrophysiologic mapping of the ventricles during sinus rhythm in patients with previous myocardial infarction. Identification of the electrophysiologic substrate of ventricular arrhythmias. Circulation 66:847
9. Ostermeyer J, Breithardt G, Kolvenbach R et al. (1979) Intraoperative electrophysiologic mapping during cardiac surgery. Thorac Cardiovasc Surgeon 27:260–270
10. Spielman SR, Untereker WJ, Horowitz LN, Greenspan AM, Simson MB, Kastor JA, Josephson ME (1981) Fragmented electrical activity—relationship to ventricular tachycardia. Am J Cardiol 47:448 (abstr)
11. Josephson ME, Horowitz LN, Farshidi A, Spielman SR, Michelson EL, Greenspan AM (1978) Sustained ventricular tachycardia: evidence for protected localized re-entry. Am J Cardiol 42:416–424
12. Berbari EJ, Scherlag BJ, Hope RR, Lazzara R (1978) Recording from the body surface of arrhythmogenic ventricular activity during the ST-segment. Am J Cardiol 41:697–702
13. Breithardt G, Becker R, Seipel L (1980) Non-invasive recording of late ventricular activation in man. Circulation 62:III–320 (abstr)
14. Breithardt G, Becker R, Seipel L, Abendroth RR, Ostermeyer J (1981) Non-invasive detection of late potentials in man—a new marker for ventricular tachycardia. Europ Heart J 2:1–11
15. Hombach V, Höpp HW, Braun V, Behrenbeck DW, Tauchert M, Hilger HH (1980) Die Bedeutung von Nachpotentialen innerhalb des ST-Segmentes im Oberflächen-EKG bei Patienten mit koronarer Herzkrankheit. Dtsch med Wschr 105:1457–1462
16. Rozanski JJ, Mortara D, Myerburg RJ, Castellanos A (1981) Body surface detection of delayed depolarizations in patients with recurrent ventricular tachycardia and left ventricular aneurysm. Circulation 63:1172–1178
17. Simson M, Horowitz L, Josephson M, Neil Moore E, Kastor J (1980) A marker for ventricular tachycardia after myocardial infarction. Circulation 62:III–262 (abstr)
18. Simson MB (1981) Use of signals in the terminal QRS complex to identify patients with ventricular tachycardia after myocardial infarction. Circulation 64:235–242
19. Uther JB, Dennett CJ, Tan A (1978) The detection of delayed activation signals of low amplitude in the vectorcardiogram of patients with recurrent ventricular tachycardia by signal averaging. In: Management of ventricular tachycardia—role of mexiletine. Amsterdam, Oxford: Excerpta Medica pp 80–82
20. Cain ME, Ambos D, Witkowski FX, Sobel BE (1984) Fast-Fourier Transform analysis of signal-averaged electrocardiograms for identification of patients prone to sustained ventricular tachycardia. Circulation 69:711–720
21. Cain ME, Ambos HD, Markham J, Fischer AE, Sobel BE (1985) Quantification of differences in frequency content of signal-averaged electrocardiograms in patients with compared to those without sustained ventricular tachycardia. Am J Cardiol 55:1500–1505
22. Haberl R, Hengstenberg E, Pulter R, Steinbeck G (1986) Frequenzanalyse des Einzelschlag-Elektrokardiogrammes zur Diagnostik von Kammertachykardien. Z. Kardiol 75:659–665

23. Zuckermann R (1960) Postexzitation. Z Kreislauf 49:654–658
24. Fontaine G, Guiraudon G, Frank R et al (1977) Stimulation studies and epicardial mapping in ventricular tachycardia: study of mechanisms and selection for surgery. In: Kulbertus HE (ed.) Reentrant arrhythmias, mechanisms and treatment. Lancaster: MTP Press, pp 333–350
25. Santipetro RF (1977) The origin and characterization of the primary signal, noise and interface sources in the high frequency electrocardiogram. IEEE Trans Biomed Eng 65:707–713
26. Breithardt G, Seipel L, Becker R, Abendroth RR (1980) Ableitung ventrikulärer Spät-potentiale von der Körperoberfläche-Methodik und erste Ergebnisse. Z Kardiol 69:698 (abstr)
27. Karbenn U, Breithardt G, Borggrefe M, Simson MB (1985) Automatic identification of late potentials. J Electrocardiology 18:123–134
28. Breithardt G, Borggrefe M, Karbenn U, Abendroth RR, Yeh HL, Seipel L (1982) Prevalence of late potentials in patients with and without ventricular tachycardia: correlation to angiographic findings. Am J Cardiol 49:1932–1937
29. Kertes PJ, Glaubus M, Murray A, Julian DG, Campbell RWF (1984) Delayed ventricular depolarization-correlation with ventricular activation and relevance to ventricular fibrillation in acute myocardial infarction. Europ Heart J 5:974–983
30. Freedman RA, Gillis AM, Keren A, Soderholm-Difatte V, Mason JW (1984) Signal-averaged ECG late potentials correlate with clinical arrhythmia and electrophysiology study in patients with ventricular tachycardia or fibrillation. Circulation 70:II-252
31. Höpp HW, Hombach V, Deutsch HJ, Osterspey A, Winter U, Hilger HH (1983) Assessment of ventricular vulnerability by Holter ECG, programmed ventricular stimulation and recording of ventricular late potentials. In: Cardiac Pacing. Darmstadt: Steinkopff Verlag, p 625–632
32. Kanovsky MS, Falcone RA, Dresden CA, Josephson ME, Simson ME (1984) Identification of patients with ventricular tachycardia after myocardial infarction: signal-averaged electrocardiogram, Holter monitoring, and cardiac catheterization. Circulation 70:264–270
33. Poll DS, Marchlinski FE, Falcone RA, Simson MB (1984) Abnormal signal averaged ECG in nonischemic congestive cardiomyopathy: relationship to sustained ventricular tachyarrhythmias. Circulation 70:II-253
34. Oeff M, Leitner v ER, Brüggemann T, Andresen D, Sthapit R, Schröder R (1982) Methodische Probleme bei der Registrierung ventrikulärer Spätpotentiale. Z Kardiol 71:204 (abstr)
35. Flowers NC, Shvartsman V, Horan LG, Palakurthy P, Sohi GS, Sridharan MR (1983) Analysis of PR subintervals in normal subjects and early studies in patients with abnormalities of the conduction system using surface His bundle recordings. JACC 2:939
36. Abboud S, Belhassen B, Laniado S, Sadeh D (1983) Non-invasive recording of late ventricular activity using an advanced method in patients with a damaged mass of ventricular tissue. J Electrocardiol 16:245
37. Denniss AR, Ross DL, Johnson DC, Nunn G, Uther JB (1984) Comparison of ventricular activation times obtained by signal averaged ECG and epicardial mapping. JACC 3:623
38. Gardner PHJ, Ursell PHC, Pham TD, Fenoglio JJ, Wit AL (1984) Experimental chronic ventricular tachycardia: Anatomic and electrophysiologic substrates. In: Tachycardias: Mechanisms, Diagnosis, Treatment. Philadelphia: Lea and Febiger, pp 29–60
39. Richards DA, Blake GJ, Spear JF, Moore EN (1984) Electrophysiologic substrate for ventricular tachycardia: correlation of properties in vivo and in vitro. Circulation 69:369–381

216

40. Kienzle MG, Miller J, Falcone R, Harken A, Josephson ME (1984) Intraoperative endocardial mapping during sinus rhythm: relationship to site of origin of ventricular tachycardia. Circulation 70:957–965.

41. Breithardt G, Schwarzmaier J, Borggrefe M, Haerten K, Seipel L (1983) Prognostic significance of ventricular late potentials after acute myocardial infarction. Eur Heart J 4:487–495

42. Simson MB, Euler DE, Michelson EL, Falcone R, Spear JF, Moore N (1981) Confirmation of a new technique for detecting slow ventricular activation on the body surface. Am J Cardiol 47:488 (abstr)

43. Simson MB, Falcone RA, Dresden CA, Josephson ME (1984) Late potentials in anterior versus inferior myocardial infarction. JACC 3:624 (abstr)

44. Rosen M, Fisch C, Hoffman B, Knoebel S (1979) Delayed after depolarizations as a mechanism for accelerated junctional escape rhythm. Circulation 60 (Suppl II):II-253

45. Moak JP, Rosen MR (1984) Induction and termination of triggered activity by pacing in isolated canine Purkinje fibers. Circulation 69:149–62

46. Denniss AR, Cody DV, Fenton SM, Richards DA, Ross DL, Russell PA, Young AA, Uther JB (1983) Significance of delayed activation potentials in survivors of myocardial infarction. J Am Coll Cardiol 1:582 (abstr)

47. Kacet S, Libersa C, Caron J, Bondoux d'Haute-Fenille B, Marchand X, Dagano J, Lekieffre J: The prognostic value of averaged late potentials in patients suffering from coronary artery disease. In: Aliot, E, Lazzara R, (eds) Ventricular Tachycardias. Dordrecht – Boston – Lancaster: Martinus Nijhoff Publishers, (In Press)

48. Kuchar D, Thorburn C, Sammel N (1985) Natural history and clinical significance of late potentials after myocardial infarction. Circulation 72:III–477

49. Höpp HW, Hombach V, Osterspey A, Deutsch H, Winter U, Behrenbech DW, Tauchert M, Hilger HH (1985) Clinical and prognostic significance of ventricular arrhythmias and ventricular late potentials in patients with coronary heart disease. In: Hombach V, Hilger HH (eds) Holter Monitoring Technique. Technical Aspects and Clinical Applications. Stuttgart – New York. FK Schattauer Verlag, pp 297–307

50. Leitner v ER, Oeff M, Loock D, Jahns B, Schröder R (1983) Value of non invasively detected delayed ventricular depolarizations to predict prognosis in post myocardial infarction patients. Circulation 68:III-83

51. Breithardt G, Borggrefe M, Haerten K (1985) Role of programmed ventricular stimulation and noninvasive recording of ventricular late potentials for the identification of patients at risk of ventricular tachyarrhythmias after acute myocardial infarction. In: Zipes DP, Jaliffe J, (eds) Cardiac Electrophysiology and Arrhythmias. New York, Grune and Stratton, pp 553–61

52. Breithardt G, Borggrefe M, Quantius B, Karbenn U, Seipel L (1983) Ventricular vulnerability assessed by programmed ventricular stimulation in patients with and without late potentials. Circulation 68:275–281

53. Jauernig RA, Senges J, Langfelder W, Rizos J, Hoffmann E, Brachmann J, Kübler W (1983) Effect of antiarrhythmic drugs on ventricular late potentials at sinus rhythm and at constant heart rate. In: Steinbach D, Glogar D, Laszkovics A, Scheibelhofer W, Weber W, (eds.) Cardiac Pacing. Darmstadt: Steinkopff Verlag, pp 767–772

54. Oeff M, Leitner V ER, Sthapit R, Breithardt G, Borggrefe M, Karbenn U, Meinertz T, Zotz R, Clas W (1983) Methods for non-invasive detection of ventricular late potentials—A comparative multicenter study. In: Steinbach K, Glogar D, Laszkovics A, Scheibelhofer W, Weber W (eds) Cardiac Pacing. Darmstadt: Steinkopff Verlag, pp 641–647

55. Davies MJ, Path FRC, Thomas AC, Path MRC, Knapman PA, Hangartner JR (1986)

Intramyocardial platelet aggregation in patients with instable angina pectoris suffering sudden ischemic cardiac death. Circulation 73:418–427

56. Patterson E, Holland K, Eller BT, Lucchesi BR (1982) Ventricular fibrillation resulting from ischemia at a site remote from previous myocardial infarction. A conscious canine model of sudden coronary death. Am J Cardiol 50:1414

57. Malliani A, Schwartz PJ, Zanchetti A (1980) Neural mechanisms in life-threatening arrhythmias. Am Heart J 100:705–715

58. Tavazzi L, Zotti AM, Rondanelli R (1986) The role of psychologic stress in the genesis of lethal arrhythmias in patients with coronary artery disease. Eur Heart J 7(suppl A):99–106

18. Dynamic behavior of ventricular late potentials

V. HOMBACH, M. KOCHS, H. W. HÖPP, U. KEBBEL,
T. EGGELING, A. OSTERSPEY, H. HIRCHE & H. H. HILGER
*Medical Clinic III and Department of Cardiology and Department of Applied Physiology,
University of Cologne, F.R.G.*

Key words: ventricular late potentials, ventricular vulnerability, high resolution electrocardiography, sudden cardiac death

Abstract

In a series of 44 patients, 5 females and 39 males, the incidence and dynamic behavior of ventricular late potentials was studied. Using a home-built high resolution electrocardiogram equipment ventricular late potentials were found within the ST segment in 27/44 patients, and in 11 patients were the late potentials observed intermittently. In 21/44 patients late potentials were also present after the T wave, in 5 individuals intermittently.

There were good correlations of the presence of late potentials within the high resolution electrocardiogram, obtained during endocardial mapping studies in 9 individuals. A statistically significant correlation was found between the incidence of ventricular late potentials, the occurrence of complex ventricular arrhythmias, and the inducibility of a repetitive ventricular response.

In 1/22 patients with single ventricular ectopic beats in the low noise electrocardiogram a Wenckebach conduction pattern was observed with fractionated activity between the preceding normal QRS complex and the following ectopic cycle, in 13/22 patients an isolated late potential preceded the ectopic ventricular complex, in 6/22 patients no late potential was present, and in 2/22 individuals an overlap of the ectopic beat with the T wave or P wave of the normal cycle was observed.

During spontaneous or pacing induced episodes of ventricular tachycardia diastolic slowly depolarizing potentials were recorded prior to each tachycardia-QRS complex in 3/4 patients, and 'stressing' of late potentials was seen in 9/15 patients on ventricular pacing.

V. Hombach, H. H. Hilger and H. L. Kennedy (eds), Electrocardiography and Cardiac Drug Therapy. ISBN 978-94-010-6976-2
© 1989, Kluwer Academic Publishers, Dordrecht –

From these results one may conclude that ventricular late potentials may serve as a marker of ventricular vulnerability, that dynamic changes may occur during sinus rhythm, and that the functional role of late potentials in the initiation, maintenance and termination of ventricular arrhythmias can be clarified by the high resolution surface electrocardiogram technique.

Introduction

In many patients with certain cardiac diseases (coronary heart disease, dilatative cardiomyopathy, hypertrophic obstructive cardiomyopathy, aortic valve disease etc.) frequent and complex forms of ventricular arrhythmias can be detected, whose exact pathophysiological mechanisms have not exactly been clarified as yet. From animal experiments and—to a limited degree—from human studies at least three basic mechanisms of ventricular ectopic activity have been discussed [1]: focal activity, triggered activity, and re-entrant mechanisms. Focal activity is present, if a certain area of atrial or ventricular tissue is capable of spontaneous distolic depolarisation, that may induce single or repetitive ectopic beats, when the depolarisation wave exceeds the threshold potential. The mechanism of triggered activity has been studied in special types of myocardial cells, e.g. from the mitral valve or the vicinity of the coronary sinus, that were partially depolarized by aconitine or by potassium depletion. Under these special conditions the cells are capable of developing oscillatory afterdepolarisations with subsequent repetitive electrical activity [2, 3]. The third mechanism, the re-entrant concept, has been studied extensively in chronic animal heart infarct models [4–7]. Due to Wenckebach-conduction delays within areas of depressed myocardial tissue re-entrant premature depolarisations of the surrounding normal myocardium may be induced, when recovered from depolarisation. Such abnormal and delayed ventricular electrical activity may be visible within the ST segment or after the T wave in electrocardiograms recorded directly from the endo- or epicardial site of the peri-infarction tissue, or within the low noise electrocardiogram, obtained from body surface by using special high resolution recording techniques [8]. In principle, these three mechanisms may be active in inducing ventricular arrhythmias within diseased human myocardium, though endocardial catheter mapping or endo-epicardial mapping studies during open heart surgery favor the re-entrant concept.

During episodes of sustained tachycardias endocardial electrogram recordings have demonstrated that the interval between the tachycardia-QRS complexes may be bridged by fractionated potentials, thus indicating a closed circuit of electrical activity within the ventricular myocardium, the so-called re-entrant circuit [4, 7, 9, 10, 11]. But during sinus rhythm delayed ventricular activation following the regular QRS complex may also be seen with endocardial electrogram recordings [9, 12, 13, 14]. Such diastolic activity may be retrieved from body surface by using the signal averaging technique [15–21], when the heart is driven by a regular sinus rhythm. However, dynamic events like transition of sinus beats into single or repetitive ventricular ectopic beats via diastolic potentials or fractionated inter-QRS activity is most commonly lost during the averaging process. Therefore special high resolution surface electrocardiogram techniques have been developed in recent years, that allow retrieval of late ventricular depolarisations on a beat-to-beat basis, particularly during periods of ventricular arrhythmias [22–25]. Studies evaluating the relationship between ventricular late potentials and ventricular ectopic beats noninvasively have not been published to our knowledge. Therefore our preliminary observations with the high resolution electrocardiogram technique are reported in documenting the full dynamic behavior of ventricular late potentials under various clinical and electrophysiological conditions.

Patients

44 patients, 5 females and 39 males, aged 17 to 67 years (mean: 50.2 + 11.2 years), were studied. 33 patients were suffering from coronary heart disease, as confirmed by left ventricular and coronary angiography in 31 individuals, another 10 patients from dilatative cardiomyopathy, also diagnosed angiographically, and one patient with recurrent attacks of ventricular tachycardias had been surgically corrected for Fallot's tetralogy. 30 individuals with coronary heart disease had experienced a previous myocardial infarction, 8 of these had a history of recurrent ventricular tachycardias, and one patient suffered from several syncopies. 4 individuals had been resuscitated from ventricular tachycardia-fibrillation. Coronary angiography performed in 31/33 patients revealed a single vessel disease in 10 patients, a double vessel disease in 12 individuals, and a triple vessel disease in 9 subjects. On left ventricular angiography normocinesis was found in one patient, anterior wall hypo-acinesia in 18 patients, inferior wall hypoacinesia in 6 individuals, and a generalized hypocinesia in 7 subjects. Left ventricular ejection fraction was lower than 30% in 5 patients, and higher than 30% in the remaining 26 individuals.

Of the 10 patients with dilatative cardiomyopathy 4 had episodes of ventricular tachycardias, 4 individuals had been resuscitated from ventricular tachycardia-fibrillation episodes. One of the cardiomyopathy patients had an embolic occlusion of the left anterior descending coronary artery, the remaining 9 individuals were free from coronary artery lesions. Left ventricular ejection fraction below 30% was found in 3 patients, and beyond 30% in 7 individuals. The patient with operated Fallot's tetralogy was only studied clinically and by means of two-dimensional echocardiography, that showed a reduced right ventricular but nearly normal left ventricular contraction pattern.

In 12 patients the high resolution surface electrocardiogram could only be recorded on oral maintenance antiarrhythmic drug therapy, that was necessary to stabilize the patients from their frequent attacks of ventricular tachyarrhythmias. The remaining patients could be studied during drug-free periods with Holter electrocardiogram monitoring, high resolution electrocardiography, and by programmed ventricular stimulation.

Methods

Our home-built high resolution electrocardiogram recording unit has been recently described in detail [23, 24]. The essential measures of noise reduction are:

1. the use of specially designed suction electrodes (4 to 16 pole) for proper contact to the skin,
2. the incorporation of special extremely low noise amplifiers (Siliconix FET 2N 5521, voltage and current noise specifications of $2\,nV/\sqrt{Hz}$ and $0.1\,pA/\sqrt{Hz}$, respectively),
3. the use of spatial averaging instead of sequential averaging of 4 electrograms (initial equipment) or 16 single electrocardiograms (more recent version) obtained from 4 or 16 pairs of bipolar electrodes,
4. the recordings are performed within a Faraday cage with the cage and the patient properly grounded, and
5. the patient is taught to keep relaxed with shallow breathing or with endexpiratory breath hold to minimize respiratory muscle interferences.

By this means noise levels of 1 to 2 μV and in rare cases of 4 to 5 μV are obtained. The low noise electrocardiogram can also be recorded and stored on a magnetic tape for a period of 4 hours (long-term high resolution electrocardiography), using an 8-channel high performance tape recorder (Gould 6500, [26]), that allows the detection of ventricular arrhythmias and the evaluation of possible ventricular late potential-ectopic beat interactions.

The bipolar surface low noise electrocardiograms are recorded using the following electrode positions: 2nd right intercostal space to the 4th left intercostal space, 4th right intercostal space at the medio-clavicular line to the 4th left intercostal space at mid-clavicular line, the 4th left intercostal space at the mid-clavicular line to a corresponding point at the mid- or posterior axillary line (thereby avoiding the apex beat of the heart that could possibly interfere with the low noise electrocardiogram recordings), and sometimes 4th intercostal space at the right mid-axillary line to the 4th intercostal space at the left mid-axillary line.

Holter longterm conventional electrocardiogram recordings were performed by using either a real-time Holter system (Quickscan, IMC corporation), or a conventional continuously recording Holter equipment (Anatec, Ela-Medical), whose performance characteristics and reliability of arrhythmia analysis have been tested previously [27]. The recording periods lasted 24 to 72 hours, and ventricular arrhythmias found within the Holter electrocardiogram were classified according to the Lown-grading system [28].

In 3 patients right ventricular and left ventricular catheter mapping was performed, using a bipolar 4F catheter electrode (USCI) within the right ventricle, and a quadripolar 5F catheter electrode (USCI) within the left ventricle. Endocardial electrocardiograms were recorded from the following sites: right ventricular inflow tract, -apex, -septal area, and right ventricular outflow tract, left ventricular diaphragmatic wall at the base, intermediate part and at the apex, left ventricular posterolateral wall, left ventricular anterior free wall at the base, intermediate area and the apical region, and the left ventricular septal area. Epiendocardial direct mapping during open heart surgery was performed in another 7 patients (including one individual with catheter mapping as well) for localization of the tachycardia origin and consequently, for antiarrhythmic surgery like endocardectomy and/or circumcision [29]. The endocardial left ventricular activation times of the anterior free wall, the lateral wall, the diaphragmatic parts and the septal area were recorded using a tripolar hand-held electrode probe during sinus rhythm and pacing induced ventricular tachycardias, measured against the activation of a reference electrode epicardially at the right ventricular outflow tract, and noted within a special grid of the endocardial left ventricular free wall and septal areas. The area of ventricular tachycardia origin was assessed by searching for the area of latest ventricular activation, grade of fractionating during sinus rhythm, and for the area of earliest ventricular activation during periods of sustained ventricular tachycardias [29].

Programmed ventricular stimulation was performed according to a standardized pacing protocol [30]. The patients were instructed about the procecure and the possible risks and gave their written consent. The right ventricle was paced with basic driven rhythms of 100, 120, 140 and 160 stimuli/min, and a single extrastimulus was delivered every 8th paced beat with steadily decreasing coupling intervals, until the right ventricular effective refractory period was reached. When a repetitive ventricular response [31] or an episode of ventricular tachycardia could not be induced by a single extrastimulus, a second pacing protocol with double extrastimuli was performed, using the same basic pacing rates. The S1–S2 interval was steadily decreased down to reaching the right ventricular effective refractory period, while the S2–S3 interval was kept constant by 10 to 20 ms above the effective refractory period. These two pacing protocols were performed with the pacing electrode positioned at the right ventricular apex and thereafter at the right ventricular outflow tract.

In 15 patients programmed ventricular stimulation or regular ventricular overdrive pacing was performed during the recording periods of the low noise electrocardiogram. The stimulation protocol was much less aggressive than that of conventional programmed stimulation, that was regularly performed within the coronary care unit. Only in patients with hemodynamically tolerable ventricular tachycardias and easy modes of termination like burst pacing or endocardial cardioversion was programmed stimulation performed on low noise electrocardiogram recordings, whereas in patients with faster tachycardia rates and hemodynamic compromise only ventricular overdrive pacing was performed without the end point of inducing the clinical ventricular tachycardia.

For identifying ventricular late potentials within the high resolution surface electrocardiogram we have used the following criteria: late potentials are additional and separate signals at the end of the QRS complex, using the conventional and low amplified low noise electrocardiograms as the reference leads, within the ST segment, and/or after the T wave with amplitudes of equal or more than twice the amplitude of the baseline noise. Questionable late potentials were those with considerably changing morphology beat-by-beat and/or with intermittent occurrence and/or with amplitudes lower than the values indicated.

The normal QRS width was measured in the conventional standard lead I from the beginning of the Q wave to the end of the S- or R-wave (45° intercept with baseline). The QRS width of the low noise electrocardiogram was measured similarly from the beginning of the Q wave to the latest deflection of the R- or S-wave (45° intercept with baseline) of the low noise electrogram lead with lowest amplification. The total QRS width, i.e. the pure QRS width plus the ventricular late potential, was measured from the beginning of the Q wave to the last portion of the late potential within the ST segment (45° intercept with baseline) of the high resolution electrocardiogram lead with highest amplification. The QT interval was measured within the standard lead I as the reference lead from the beginning of the Q wave to the end of the 45°-intercept of the downsloping T signal with baseline. The QT interval of the low noise electrocardiogram was determined in a similar manner, using the high resolution electrocardiogram lead with lowest amplification. The total QT interval, i.e. the pure QT time plus the post T late potential, was taken from the high resolution lead with highest amplification by measuring the interval from the beginning of the Q wave to the end of the last deflection of the post T late potential (45° intercept with the baseline).

The statistical significance of the correlations between the various electrophysiological parameters was calculated according to the X^2-test using Yates' correction, and statistical significance was accepted when $p < 0.05$. The values are given as the mean ± standard deviation.

Results

Incidence of ventricular late potentials

In 27/44 patients ventricular late potentials were found within the ST segment, clearcut late potentials in 11, and doubtful in 16 patients. These late depolarisations were observed intermittently in 11 individuals. The QRS width within the standard electrocardiogram was 95–120 ms (mean: 112.3 ± 5.6 ms), the QRS width of the low noise electrocardiogram was 100–150 ms (mean: 131.4 ± 21.5 ms), whereas the total QRS width amounted to 110–380 ms (mean: 201.3 ± 65.1 ms). Ventricular late potentials were retrieved after the T wave in 21/44 patients, clearcut late potentials in 7, and doubtful in 14 patients. In 5 individuals these late potentials were found to occur intermittently (Figure 1). The QT interval within the standard electrocardiogram ranged from 340 to 460 ms (mean: 436.3 ± 12.4 ms), the QT interval of the low noise electrocardiogram was 360–615 ms (mean: 465.4 ± 72.9 ms), and the total QT interval of the low noise electrocardiogram amounted to 370–660 ms (mean: 518.6 ± 87.3 ms). The amplitudes of ventricular late potentials within the ST segment ranged from 5 to 15 μV, and those after the T wave from 3 to 20 μV.

Correlations of late potentials with endocardial mapping results

In 3 patients endocardial cathether mapping, and in 7 individuals left ventricular endocardial mapping during heart surgery was performed (Table 1). In 2 patients singular potentials were found after the end of the corresponding T wave, when using left ventricular endocardial catheter mapping. In the remaining patients fractionations of the QRS complex, that exceeded the terminal part of the conventional surface electrocardiogram

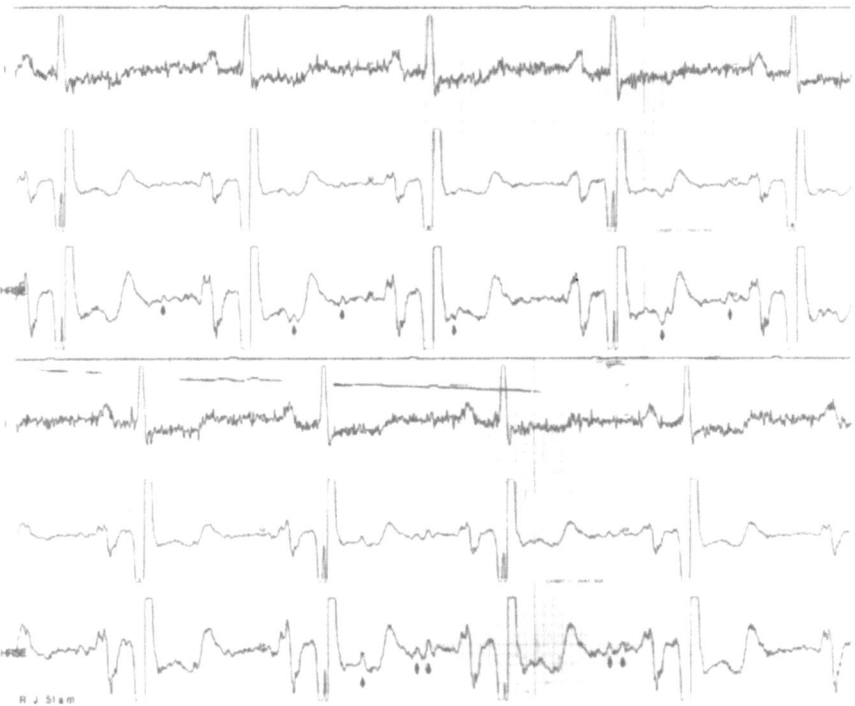

Figure 1. Surface low noise electrocardiogram (HRSE) in a patient with anterior wall aneurysm and recurrent attacks of ventricular tachycardias. Note the considerable variability in the occurrence, amplitude and timing of ventricular late potentials (arrows) during regular sinus rhythm. I: Conventional Einthoven lead I.

QRS complex, together with a reduction of the QRS amplitudes were recorded from different left ventricular endocardial areas, as indicated in Table 1. In all of these 9 patients were late potentials found within the ST segment and/or after the T wave within the surface high resolution electrocardiogram, and in 3 patients 'stressing' of the late potentials, i.e. lengthening of base width and/or increase of fragmentation, was observed on right ventricular high rate or programmed stimulation. Figure 2 shows an example of the good correlation of late potential recording from body surface by low noise electrocardiography and from the left ventricular endocardial mapping. In 6 of these 9 patients areas of the origin of the ventricular tachycardia could be localized, and these foci were subsequently inactivated by aneurysmectomy plus endocardectomy and/or endocardial circumcision.

Table 1. Correlation of endocardial mapping findings with late potential detection within the high resolution surface ECG. **Abbreviations:** Cath: LV-endocardial catheter mapping, Endo: LV-endocardial mapping using a hand held probe, VLP: ventricular late potentials (area of late depolarisation, area of VT re-entry), HRSE: high resolution surface ECG, AW: anterior wall, ST: ST segment, post-T: post-T interval, interm: intermittently occurring late potentials, const: constantly beat-by-beat occurring late potentials, VLP stressing on programmed or high rate ventricular pacing, +: positive, 0: stimulation not performed, Lead position (of HRSE) showing late potentials: 1: 2nd right ICS parasternal to 4th left ICS parasternal, 2: 4th right ICS-mid-clavicular line to 4th left ICS-mid-clavicular line, 3: 4th left ICS-mid-clavicular line to a corresponding point at the left mid-axillary line.

Patient	Type of mapping	Fractionation of QRS-complex	Amplitude reduction of QRS	LV-endocardial localization of VLP	VLP within HRSE	VLP type	VLP-stressing	Lead position
S.W.	Cath	−	−	postero-lateral-wall	ST, post-T	interm	0	1
M.H.	Endo	+	+	anterior-aneurysm, septum	ST, post-T	const interm	0	2
L.H.	Endo Cath	+	+	inferior wall (peri-aneurysm)	ST	const	+	1, 2
W.K.	Endo	+	+	AW-apex, septum-apex	ST, post-T	interm	0	1, 2
E.G.	Cath	−	−	AW-apex	post-T	interm	0	2
M.W.	Endo	+	+	inferior wall	ST, post-T	const interm	+	2, 3
R.J.	Endo	+	+	diaphrag-matic wall septum	ST, post-T	interm	0	1, 3
P.W.	Endo	+	−	anterior wall (diffuse)	ST, post-T	interm	0	1, 3
B.F.	Endo	+	+	inferior wall-septum	ST	const	+	2, 3

227

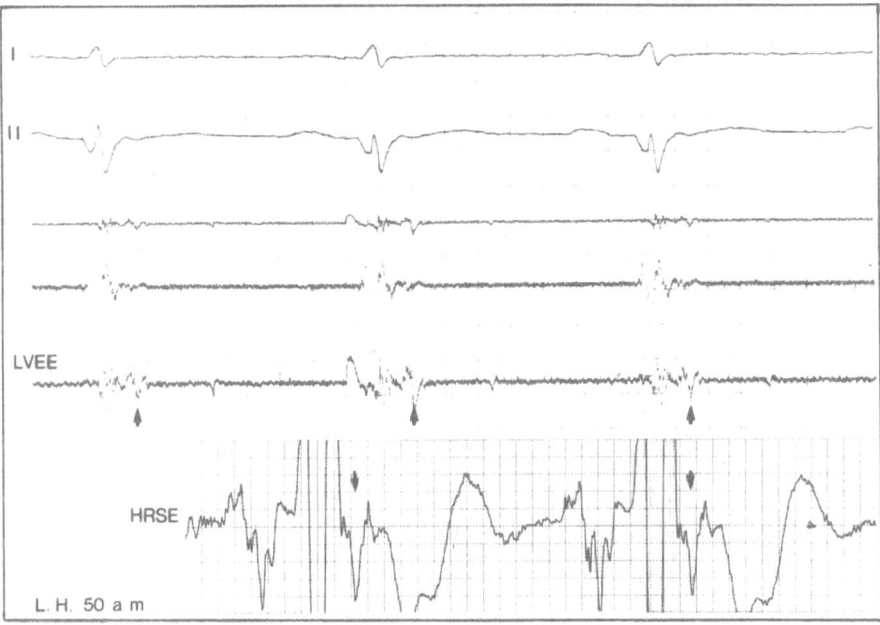

Figure 2. Left ventricular endocardial catheter recording from the anterior border of a large inferior wall aneurysm (top), and non-invasive high resolution ECG (bottom) in a patient with coronary heart disease and recurrent attacks of ventricular tachycardias. Note the stable and large ventricular late potential within the ST segment of the endocardial and surface low noise ECG (arrows). LVEE: left ventricular endocardial electrogram, HRSE: high resolution surface electrogram.

Incidence of ventricular arrhythmias

In 41 patients conventional Holter electrocardiogram recordings were available, the following spectrum of ventricular arrhythmias was found (all Lown-grades seen in each patient totaling 70 grades of ventricular arrhythmias): grade 0: 2 patients, grade I: 10 patients, grade II: 5 patients, grade III: 19 patients, grade IVa: 21 patients, grade IVb: 13 patients. When only considering the highest Lown-grade of ventricular arrhythmias, the following distribution was found: grade 0: 2 patients, grade I: 10 patients, grade II: 0 patients, grade III: 3 patients, grade IVa: 14 patients, garde IVb: 13 patients. When comparing the number of patients with either simple (Lown-grade 0-II) or complex (Lown-grade III–IVb) forms of ventricular arrhythmias to the number of patients without or with ventricular late potentials, the following correlation was found (Table 2): of the

228

Table 2. Correlation between the incidence of ventricular late potentials (VLP) within the high resolution surface ECG and the incidence of ventricular arrhythmias (VEA), as graded according to Lown's scheme. $X^2 = 4.731$, $p < 0.03$

	VEA-Lown 0–2	VEA-Lown 3–4b	Sum
VLP absent	5	1	6
VLP present	7	20	27
Sum	12	21	33

6 patients without late potentials 5 had simple, and one had complex ventricular arrhythmias, in contrast to 27 patients with late potentials, of whom 7 had simple, but 20 had complex forms of ventricular arrhythmias (statistically significant with $p < 0.03$).

Left ventricular vulnerability on programmed right ventricular stimulation

In 36/44 patients programmed ventricular stimulation could be performed as described above in order to evaluate ventricular vulnerability. At control states without antiarrhythmic drugs the following grades of repetitive response were found: grade I (0–2 echo beats): 8 patients, grade II (3–5 echo beats): 2 patients, grade IIIa: (ventricular tachycardia shorter than 15 s): none, grade IIIb (ventricular tachycardia longer than 15 s): 25 patients, grade IV (primary ventricular flutter-fibrillation): one patient. When only taking 3 or more ventricular echo beats as a positive result, i.e. as true repetitive response indicating ventricular vulnerability, a total of

Table 3. Correlation of the incidence of ventricular late potentials (VLP) to the inducibility of repetitive ventricular response (RVR) on programmed ventricular stimulation. $X^2 = 5.796$, $p < 0.02$

	VLP absent	VLP present	Sum
RVR negative	5	3	8
RVR positive	4	21	25
Sum	9	24	33

30/36 patients revealed a positive result. When comparing the presence or absence of a repetitive response to the presence or absence of ventricular late potentials, the following correlation was found (Table 3): of the 8 patients with negative repetitive ventricular response 5 patients did not have late potentials, while 3 had late potentials, in contrast to 25 patients with a positive repetitive ventricular response, 4 of whom did not have late potentials, but 21 patients had late potentials within the low noise electrocardiogram (statistically significant with $p < 0.02$).

Ventricular arrhythmias within the high resolution surface electrocardiogram

In 22/24 patients ventricular ectopic beats were observed during the recording period of the high resolution electrocardiogram, either during shortterm (12/17) or longterm recording (11/15). In general, 4 different types of ventricular late potential-ectopic beat interaction were observed:

type 1: more or less fractionated late potentials within the ST segment of the preceding normal beat, extending the T wave and merging into the following ventricular ectopic complex,

type 2: an isolated ventricular late potential after or at the end of the T wave of the preceding normal QRS complex with immediate merging into the ventricular ectopic beat,

type 3: no visible late potential preceding the ventricular ectopic complex, and

type 4: interference of the beginning of the ventricular ectopic complex with a physiological depolarisation like the T wave of the preceding normal QRS complex (so-called early cycle ectopic beat), or with the P wave of the following expected QRS complex (so-called late cycle ectopic beat).

The following distribution of late potential-ectopic beat interactions was found:

type 1: in one patient, type 2: in 13 patients, type 3: in 6 patients, and type 4: in 2 patients (examples in Figures 3, 4).

In 4 patients the low noise electrocardiogram could be recorded during a run of sustained ventricular tachycardia. In 2 patients the tachycardia started out of a ventricular late potential, that was located after the T wave of the preceding normal QRS complex, and in 3/4 tachycardia episodes distinct slowly depolarizing potentials within the last third of the intertachycardia QRS interval were observed. In one of these patients the tachycardia terminated spontaneously together with a decrease of the amplitude and duration of the pre-QRS signal for two sinus beats, and spontaneously started again with an increase of the amplitude and duration

Table 4. Results of ventricular stimulation (high rate or programmed) during registration of the high resolution ECG. Induction of VLP: appearance of late potentials within the ST Segment or after the T wave in the first spontaneous beat following ventricular pacing, Stressing of VLP: widening of basewidth and/or change in amplitude and configuration of late potentials following ventricular stimulation, Induction of VEA: induction of single or repetitive ventricular ectopic beats following the last extrastimulus or high rate paced ventricular complex, Type of VLP-VEA interaction: Type 1: fractionated late potentials within the ST segment of the last paced beat merging into the ventricular ectopic complex, Type 2: single late potential within the ST segment of the last paced beat merging into the ventricular complex, Type 3: no late potential preceding the induced ectopic beat. 0: not performed. Abbreviations: VLP: ventricular late potential, VEA: ventricular ectopic activity, VP: ventricular pacing, PVS: programmed ventricular stimulation, RVR: repetitive ventricular response, CHD: coronary heart disease, COCM: congestive cardiomyopathy, TET: tetralogy, VT: ventricular tachycardia

Patient	Heart disease	Type of stimulation	Induction of VLP	Stressing of VLP	Induction of VEA	Type of VLP-VEA on VP	RVR on conventional PVS
B.F.	CHD	VVI	+	+	+	1, 2	+ VT
S.L.	COCM	PVS	-	+	+	1, 2	+ VT
S.J.	CHD	PVS	(+)	-	+	3	-
R.J.	CHD	PVS	(+)	+	+	1, 2	0
C.G.	CHD	VVI	-	-	-	-	0
F.R.	CHD	PVS	+	+	+	1	+ VT
L.H.	CHD	VVI	-	+	-	-	+ VT
R.B.	CHD	PVS	+	+	-	-	0
L.P.	CHD	PVS	+	-	-	-	+
D.A.	OP-FALLOT TET	PVS	(post-T) (+)	(post-T) +	+	2	+ VT
M.W.	CHD	VVI	-	+	-	-	+ VT
C.A.	CHD	PVS	-	-	+	2, 3	-
F.F.	CHD	PVS	+	+	-	-	+ VT
M.M.	COCM	PVS	(+)	+	-	-	+ VT
S.W.	COCM	PVS	+ (post-T)	-	-	-	+ VT

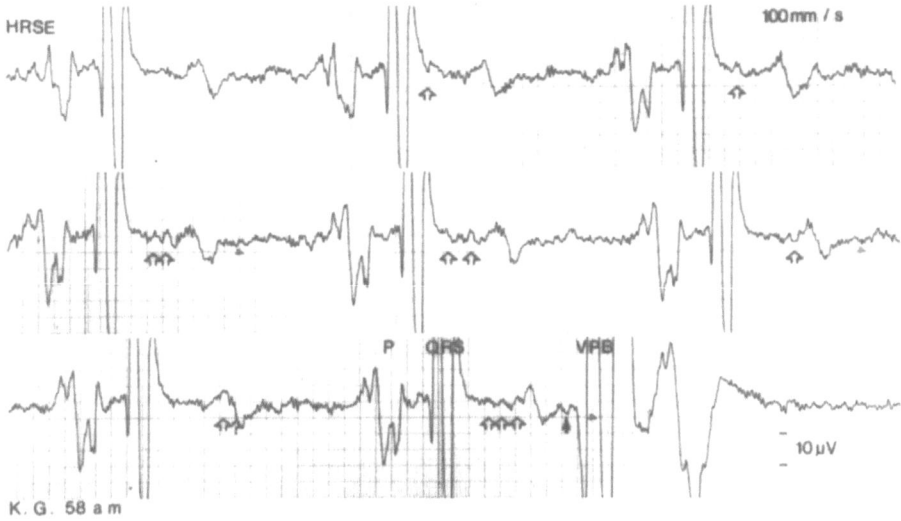

Figure 3. Wenckebach conduction pattern of delayed ventricular activation resulting in a single ventricular premature beat (VPB). Note increase of fractionation of ventricular depolarisation (arrows) with continuous electrical activity throughout ST segment and post-T interval prior to the occurrence of the premature beat (one re-entrant cycle). HRSE: high resolution surface electrocardiogram.

of the pre-QRS signal (Figure 5). Following iv.-administration of a bolus of 100 mg of Lidocaine the pre-QRS signal decreased with amplitude and base width, and soon after this observation the ventricular tachycardia terminated spontaneously.

Programmed or high rate ventricular pacing and ventricular late potentials

In 11 patients programmed ventricular pacing and in 4 individuals ventricular high rate pacing could be performed during the registration of the high resolution surface electrocardiogram (Table 4). New pacing induced ventricular late potentials were observed in 4 individuals within the ST segment (Figure 6), and in 2 patients after the T wave of the low noise electrocardiogram. 'Stressing' of late potentials on ventricular pacing, i.e. variable prolongations of the base width with continuously decreasing duration to the pre-pacing values within 2 to 5 sinus beats post-pacing, was seen in 10/15 individuals paced, and in 9 patients these changes were related to late potentials within the ST segment, and in one patient after T wave of the low noise electrocardiogram. Augmentation of the amplitude of a post T late potential by ventricular pacing was observed in 3 patients.

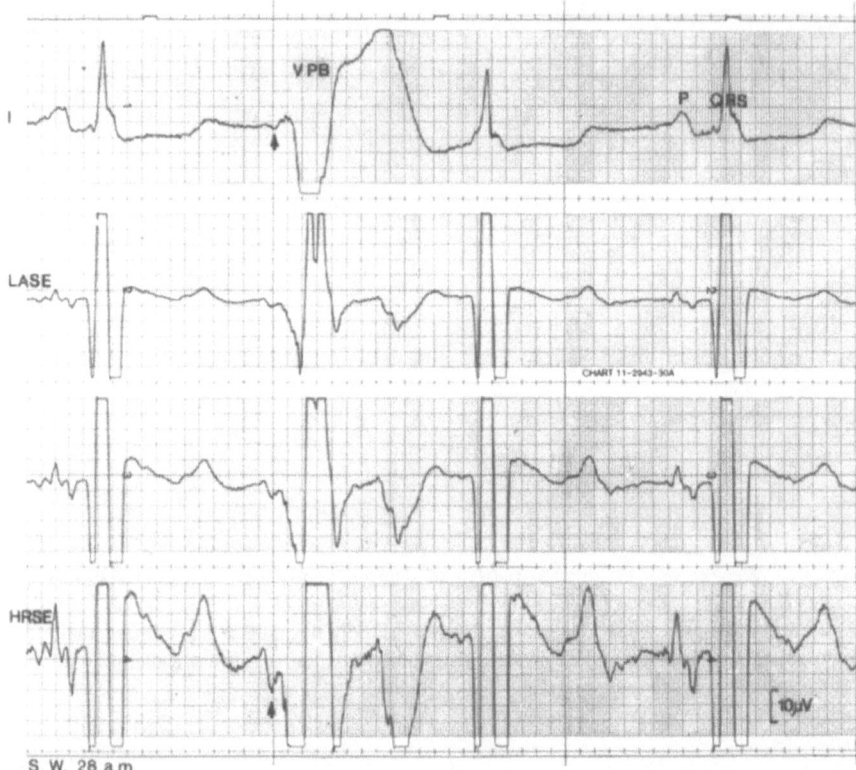

Figure 4. 'Focal' type of ventricular ectopic activity. Note a single biphasic signal following the T wave of the normal pre-ectopic QRS complex, which merges into the ectopic ventricular complex (VPB). I: conventional Einthoven lead I, LASE: low amplified surface ECG, HRSE: high resolution surface electrocardiogram.

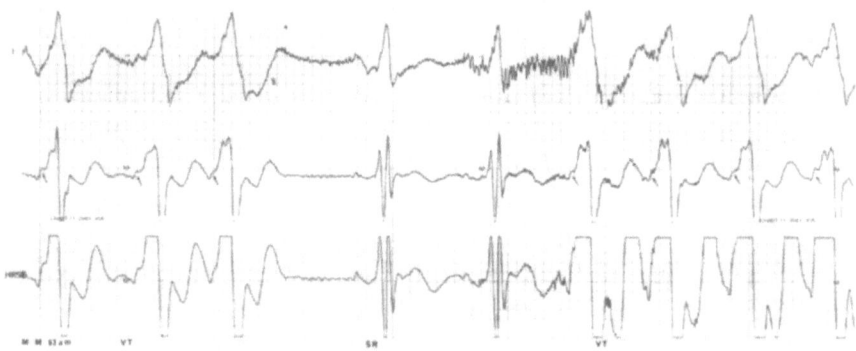

Figure 5. Low noise electrocardiogram in a patient with dilative cardiomyopathy during a run of ventricular tachycardia (VT). Note a slowly depolarizing potential prior to the onset of the VT-QRS compleses (arrows, strip in the middle). With decreasing amplitude the VT spontaneously ceases (left panel) and sinus rhythm occurs for two beats (SR, center), with increasing amplitude of these potentials ventricular tachycardia starts again (VT, right panel). I: regular Einthoven lead I, HRSE: high resolution surface electrocardiogram.

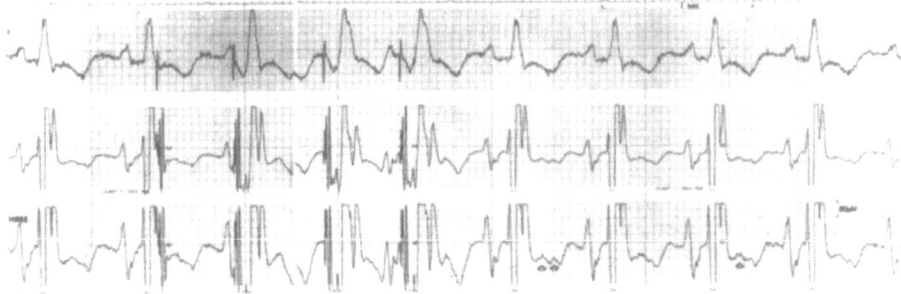

Figure 6. Induction of 'new' ventricular late potentials by regular right ventricular high rate pacing. Note regular sinus beats (first two) on the left, first paced beat (third QRS complex), last two paced beats (center), and following 4 sinus beats (right panel). During sinus rhythm before pacing no late potentials are visible within the ST segment and the post-T interval. After cessation of pacing late potentials are seen within the ST segment of the first and third post-pacing sinus beat (arrows). I: regular Einthoven lead I, HRSE: high resolution surface electrocardiogram.

Discussion

Clinical assessment of ventricular vulnerability

Several clinical studies have shown that non-invasively detected ventricular late potentials (by use of the signal averaging technique) may indicate ventricular vulnerability, at least in patients with coronary heart disease. The detection of certain types of ventricular arrhythmias is also considered as an indicator of ventricular electrical instability. However, the prognostic stratification of ventricular ectopic beats bears the weakness that the underlying electrophysiologic mechanisms are not taken into consideration. The third indicator of ventricular vulnerability, the repetitive ventricular response, can only be obtained by the invasive approach of programmed ventricular stimulation, that renders this method less suitable for repeat follow-up studies of high risk patients. Moreover, in a group of 40 patients with coronary heart disease and documented ventricular electrical in-stability (all of these patients had had at least one attack of ventricular tachycardia or more) the sensitivity of each of the parameters of ventricular electrical instability was found to be well below 100%: complex ventricular arrhythmias within the Holter electrocardiogram: 55%, ventricular late potentials within the averaged surface electrocardiogram: 75%, repetitive ventricular response on programmed ventricular stimulation: 72%. And in addition there was no uniform distribution of the presence or absence of these three parameters in the individual patient: concordant positive findings in 13/40 patients, concordant negative results in 4/40 patients, and discrepant findings in 23/40 patients [32]. The predictive value of these vulnerability parameters in identifying candidates at risk of sudden arrhythmic death ranges between 25 to 50%, depending on the population studied [33–36]. Therefore as yet the possible risk of an individual patient prone to sudden cardiac death can only be assessed by a risk profile encompassing clinical and angiographic signs of left ventricular dysfunction, certain types of ventricular arrhythmias (complex arrhythmias), and probably the detection of ventricular late potentials and provocation of repetitive ventricular response. Thus, no single non-invasive parameter exists that could differentiate between a high or low risk of an individual to die suddenly from ventricular tachycardia-fibrillation, based on one single examination period.

Ventricular late potentials and arrhythmias—mechanisms

Focal as well as triggered activities are characterized as single slowly depolarizing low voltage deflections, that induce single or repetitive forms of ventricular ectopic beats, when reaching the threshold potential [2, 3]. On the other hand, re-entrant exitations are electrocardiographically characterized as continuous electrical activity between the last normal beat and the following ectopic beat, and in case of ventricular tachycardia continuous electrical activity should be present between the tachycardia-QRS complexes [37]. The former mechanisms have—as yet—only been demonstrated in electrophysiological experiments with single myocardial fibers, whereas the latter could be confirmed in the human heart in vivo by endocardial catheter recordings or in animal preparations by epicardial composite electrode recordings. The two types of pre-ectopic diastolic potentials, as found in our patients, closely resemble the single ecotopic depolarisation (probably focal or triggered activity) or the Wenckebach conduction pattern (probably re-entrant excitation) known from animal experiments. Thus, the differentiation between focal and re-entrant ventricular arrhythmias in man may probably be assessed by the completely non-invasive high resolution electrocardiogram recording technique. However, these preliminary results have to be confirmed in a larger series of studies, in which direct endocardial catheter recording results have to be correlated with the findings of surface low noise electrocardiograms during periods of single and particularly repetitive ventricular ectopic depolarisations. The clinically most important suggestion that focal rhythms may be more 'benign' than the 'malignant' reentrant mechanisms, as recently discussed by El-Sherif and coworkers [37], may also be elucidated by prognostic studies, using the high resolution electrocardiogram recording technique described above.

Pathophysiological role of ventricular late potentials

The percentage incidence of late potentials, found in this study by using the high resolution beat-to-beat technique, is in accordance with the results recently published in the literature [22, 23, 24, 37]. From the reasonably good concordance of late potential detection with the low noise electrocardiogram technique compared to the endocardial mapping technique, as found in our 9 patients, we suppose that the diastolic potentials within the ST segment and after the T wave of the low noise electrocardiogram are really existing electrophysiologic phenomena (see Figure 2). The significant correlations between the presence or absence of late potentials and the incidence of simple or complex ventricular arrhythmias, and also the inducibility of a repetitive ventricular response suggest that late potentials within the low noise electrocardiogram represent indeed a separate parameter of increased ventricular electrical instability. But the findings of dynamic changes of late potentials like intermittent occurrence or change of amplitude and base width during sinus rhythm or on programmed stimulation deserve attention. In chronic dog heart infarct models intermittent Wenckebach conduction patterns with fractionations of the QRS complex and parts of the ST segment have been found, that are reflecting a conduction delay within areas of depressed and partially depolarized ventricular myocardium. And a gradual increase of fractionation and conduction delay has been observed as well, when the heart rate was increased by ventricular high rate pacing (= rate dependent conduction block, 4–7, 37). Similar conduction patterns, i.e. ventricular late depolarisations with varying intervals to the corresponding QRS complex, or intermittent occurrence during sinus rhythm, and 'stressing' of late potentials on ventricular programmed or high rate pacing, could be documented in this limited series of patients. We gained the impression that patients with considerable variability of late potentials within the low noise electrocardiogram, whose characterization as being true signals is of course more crucial than their stable beat-by-beat occurrence, may have the highest degree of ventricular vulnerability, as evidenced by the response to programmed stimulation, the findings during intraoperative mapping, and by further follow-up studies of these patients. However, our experience at present is too limited to draw valid conclusions from the observation of "unstable" late potentials within the low noise electrocardiogram, particularly with regard to their prognostic significance.

The pathophysiological role of late potentials during ventricular tachycardia in man is as yet relatively unclear. The observation of diastolic potentials within the low noise electrocardiogram prior to each tachycardia-QRS complex in 3/4 patients with dilated cardiomyopathy suggests a

236

focal or triggered activity mechanism of the ventricular tachycardia. On the other hand, possible continuous electrical activity in between the tachycardia-QRS complexes, that would indicate a re-entrant mechanism operating, may have been lost by the use of relatively flat (6 db/octave) 20-Hz high pass filters and by interference of these small amplitude diastolic potentials with the huge T wave of the corresponding tachycardia-QRS complex. Our new generation of 16-channel equipment now provides the facility of recording the low noise electrocardiogram with different filter settings (flat and sharp cut-offs), thus probably allowing the retrieval of continuous diastolic electrical activity. And this can be performed most conveniently in a larger series of sampling ventricular tachycardia episodes by longterm recordings of the low noise electrocardiogram, and/or by recording the low noise electrocardiogram during pacing induced ventricular tachycardias. By this means it may be expected that the pathophysiological role of late potentials in the initiation, maintenance, and termination of ventricular tachycardias in man can be further clarified.

References

1. El-Sherif N (1980) The ventricular premature complex: mechanisms and significance. In: Mandel WJ (ed.) Cardiac arrhythmias, their mechanisms, diagnosis and management. Philadelphia – Toronto: JB Lippincott Company, pp 288–319
2. Gadsby DC, Witt AL (1980) Normal and abnormal electrophysiology of cardiac cells. In: Mandel WJ (ed.) Cardiac arrhythmias, their mechanisms, diagnosis and management. Philadelphia – Toronto: JB Lippincott Company, pp 55–82
3. Bonke FIM, Alessie MA (1803) Electrophysiological mechanisms underlying tachyarrhythmias. In: Breithardt G, Loogen F (eds) New aspects in the medical treatment of tachyarrhythmias. München – Wien – Baltimore: Urban and Schwarzenberg, pp 2–9
4. El-Sherif N, Scherlag BJ, Lazzara R, Hope RR (1977) Reentrant ventricular arrhythmias in the late myocardial infarct period. I. Conduction characteristics in the infarction zone. Circulation 55:686–702
5. El-Sherif N, Hope RR, Scherlag BJ, Lazzara R (1977), Reentrant ventricular arrhythmias in the late myocardial infarction period. II. Pattern of initiation and termination of reentry. Circulation 55:702–719
6. El-Sherif N, Lazzara R, Hope RR, Scherlag BJ (1977) Reentrant ventricular arrhythmias in the late myocardial infarction period. III. Manifest and concealed extrasystolic grouping. Circulation 56:225–234
7. Scherlag BJ, Brachmann J, Harrison L, Lazzara R (1985) Mechanisms of chronic ventricular arrhythmias: The concept of latent ischemic damage. In: Hombach V, Hilger HH (eds) Holter Monitoring Technique, Technical Aspects and Clinical Application. Stuttgart–New York: FK Schattauer-Verlag, pp 273–284
8. Hombach V, Braun V, Höpp HW, Gil-Sanchez D, Scholl H, Behrenbeck DW, Tauchert M, Hilger HH (1982) The applicability of the signal averaging technique in clinical cardiology. Clin Cardiol 5:107–124

9. Klein H, Werner P, Frank G, Bethge KP, Lichtlen PR (1981) Value of left ventricular endocardial catheter mapping in patients with ventricular arrhythmias. Europ Heart J (Suppl A) 2:42

10. Josephson ME, Seides SF (1979) Clinical Cardiac Electrophysiology Techniques and Interpretations. Philadelphia: Lea and Febiger

11. Josephson ME, Horowitz LN, Spielman SR, Greenspan AM, Van de Pol C, Harken AH (1980) Comparison of endocardial catheter mapping with intraoperative mapping of ventricular tachycardia. Circulation 61:395–404

12. Ostermeyer J, Breithardt G, Kolvenbach, Borggrefe M, Seipel L, Schulte HD, Bircks W (1982) The surgical treatment of ventricular tachycardias. Simple aneurysmectomy versus electrophysiologically guided procedures. J Thorac Cardiovasc Surg 84:704–715

13. Fontaine G, Guiraudon G, Frank R (1978) Intramyocardial conduction defects in patients prone to chronic ventricular tachycardia, I, II, III. In: Sandoe E, Julian D, Bell G (eds) Management of ventricular tachycardia-role of mexiletine. Amsterdam – Oxford: Excerpta Medica, pp 39–55, 56–66, 67–79

14. Josephson ME, Miller JM, Kienzle G, Kempf FC, Marcus NH, Harken AH, Marchlinski FE (1985) Electrical and surgical therapy to prevent sudden death. In: Hombach V, Hilger HH (eds) Holter monitoring technique—technical aspects and clinical application. Stuttgart – New York: FK Schattauer-Verlag, pp 333–353

15. Berbari EJ, Scherlag BJ, Hope RR, Lazzara R (1978) Recording from the body surface of arrhythmogenic ventricular activity during the ST segment. Amer J Cardiol 41:697–708

16. Rozanski JJ, Mortara D (1981) Delayed depolarizations in patients with recurrent ventricular tachycardia and left ventricular aneurysm. In: Hombach V, Hilger HH (eds) Signal averaging technique in clinical cardiology. Stuttgart – New York: FK Schattauer-Verlag, pp 205–218

17. Simson MB (1981) Use of signals in the terminal QRS complex to identify patients with ventricular tachycardia after myocardial infarction. Circulation 64:235–242

18. Hombach V, Höpp HW, Braun V, Behrenbeck DW, Tauchert M, Hilger HH (1980) Die Bedeutung von Nachpotentialen innerhalb des ST-Segments im Oberflächen-EKG bei Patienten mit koronarer Herzkrankheit. Deutsch Med Wochenschr 105:1457–1466

19. Höpp HW, Hombach V, Braun V, Behrenbeck DW, Tauchert M, Hilger HH: (1981) Ventricular delayed depolarizations in patients with chronic stable coronary heart disease and with acute myocardial infarction. In: Hombach V, Hilger HH (eds) Signal averaging technique in clinical cardiology. Stuttgart – New York: FK Schattauer-Verlag, pp 233–252

20. Breithardt G, Becker R, Seipel L, Abendroth RR, Ostermeyer J (1981) Noninvasive detection of late potentials in man—a new marker for ventricular tachycardia. Europ Heart J 2:1–11

21. Leitner ERv, Oeff M, Sthapit R, Schröder R (1983) Nicht-invasive Registrierung ventrikulärer Spätpotentiale bei Herzgesunden und Patienten mit koronarer Herzkrankheit—Beziehung zu Langzeit-EKG und Ventrikulographiebefunden. Z Kardiol 72:106 (Suppl 1)

22. El Sherif N, Mehra R, Gomes JAC, Kelen G (1983) Appraisal of a low noise electrocardiogram. J Amer Coll Cardiol 1:456–467

23. Hombach V, Kebbel U, Höpp HW, Winter UJ, Braun V, Deutsch H, Hirche H, Hilger HH (1982) Continuous registrating of micropotentials of the human heart: preliminary results with a new high-resolution ECG-amplifier system. Deutsch Med Wochenschr 107:1951–1956

24. Hombach V, Kebbel U, Höpp HW, Winter U, Hirche H (1984) Noninvasive beat-by-beat registration of ventricular late potentials using high resolution electrocardiography. Intern J Cardiol 6:167–183

238

25. Oeff M, Leitner ERv, Erné NS, Halbohm HP, Lehmann HP, Schröder R (1982) Einzelschlagregistrierung ventrikulärer Spätpotentiale von der Körperoberfläche koronarkranker Patienten. Z Kardiol 71:627 (Suppl)
26. Hombach V, Kebbel U, Höpp HW, Osterspey A, Eggeling T, Winter U, Hirche H, Hilger HH (1984) Longterm recording of the low noise ECG from body surface-technical development and clinical significance. Herz/Kreisl 12:620–626
27. Osterspey A, Höpp HW, Hombach V, Braun V, Schulz P, Hilger HH (1985) Evaluation of discontinuous and continuous Holter ECG systems. In: Hombach V, Hilger HH (eds) Holter monitoring technique—technical aspects and clinical applications. Stuttgart – New York: FK Schattauer-Verlag, pp 51–63
28. Lown B, Wolf M (1971) Approaches to sudden death from coronary heart disease. Circulation 44:130–142
29. Josephson ME, Harken AH, Horowitz LN (1979), Endocardial excision: A new surgical technique for the treatment of recurrent ventricular tachycardia. Circulation 60:1430–1439
30. Greene HL, Reid PR, Schaeffer AH (1978) The repetitive ventricular response in man. A predictor of sudden death. N Engl J Med 299:729–734
31. Naccarelli GV, Prystowsky EN, Jackmann WM, Heger JJ, Rinkenberger RL, Zipes DP (1981) The repetitive ventricular response. Prevalence and prognostic significance. Br Heart J 46:152–158
32. Höpp HW, Hombach V, Deutsch H-J, Osterspey A, Winter U, Hilger HH (1983) Assessment of ventricular vulnerability by Holter ECG, programmed ventricular stimulation and recording of ventricular late potentials. In: Steinbach K, Glogar D, Laszkovics A. Scheibelhofer W, Weber H (eds) Cardiac pacing, proceedings of the VIIth world symposium on cardiac pacing. Darmstadt: Steinkopff-Verlag, pp 625–632
33. Hombach V, Höpp HW, Osterspey A, Winter U, Deutsch H-J, Hilger HH (1984) Ambulatory ECG monitoring in the detection of patients at risk of sudden cardiac death. Herz 9:6–25
34. Osterspey A, Höpp HW, Hombach V, Deutsch H-J, Winter U, Behrenbeck DW, Tauchert M, Hilger HH (1983) Diagnostic and prognostic significance of ventricular late potentials in patients with coronary heart disease. In: Steinbach K, Glogar D, Laszkovics A, Scheibelhofer W, Weber H (eds) Cardiac pacing, proceedings of the VIIth world symposium on cardiac pacing. Darmstadt: Steinkopff-Verlag, pp 663–670
35. Zimmermann M, Adamec R, Simonin P, Richez J (1985) Prognostic significance of ventricular late potentials in coronary artery disease. Amer Heart J 109:725–732
36. Breithardt G, Seipel L, Meyer J, Abendroth PR (1985) Prognostic significance of repetitive ventricular response during programmed ventricular stimulation. Amer J Cardiol 49:693–698
37. El-Sherif N, Gomes JAC, Restivo M, Mehra R (1985) Late potentials and arrhythmogenesis. PACE 8:440–462
38. Janse M (1985) The acute phase of experimental myocardial ischemia. Electrophysiology and mechanisms of arrhythmias. In: Hombach V, Hilger HH (eds) Holter monitoring technique, technical aspects and clinical application. Stuttgart – New York: FK Schattauer-Verlag, pp 257–272

19. Clinical value of magnetocardiography

R.R. FENICI, M. MASSELLI, L. LOPEZ & G. MELILLO

Clinical Physiology—Cardiovascular Biomagnetism Unit C.N.R. Catholic University of S. Heart, L. go A. Gemelli, Rome, Italy

Key words: magnetocardiography, localization of accessory pathways, ablation of cardiac arrhythmias, biomagnetism.

Introduction

Magnetocardiography, that is to say the recording of the magnetic field generated by the electrical activity of the heart, was born in 1963 when Baule and McFee, using an induction coil, measured for the first time magnetic signals produced by a human heart [2]. Since then, the evolution from a pioneering experimental observation to the present state of art has passed through fundamental technological progress. First, in 1970, the introduction of superconducting instrumentation in the MIT shielded room demonstrated that magnetocardiograms of quality comparable with that of standard electrocardiograms could be recorded [6, 8, 36]. The next important step was the adoption of gradiometric detection coils which allowed MCG recording in unshielded laboratories [1, 3, 33, 44, 47] and opened the way to pioneering clinical measurements [4, 16, 18]. During the same years MCG were also recorded without a superconducting instrumentation [9]. Since the beginning the question arose whether or not magnetic measurements could increase the diagnostic capability of cardiologists in respect to more conventional methods. Several different approaches were used to quantify the information [5, 8, 33, 39] and, although some authors still favour analysis of MCG signal in the time domain both at standard [7, 28, 49] as well as at high resolution [38] isofield contour maps are nowadays preferred to give images of the magnetic field distribution during depolarization and repolarization [10, 11, 13, 21, 22, 27, 29]. More recently different kinds of inverse solution have been developed to compute and three-dimensionally localize cardiac equivalent sources [11, 12, 43, 46]. The latter approach has proven to be effective for 'functional localization' in cardiac investigation and is the first step forward to provide 'functional imaging' of cardiac electrophysiological phenomena.

V. Hombach, H. H. Hilger and H. L. Kennedy (eds), Electrocardiography and Cardiac Drug Therapy. ISBN 978-94-010-6976-2
© 1989, Kluwer Academic Publishers, Dordrecht –

As it is not possible in this brief review to discuss all the theoretical and technological aspects related to magnetocardiography, the interested reader is addressed to the proceedings of an Advanced Nato Institute [51] and to recent more detailed review articles [11, 19, 45, 46].

A clearcut clinical validation of the method has not been given so far, mostly because presently available equipment is not medically-oriented and its set up in hospitals has been delayed by the lack of demonstration of fundamental advantages of the magnetic approach over more standardized and less expensive electrical methods.

Since the end of 1979 we have had the unique opportunity to cooperate with the physicists of the Istituto di Elettronica dello Stato Solido of the C.N.R. in Rome, who were able to design a superconducting instrumentation capable of working in an unshielded noisy environment with sufficient sensitivity to record good quality MCG [4, 18]. At the end of 1980 this equipment was for the first time transferred to the department of Internal Medicine of the Catholic University and first magnetocardiograms as well as magnetomyograms were recorded under real clinical conditions [4, 18].

In early 1982 the first prototype of a commercial instrumentation (BIOMAG I. Elettronica S.p.A., Rome, Italy) was permanently set up in the hospital and clinical magnetocardiography was initiated. In 1984 the first MCG recording in a patient with cardiac preexcitation was reported, and it was seculated that MCG source localization could have been useful to localize accessory pathways [11]. A step forward toward the understanding of the electrogenesis of the MCG patterns was accomplished when simultaneous MCG and invasive electrophysiology became possible [22, 23, 26, 27]. Direct recording of His and Kent bundles electrograms as well as magnetic mapping during reciprocating tachycardias or pacing of the preexcitation area were used to validate the accuracy of MCG localization of accessory pathways [24, 26]. Magnetic mapping under cardiac pacing was also proposed as a calibration method to quantify the accuracy and reliability of functional localization of cardiac sources by the magnetic equivalent current dipole inverse (ECD) solution [25].

Until 1983, most of the published work on magnetocardiography has been mainly carried out in laboratories or shielded rooms located in physics departments, therefore not adequate to work on critical patients and with diagnostic finality. On the contrary, our approach has been to introduce magnetocardiography in the hospital as one of the diagnostic tools available for the clinical electrophysiologist. This has been useful to learn and overcome many technical problems linked to the use of a biomagnetic instrumentation in an hospital laboratory. Here our five years of experience will be summarized, which, through a progressive evolution of both the investigation procedures and interpretative approaches, has led to present use of magnetocardiography as a unique, non invasive clinical method for electrophysiological functional localization and imaging technique.

Instrumentation

Any clinician willing to measure biomagnetic fields has to face a fundamental problem: the signals are several orders of magnitude weaker than the environmental noise.

Working in an unshielded hospital laboratory and willing to perform simultaneous magnetocardiographic and invasive electrophysiological measurements, the major difficulty was represented by the need to couple in close proximity highly noisy fluoroscopic and poligraphic equipments with the biomagnetic sensor obviously sensitive to any kind of environmental, electromagnetic and ferromagnetic noise. A solution was achieved by using a specially designed superconducting instrumentation for MCG measurements [4], by customizing other components like the catheterization table, recording and pacing catheters and by using equipment which can be wheeled away during MCG recordings [22–27]. The experimental measurements here reported were possible only after the availability of present laboratory configuration which takes into account the different needs of a biomagnetic facility and of a cardiac catheterization room (Figure 1).

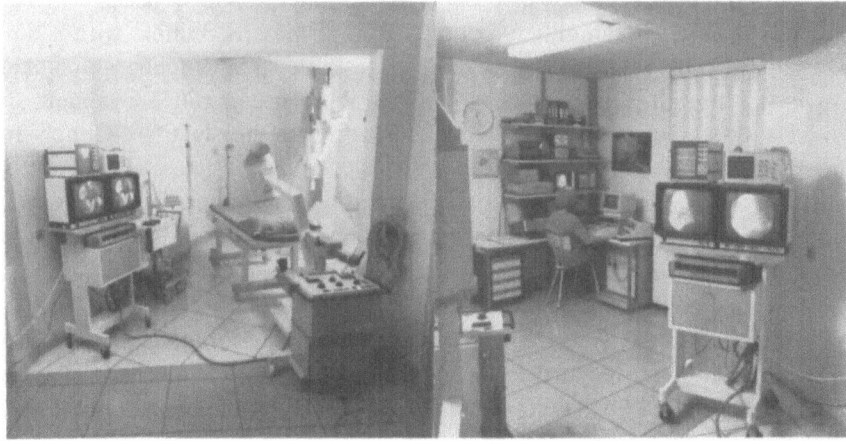

Figure 1. Overview of the Cardiovascular Biomagnetism Unit at the Catholic University of Rome.

The recording equipment consists of

1) The prototype of a commercial biomagnetic instrumentation (BIOMAG I) which is based on a superconducting circuitry. Schematically it consists of a cryogenic part contained in a superinsulated fiberglass dewar filled with liquid Helium to keep the temperature as low as 4.2 K. At that temperature the detection coil becomes intrinsically noise-free. The magnetic field sensed by the detection coil generates a proportional current in the superconducting flux transporter which, by means of an input coil, imposes a magnetic flux to an RF SQUID (Superconducting QUantum Interference Device) that converts it into a voltage. The output voltage is proportional to the magnetic field over a frequency range between 0 and 10 KHz.

In order to reduce the ambient noise working in an unshielded room, the detection coil has to be shaped in such a way as to be insensitive to fields generated by sources far and different from the patient's heart. This result can be obtained using a particular geometry of the detection coil named 'gradiometer' [44, 46].

Two different symmetric second order gradiometers have been subsequently used in our laboratory, the diameter of the pick-up coil being respectively 3 or 1.5 cm. In both gradiometers a baseline of 5 cm was adopted as the best compromise between optimal sensitivity to the investigated field and rejection of the environmental noise [4, 46].

2) The output of the SQUID is preamplified and coupled to a COMB filter to reject power line interferences (50 Hz) and harmonics. The final amplification and filtering before A/D conversion is provided by a custom made four channel signal conditioning unit for both the magnetocardiographic and three surface electric signals. This system consists of three optically isolated preamplifiers coupled to high pass RC filters with a time constant of ten seconds, intermediate adjustable gain amplifiers and final low pass filters (8 poles Bessel type). The three preamplified channels are used for surface electrical recordings. The input to the electric channels are three couples of Ag/AgCl surface chest electrodes. Their outputs can be electronically added to obtain a single, spatially averaged, high resolution bipolar ECG (HR ECG). The fourth channel is used to handle the magnetic signal in the same way (bandwidth 0.016–250 Hz).

3) A programmable four channel MINGOGRAF 4 (Siemens-Elema AB, Sweden) is used for intracardiac electrophysiological and hemodynamic as well as standard ECG recordings.

4) A custom DC differential amplifier (input impedance > than 10^{11} ohms; common rejection mode = 120 db) for monophasic action potential recording [17].

5) A 14 channel Racal FM tape recorder is used to simultaneously store

in analog form at least three standard ECG, one MCG and up to four intracavitary signals.

The computer processing is performed, after 12 bits resolution A/D conversion, with an HP A700 minicomputer. The software programs, previously described in detail [10, 11], allow high resolution analysis of the recordings in the time domain, isofield contour map drawing and automatic computation of the equivalent current dipole (ECD) parameters, when a magnetic field distribution of dipolar configuration is experimentally found [11, 12, 20, 21, 22]. Further off-line processing provides a three-dimensional display of the cardiac activation pathways.

Fluoroscopic imaging of the heart in any projection is provided by a mobile X-ray unit with image intensifier and double digital memory TV (SIAS 9C1/U Bologna, Italy). All cardiac images are stored on video tape and multiformat films to define, in individual patients, the position and size of the heart as well as that of the catheters, with respect to the MCG recording grid [25, 26, 27].

Cardiac pacing is performed with a programmable stimulator SAP 40 (cb Bioelettronica S.p.A. Firenze, Italy). Due to the presence of ferromagnetic material, commercial intracardiac electrocatheters induced rhythmic, rate-dependent artefacts which increased when the sensor was moved closer to the catheter. This drawback, which obviously impeded good quality MCG recording, was overcome by manufacturing custom non ferromagnetic electrocatheters differently designed for pacing or monophasic action potential recordings.

Recording procedures

Since present laboratory configuration has been available 64 subjects (49 males and 15 females) were studied. 40 were studied with a 1.5 cm pick-up coil diameter, 24 with a 3 cm pick-up coil. In 23 patients more than one recording was performed to test the reproducibility of the measures. 12 were normal according to clinical history, physical examination, ECG and echocardiographic findings and constitute the normality standard for our laboratory. The others were affected by various cardiac arrhythmias, ischemic or other organic cardiomyopaties. The localization of arrhythmogenic areas was attempted in patients with cardiac preexcitation, focal atrial tachycardia and ventricular tachycardia.

In all subjects MCG recordings were performed in supine position mapping the signal sequentially from 36 positions over the anterior chest wall according to the standard grid proposed by Karp et al. [33] which is normalized to the size of the subject's chest. However the recording grid

244

has been shifted to the left to obtain a more appropriate window for the study of specific abnormalities. According to a semplified model [12, 20, 46] the chest is assumed as flat, and the magnetic sensor is oriented perpendicularly to it. The magnetic signal was recorded for 80 seconds for each position.

When indicated, MCG mapping was repeated after administration of cardioactive drugs.

In patients invasively studied for clinical reasons, magnetic mapping under cardiac pacing was performed as well [23, 25, 27]. In order to minimize the investigation time only 16 to 25-point maps were recorded during pacing for only 10 to 20 seconds for each position.

Signal processing and interpretation

As mentioned in the introduction the quality of a low resolution magnetocardiogram, even if recorded in the hospital, is comparable with that of the standard ECG (Figure 2). However, as the simplicity, low cost and diagnostic capability of electrocardiography are well established, it is

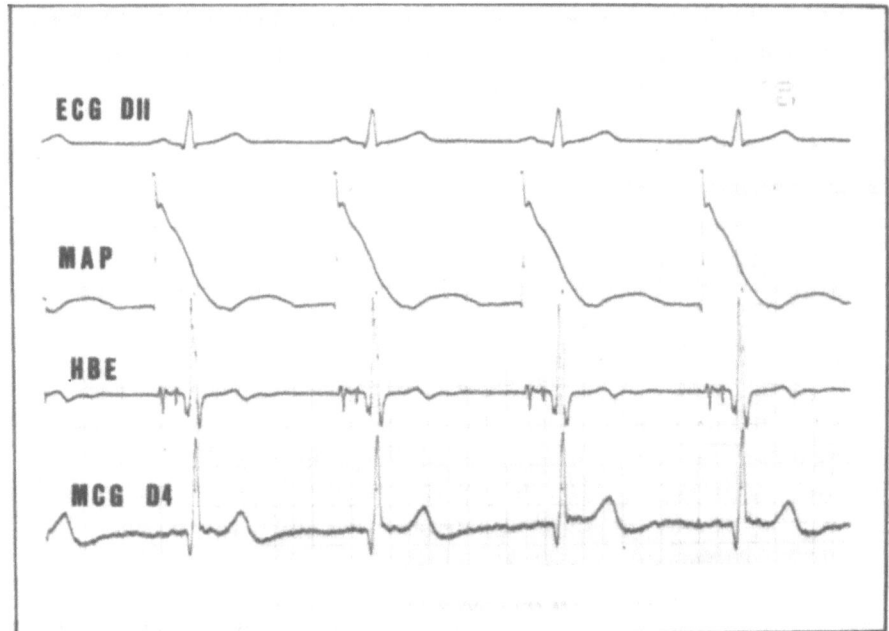

Figure 2. Simultaneous ECG, Right Atrial Monophasic Action Potential (MAP), His Bundle Electrogram (HBE) and Magnetocardiographic (MCG) recording.

necessary to demonstrate that magnetocardiography can provide new or different information of potential clinical use before it can be accepted.

In theory [46, 50, 51] the major advantage in measuring magnetic fields is that the normal component of the magnetic field is directly linked to the intracellular currents (the primary source) of fibers tangential to the chest surface and unaffected by the volume currents (secondary sources) which, on the contrary, strongly affect the surface potential distribution.

Thus, theoretically magnetocardiography provides more direct information about the cardiac generators in respect to potential measurements. On the other hand as magnetic measurements are not sensitive to the component of the primary sources which are perpendicular to the chest, there is a loss of information on part of the generators. However the advantage is that the field generated by the tangential component will maintain a symmetric pattern even in the case of obliquely oriented cardiac sources. This would still allow a magnetic localization of sources which, on the contrary, would generate only monopolar potential distribution on the anterior chest wall and therefore cannot be electrically localized.

In this view it is evident that the major advantage which MCG measurements can provide is to localize cardiac sources. This, in turn,

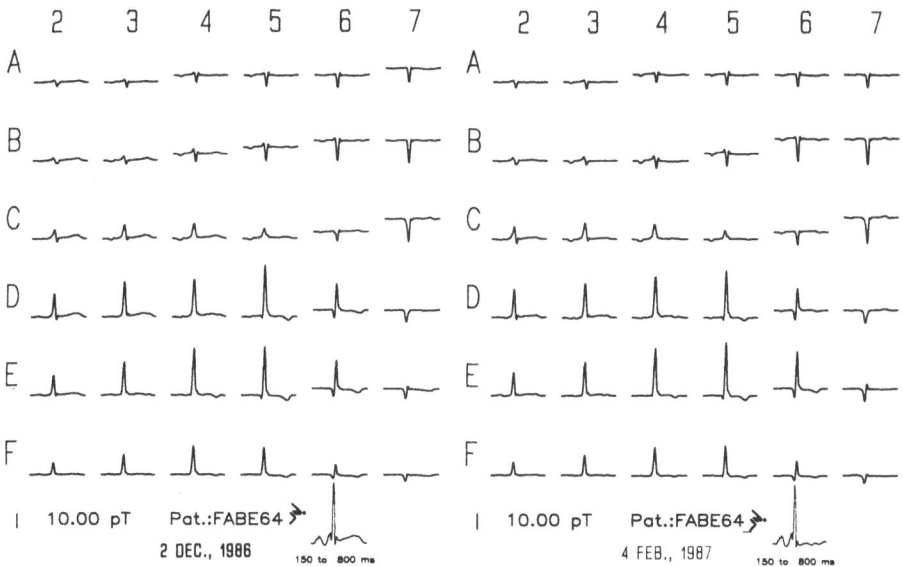

Figure 3. Reproducibility of MCG waveforms recorded in the same patient, affected by WPW syndrome, two months apart with the same sensor (pick-up coil diameter: 1.5 cm). The MCG signals are mapped according to the standard 36 point grid [33] shifted to the left, by omitting column 1 and adding column 7, to obtain a better centering of the preexcited area.

246

suggests that the analysis of MCG signals in the time domain, both at low as well as at high resolution [15, 16, 18], although having been important intermediate steps for reaching the present state of art, are mainly depleted of clinical significance. However an exception is represented by direct current (DC) magnetocardiography which, although still confined in the shielded room, could be invaluable in the study of cardiac ischemia [7]. Mapping of the magnetic field distribution and automatic computation of the intensity and localization parameters of equivalent cardiac sources is an important step forward to provide a functional imaging of both normal and abnormal cardiac electrogenic phenomena. In Figure 3, the reproducibility of MCG signals mapped in the same subject in different recording sessions, is shown. Such time recordings are the basis for the computation of the magnetic field distribution and equivalent source localization. In Figure 4 an example of magnetic reconstruction of the conduction system activation pathway is shown. This level of resolution has been achieved in the hospital

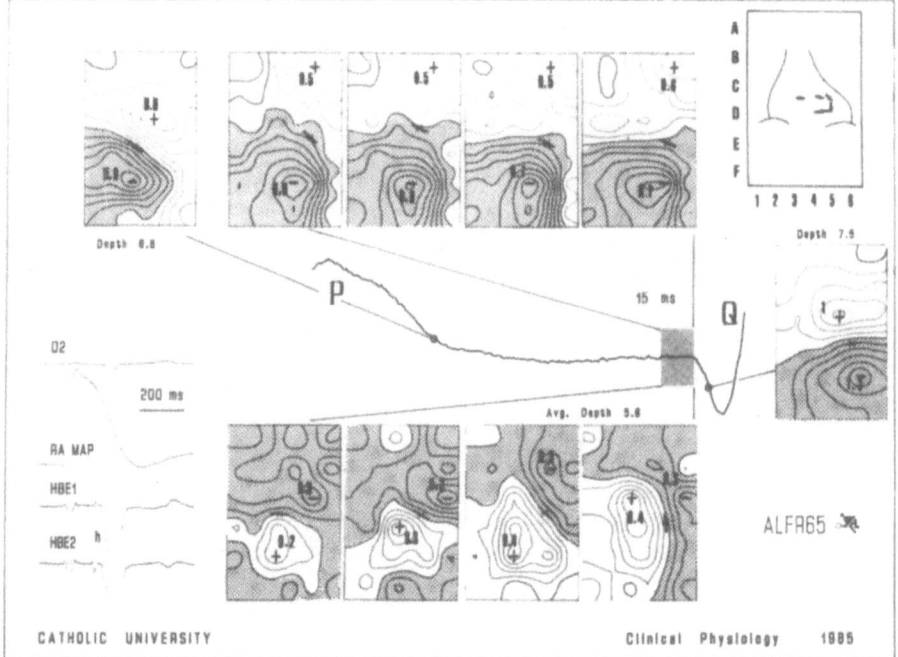

Figure 4. Magnetic field distribution during atrial repolarization (upper maps), His Purkinje System activation (lower maps) and interventricular septum depolarization (middle map). The bidimensional ECD localization depicts on the patient heart silhouette the activation pathway during the last 25 msec of the P–Q interval. On the lower left, invasive HBE recording demonstrates that the MCG is only sensitive to the terminal part of the His Bundle activation, being the measured H–V interval 40 msec.

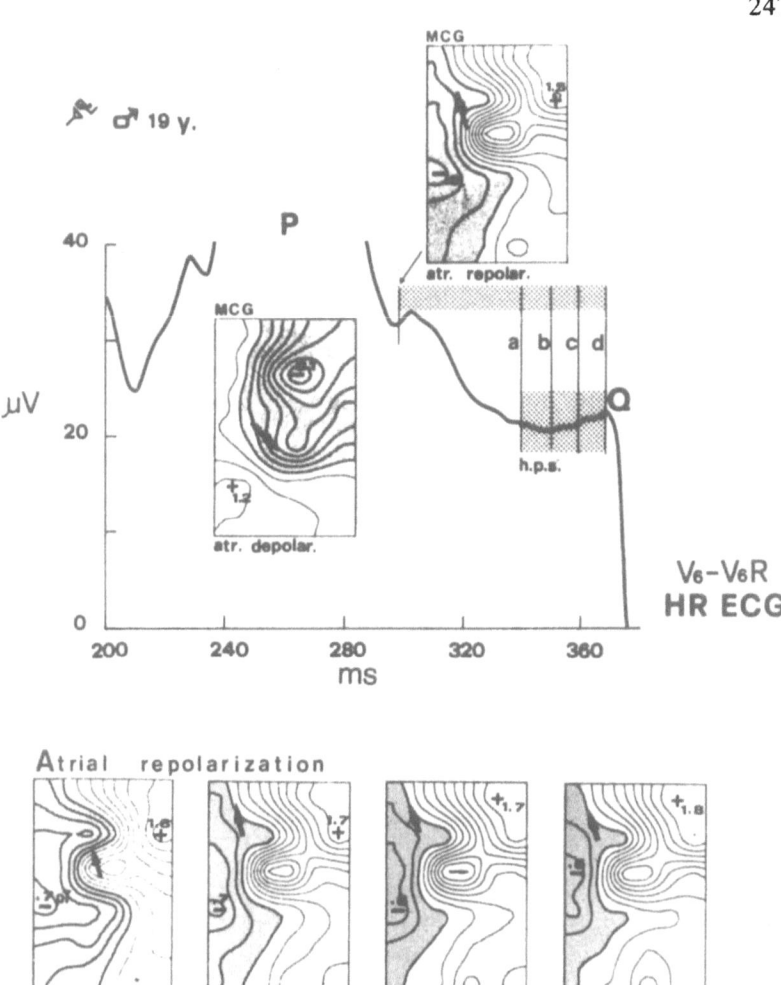

Figure 5. Comparison between High Resolution Electrocardiography (HR ECG) and MCG mapping during the P–R interval of a normal subject. The different magnetic field distribution and ECD localization both during atrial depolarization and repolarization as well as His bundle activation is evident. MCG atrial repolarization pattern begins during the descending limb of the P wave and reproducibly coincides with electric deflection appreciable only at high resolution.

248

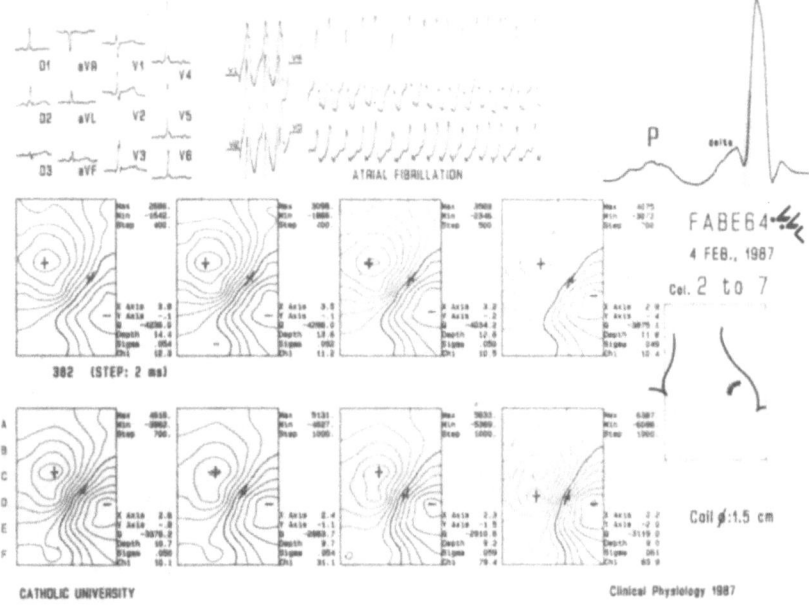

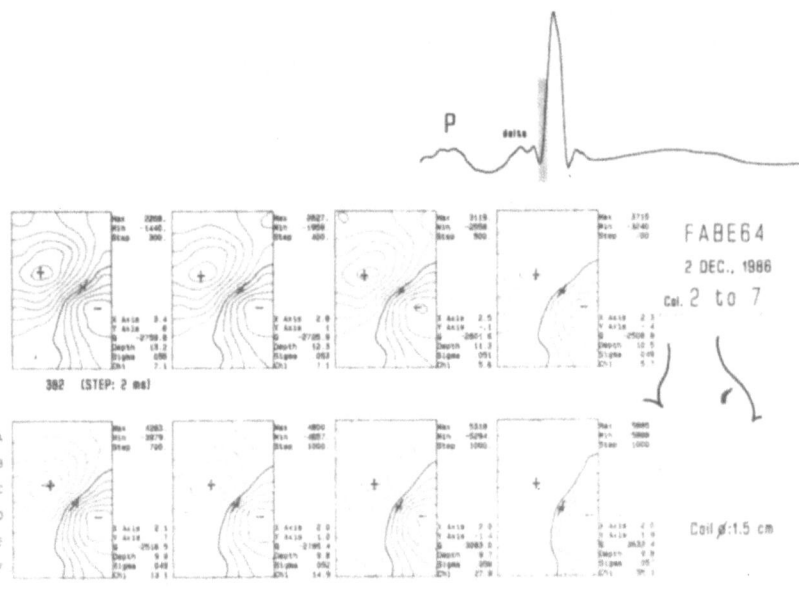

Figure 6. Same patient as in Figure 3. Reproducibility of the magnetic field distribution and ECD localization in coincidence with the delta wave (shaded bar on the reference ECG), which unequivocally localize a postero-left sided accessory pathway. Surgical ablation of the Kent bundle has fully validated the magnetic data in this case (R.R. Fenici, unpublished).

only in a limited number of normal subjects. However the identification, after proper subtraction of atrial repolarization, of magnetic fields time correlated with the activation of the His-Purkinje System, was probably the first important finding suggesting that magnetocardiography could be sensitive enough to provide localization of weak sources [16, 20, 21]. Moreover it has been useful to interpret the electrogenesis of high resolution electric waveforms (Figure 5). Even at the high level of time and field intensity resolution necessary for the localization of the site of ventricular preexcitation (Figure 6), the reproducibility of both the field distribution and ECD localization is impressive. A similar degree of reproducibility was appreciable also using different pick-up coil's diameters, and independently from changes of the size of the patient's heart (Figure 7).

In Figure 8 an example is given of proper localization of a right-sided paraseptal Kent bundle. The field distribution during preexcitation is opposite to that observed in the same subject during normal septal activation achieved after ajmaline administration.

Localization of focal arrhythmias, originating both at atrial (Figure 9) and ventricular level (Figure 10), has been attempted as well.

In the former case, a persistent form of focal atrial tachycardia, the MCG localization of the ectopic focus in the lateral wall of the left atrium is consistent with the morphology of the P wave in the 12 leads ECG. On the contrary, while the electrocardiographic morphology should suggest an apical origin of the ventricular tachycardia, MCG localization is more consistent with a focus originating in the right ventricular outflow tract. This wide discrepancy rises the question of whether or not MCG localization, although qualitatively suggestive, is quantitatively acceptable and consistent with the anatomic and pathophysiologic substrate of the individual patient. In other words the question is how to validate the accuracy of MCG functional localization. The approach to this problem has been two-fold. The physicists community has attempted an interpretation of some experimental patterns by reproducing similar field distributions on the basis of mathematical models. This was first used to validate the interpretation of fields generated by the HPS [11, 12, 14, 20, 35], by atrial repolarization [37] and, more recently by cardiac preexcitation [12]. A clinical validation is possible by comparison with other localization procedures, mainly invasive, like endocardial catheter mapping, direct recording of signal generated by accessory pathways, epicardial mapping during surgery and the results of ablation procedures [30, 31, 34, 48]. However the question is which method could be assumed as a gold-standard for validation, the range of error of all of them being still not well defined and surely in the order of tens of millimeters. For instance, catheter mapping is a precise method to localize left sided free wall accessory pathways, but its

250

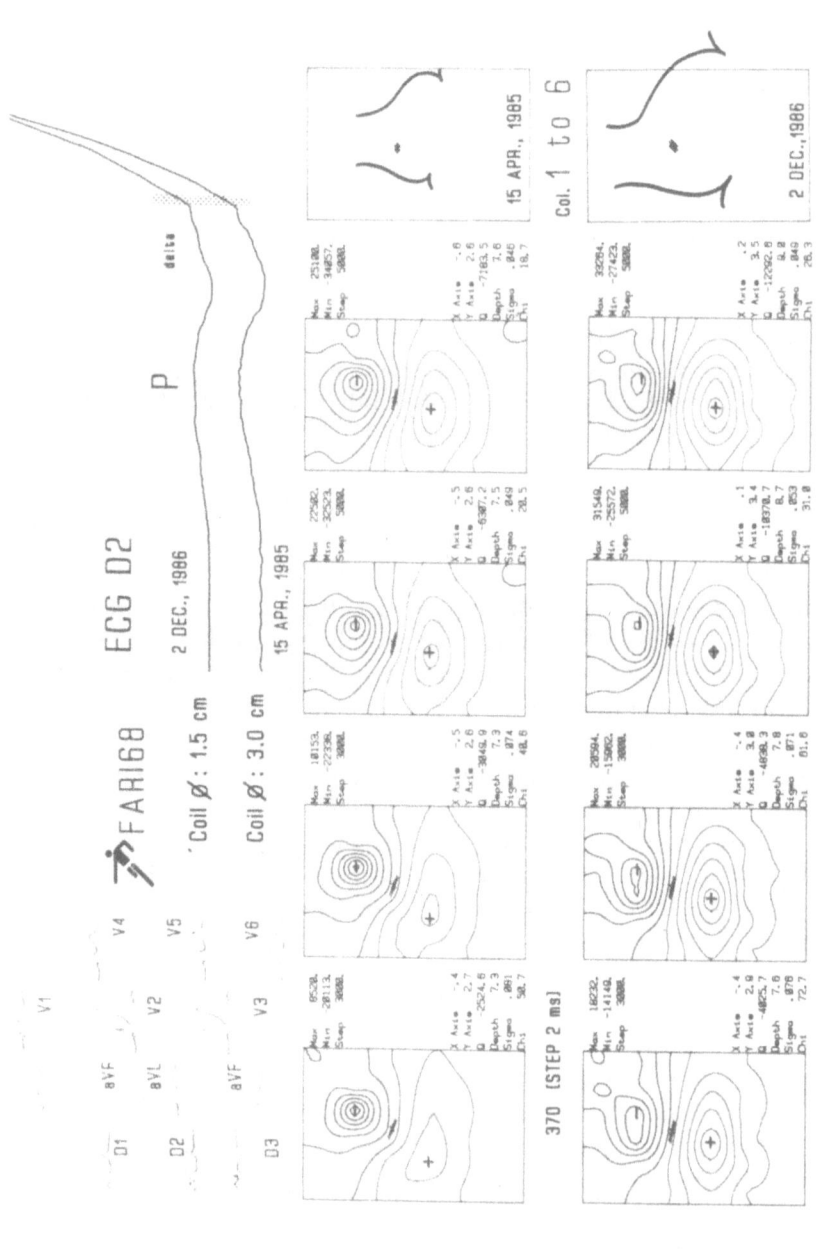

Figure 7. WPW syndrome. In spite of the use of different pick-up coil diameters, different recording sessions (about eight months apart) and different size of the heart due to the patient's growth and different degree of physical conditioning, the preexcited area is reproducibly localized.

251

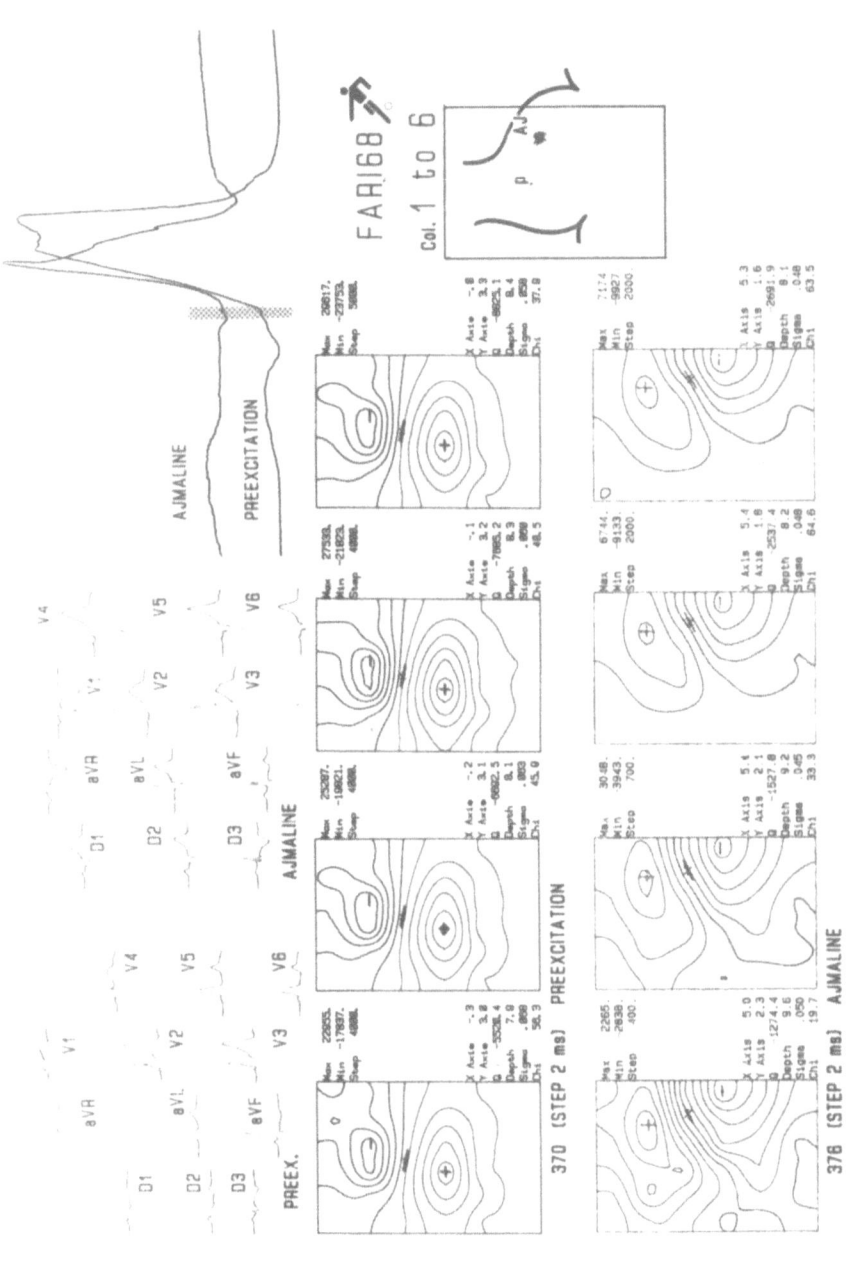

Figure 8. Same patient as in Figure 7. The comparison between magnetic field distribution during preexcitation (upper maps) and after ajmaline-induced normalization of the A–V conduction clearly localizes preexcitation in the right paraseptal area.

252

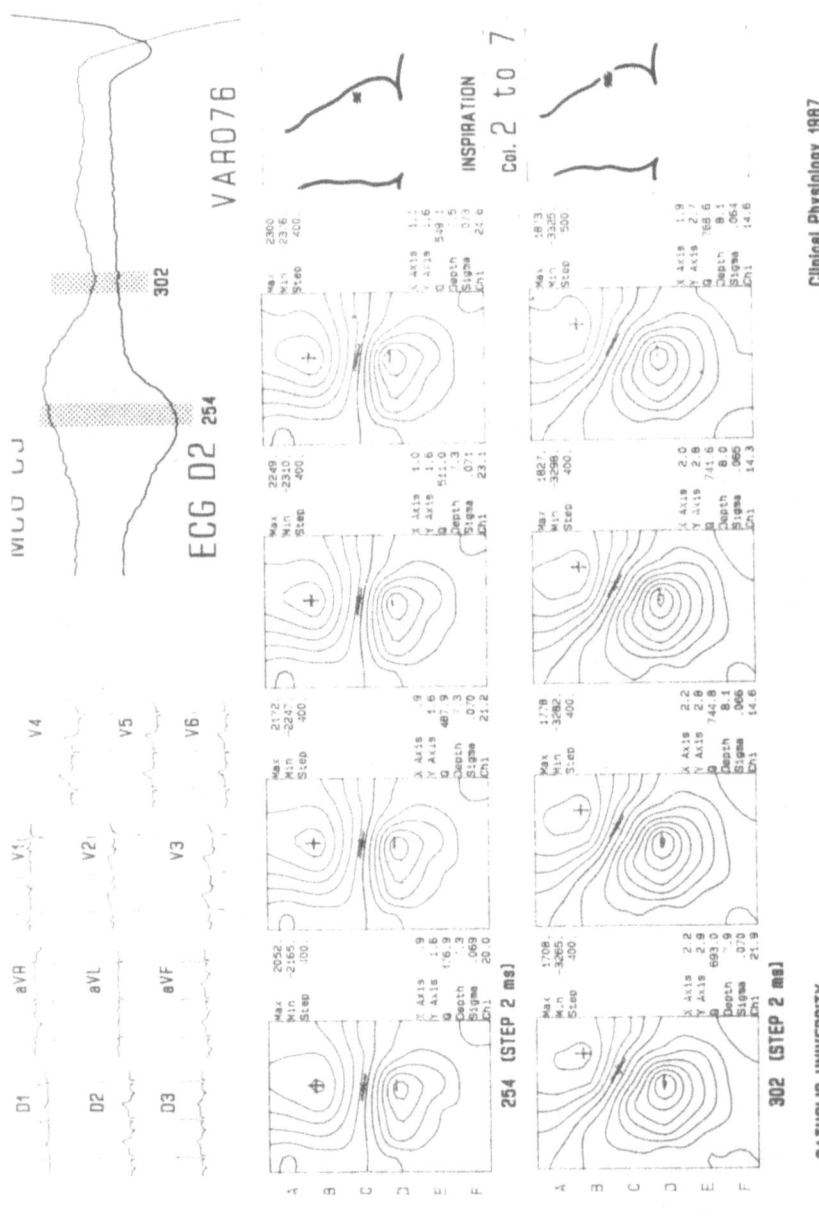

Figure 9. Focal atrial tachycardia. Magnetic localization of the arrhythmia has been calculated both at the peak of the electric P wave (upper maps), and later, when the MCG P wave still indicates atrial depolarization (lower maps). Ectopic atrial focus is localized in an area consistent with the left lateral A–V groove.

253

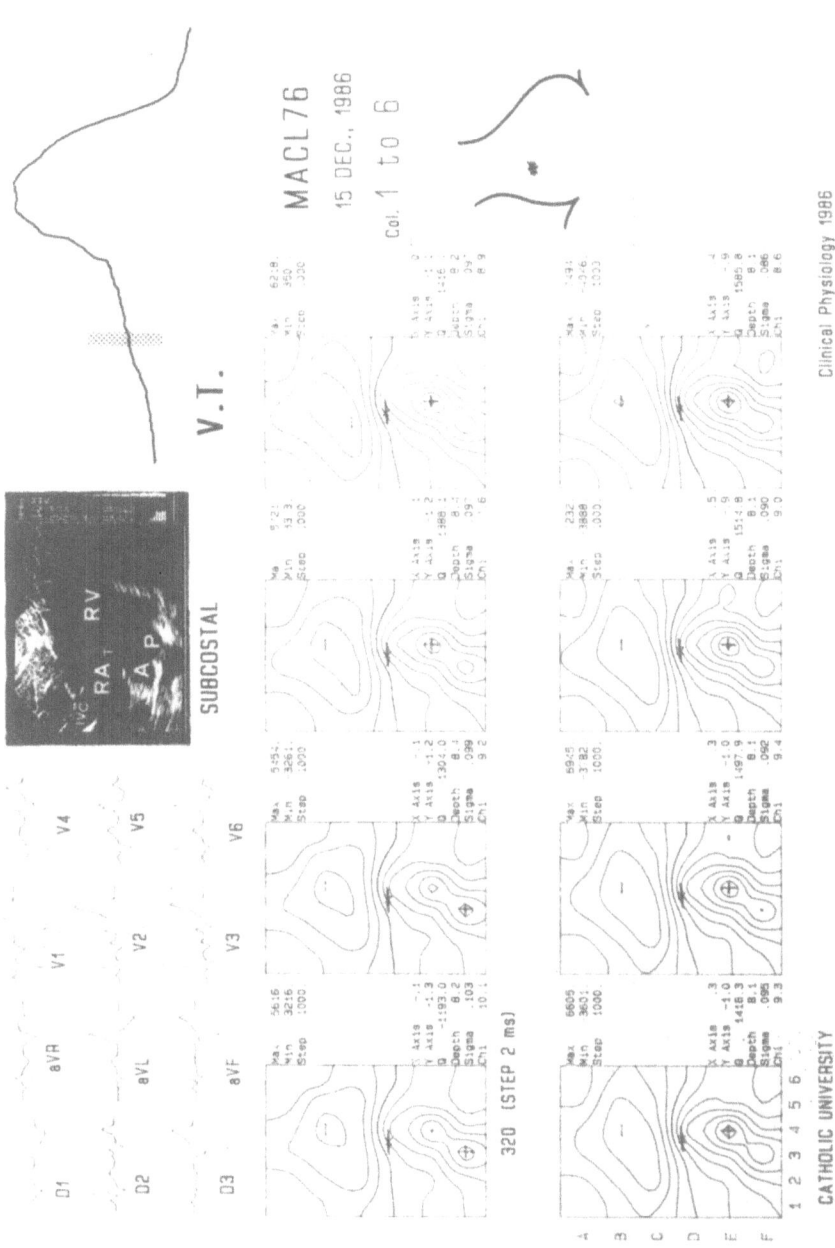

Figure 10. **Right ventricular dysplasia. MCG localization is consistent with an origin of ventricular tachycardia in the outflow tract of the right ventricle, which appears severely enlarged at the echocardiogram. However the morphology of the electric PVC is more consistent with a right apical origin of the arrhythmia. One possible explanation for this discrepancy could be a wrong automatic pattern recognition of the tachycardia, or the simultaneous occurrence of multiple wavefronts, poorly representable with a single ECD model.**

precision in the case of a right sided by-pass is less, being sometimes difficult to achieve a stable reproducible mapping of the right atrioventricular ring. On the other hand MCG mapping is probably even more accurate than catheter mapping to immediately define the side of insertion of a paraseptal accessory pathway [22]. Even the accuracy of manual epicardial mapping is relative, as the probe is usually moved in steps of about one centimeter.

At present the best method to provide a quantitative calibration of the MCG localization accuracy is to map the field generated by an electric source of dipolar configuration placed in a preknown area of the heart, define with the MCG inverse procedure the localization of the pacing dipole and compare it with the actual three-dimensional position of the electrodes inferred by radiologic imaging. Our experience with this method gives an amount of localization error of the pacing dipole which can be represented with a sphere of diameter ranging between 0.8 and 2 cm, widely changing with the position of the pacing catheter. Certainly it could be improved if a fixed position of the pacing dipole could be assured and if the mapping procedure could be performed in a single shoot using a multisensor device [46].

Perspectives

Nowadays the treatment of cardiac arrhythmias is widely changing as surgical and even closed chest ablation techniques are more frequently proposed as alternative to inefficient or chronic and poorly tolerated drug therapy. In this view a precise localization of arrhythmogenic structures is obviously mandatory to warrant successful interventions, and represents the new challenge for the clinical electrophysiologist. Perspectively magnetocardiography can be considered clinically useful for a reproducible, non invasive, localization of arrhythmogenic structures, preliminary to any invasive method. Such an approach would be invaluable in improving the accuracy and reducing the time required for other invasive localization procedures, especially when more refined closed chest ablation intervention will be applied [32, 40, 41, 42].

Still the accuracy of MCG localization of spontaneous activity cannot be quantitatively defined especially taking into account that simultaneous activation wavefronts, like for instance during incomplete ventricular pre-excitation, cannot be optimally modelled by a single ECD inverse solution. In such situations other kinds of inverse solution, like current multipole expansion, could be more appropriate [43].

In spite of the primitive instrumentation used and the experimental character of the measurements here reported, the amount of uncertainty is already relatively low, and well within the resolution needed with the current surgical procedures for antiarrhythmic surgery. It seems therefore reasonable to predict that, as technological progress will improve the resolution of magnetic recordings, in a near future magnetocardiography, magnetic resonance imaging and spectroscopy will provide the cardiologist with a complete, noninvasive, imaging of cardiac electrogenesis in direct correlation with its anatomical, metabolic and functional substrates.

Acknowledgements

The authors are indebted to Prof. G.L. Romani for his continuous and helpful support to resolve any problem arising from the use of his especially designed cryogenic instrumentation and to Ing. G. Salcito for his valid and appreciated collaboration. The authors are also thankful to R. Frattin, C. Gobbi, A. Maiolo and M. Pratarolo for their efficient technical and professional assistance.

The work was partially supported by National Research Council (CNR) contracts N. PF 85.01473.57, 85.00462.04, 86.00062.04, and by a grant (60%) from the Italian Ministry of Education.

References

1. Awano N, Owada K, Machip K, Kariyone S, Awano I (1982) A study on magnetocardiograms of normal subjects. Japan Circulation J 46:870. Proceedings of the 46th Annual Meeting
2. Baule GM, McFee R (1963) Detection of the magnetic field of the heart. Am Heart J 66:95–96
3. Barbanera S, Carelli P, Leoni R, Romani GL, Bordoni F, Modena I, Fenici RR, Zeppilli P (1981) Biomagnetic measurements in unshielded, normally noisy environments. In: Erne SN, Hahlbohm HD, Lubbig H (eds) Biomagnetism. Berlin – New York: Walter de Gruyter, pp 139–149
4. Barbanera S, Carelli P, Fenici RR, Leoni R, Modena I, Romani GL (1981) Use of superconducting instrumentation for biomagnetic measurements performed in a hospital. IEEE Trans Magn MAG-17:849–852
5. Barry WH, Fairbank WM, Harrison DC, Lehrman KL, Malmivuo JAV, Wikswo JP (1977) Measurements of the human magnetic heart vector. Science Vol 198:1159–1162
6. Cohen D, Edelsack EA, Zimmerman JE (1970) Magnetocardiograms taken inside a shielded room with a superconducting point-contact magnetometer. Appl Phys Lett 16:278–280
7. Cohen D, Kaufman LA (1975) Magnetic determination of the relationship between the ST segment shift and the injury current produced by coronary artery occlusion. Circulation Res 36:414–424

256

8. Cohen D, Lepeschkin E, Hosaka H, Massell B, Myers G (1976) Abnormal patterns and physiological variations in magnetocardiograms, J Electrocardiology 9(4):398–409

9. Denis B, Matelin D, Favier Ch, Tanche M, Martin-Noel P (1976) L'enregistrement du champ magnétique cardiaque. Considérations techniques et premiers résultats en milieu hospitalier. Arch Mal Cœur, 69 année, 3:299–304

10. Erne' SN, Fenici RR, Hahlbohm HD, Jaszczuk W, Lehmann HP, Masselli M (1983) High resolution isofield mapping in magnetocardiography. In: Il nuovo cimento, Vol 2D:291–300

11. Erne' SN, Fenici RR (1984) The present state of magnetocardiography. In: Collan H, Berglund P, Krusius M (eds) Proc of the Tenth International Cryogenic Engineering Conference. Helsinki: Butterworth, Westbury House, pp 329–338

12. Erne' SN (1985) High resolution magnetocardiography: modelling and sources localization. In: Proc of the XIV ICMBE and VII ICMP. Espoo, Finland

13. Erne' SN, Fenici RR, Hahlbohm HD, Korsukewitz P, Lehmenn HP, Uchigawa Y (1985) Magnetocardiographic study of the PR segment of normals. In: Weinberg H, Stroink G, Katila T (eds) Biomagnetism, application and theory. New York: Pergamon Press, p 132

14. Erne' SN, Lehmann HP, Masselli M, Uchigawa Y (1985) Modelling of the His-Purkinje heart conduction system. In: Weinberg H, Stroink G, Katila T (eds) Biomagnetism, application and theory. New York: Pergamon Press, p 126

15. Farrell DE, Tripp J, Norgren R (1978) Non-invasive information on the PR segment of the cardiac cycle: an assessment of the clinical potential of the electric and magnetic methods. Proc. SPIE 167:173–177

16. Fenici RR, Romani GL, Barbanera S, Zeppilli P, Carelli P, Modena I (1980) High resolution magnetocardiography: non-invasive investigation of His-Purkinje system activity in man. G Ital Cardiol 10:1366–1372

17. Fenici RR, Masselli M, Zeppilli P, Baltaro RJ (1982) Clinical demonstration of intraatrial disturbances by means of monophasic action potential recording in man. Jpn Heart J Vol 23, supp 1:189–191

18. Fenici RR, Romani GL, Leoni R, Masselli M, Modena I (1982) Magnetocardiographic recording of the His-Purkinje system activity in man. Jpn Heart J, Vol 23, supp 1:728–730

19. Fenici RR (1982) Clinical assessment of the megnetocardiogram. In: Williamson SJ, Romani GL, Kaufman L, Modena I (eds) Biomagnetism. An interdisciplinary approach. NATO ASI series vol 66:287–298

20. Fenici RR, Romani GL, Leoni R (1983) Magnetic measurements and modelling for the investigation of the human heart conduction system. In Il nuovo cimento vol 2D, n 2:280–290

21. Fenici RR, Masselli M, Erne' SN, Hahlbohm HD (1985) Magnetocardiographic mapping of the PR interval phenomena in an unshielded laboratory. In: Weinberg H, Stroink G, Katila T (eds) Biomagnetism: Applications and theory. New York – Toronto: Pergamon Press, pp 137–141

22. Fenici RR, Masselli M, Lopez L, Sabetta F (1985) High resolution magnetocardiography: electrophysiological and clinical findings. In: Proc of the XIV ICMBE and VII ICMP, Espoo, Finland, 1475–1478

23. Fenici RR, Masselli M, Lopez L, Sabetta F (1985) First simultaneous magnetocardiographic and invasive recordings of the PR interval electrophysiological phenomena in man. In: Proc. of the XIV ICMBE and VII ICMP, Espoo, Finland, 1483–1484

24. Fenici RR, Masselli M, Lopez L, Sabetta F (1985) First simultaneous MCG and invasive Kent bundle localization in man. New trends in arrhythmias 1:455–460

25. Fenici RR, Masselli M, Lopez L, Sabetta F (1986) Simultaneous MCG mapping and invasive electrophysiology to evaluate the accuracy of the equivalent current dipole

inverse solution for the localization of human cardiac sources. New trends in arrhythmias 2:357–369

26. Fenici RR, Masselli M (1986) Magnetocardiography: localization of accessory pathways (WPW). In: Proc of the IEEE Engineering in Medicine and Biology Society 8th Annual Conference, 437–438, Dallas, Nov. 7–10

27. Fenici RR, Masselli M (1986) Magnetocardiography: Perspectives in clinical application. In: Proc of the IEEE Engineering in Medicine and Biology Society 8th Annual Conference, 439–440, Dallas, Nov 7–10

28. Fujino K, Sumi M, Saito K, Murakami M, Higuchi T, Nakaya Y, Mori H (1984) Magnetocardiograms of patients with left ventricular overloading recorded with a second-derivative SQUID gradiometer. J Electrocardiology 17(3):219–228

29. Gonnelli R, Galeone P, Sicuro M (1985) A biomagnetic approach to the localization of the necrotic area in inferior myocardial infarction. In: Proc of the XIV ICMBE and VII ICMP, Espoo, Finland

30. Guiraudon GM, Klein GJ, Gulamhusein S, Jones DL, Yee R, Perkins DG, Jarvis E (1984) Surgical repair of Wolff–Parkinson–White syndrome: a new closed heart technique. Ann Thorac Surg 37:67

31. Guiraudon GM, Klein GJ, Sharma A, Jones D, McLellan D (1986) Surgery for Wolff–Parkinson–White syndrome: further experience with an epicardial approach. Circulation 74:525

32. Huang SKS (1987) Use of radiofrequency energy for catheter ablation of the endomyocardium: a prospective energy source. J Electrophysiology 1(1):78–91

33. Karp PJ, Katila TE, Saarinen M, Siltanen P, Varpula TT (1978) Etude Comparative de magnétocardiogrammes normaux et pathologiques, Ann Cardiol Angeiol 27(1):65–70

34. Klein GJ, Guiraudon GM, Perkins DG, Jones DL, Yee R, Jarvis E (1984) Surgical correction of the Wolff–Parkinson–White syndrome in the closed heart using cryosurgery: a simplified approach. JACC 3:405

35. Leoni R, Romani GL (1982) Computer simulation of magnetic field patterns from the human cardiac conduction system. Nuovo Cimento 1D:737–750.

36. Lepeschkin E (1974) Tentative analysis of the normal magnetocardiogram. Adv Cardiol Vol 10:325–332

37. Lorenzana HE, Pipes PB, Zaitlin MP, James D (1985) Structures in the PR interval of the human magnetocardiogram. In: Weinberg H, Stroink G, Katila T (eds) Biomagnetism: applications and theory. New York: Pergamon Press, p 142

38. Makijarvi M, Maniewski R, Derka I, Puurtinen J, Katila T, Siltanen P (1985) High resolution MCG study on heart conduction system. In: Proc of the XIV ICMBE and VII ICMP, Espoo, Finland, 1485–1486

39. Malmivuo JAV, Wikswo JP Jr (1977) A new practical lead system for vector magnetocardiography. Proceedings of the IEEE:810–822

40. Narula OS, Boveja BK, Cohen DM et al (1985) Laser catheter-induced atrioventricular nodal delays and atrioventricular block in dogs: acute and chronic observations. J Am Coll Cardiol 5:259

41. Narula OS, Bharati S, Chan MC et al. (1986) Microtransection of the His bundle with laser radiation through a pervenous catheter: correlation of histologic and electrophysiologic data. Am J Cardiol 54:186

42. Narula OS, Boveja BK, De Coriolis PE, Tarjan PP (1986) Induction of AV nodal (AVN) delays and block by a thermal catheter technique: acute and chronic studies JACC 7:132A (abstract)

43. Nenonen J, Salkola M, Katila T (1985) On the current multipole expansion of biomagnetic fields. In: Proc of the XIV ICMBE and VII ICMP, Espoo, Finland, 20–21

258

44. Opfer JE, Yeo YK, Pierce JM, Rorden LH (1974) A superconducting second-derivative gradiometer. IEEE Trans Mag MAG-9:536–539
45. Romani GL: Biomagnetism (1984) An application of SQUID sensors to medicine and physiology. Physica 126 B:70–81
46. Romani GL, Narici L (1986) Principles and clinical validity of the biomagnetic method. In: Medical Progress through Technology 11:123–159. Boston – Netherlands: Martinus Nijoff
47. Saarinen M, Karp PJ, Katila TE, Siltanen P (1974) The magnetocardiogram in cardiac disorders. Cardiovascular Res 8:820–834
48. Salerno JA, Chimienti M, Vigano' M, Bobba P (1982) Focal supraventricular tachycardia: clinical electrophysiological and therapeutic aspects. In: Masoni A, Alboni P (eds) Cardiac Electrophysiology today. London – New York: Academic Press, p 203
49. Weinberg H, Stroink G, Katila T (eds) (1985) Biomagnetism: applications and theory. New York – Toronto: Pergamon Press
50. Williamson SJ, Kaufman L (1981) Biomagnetism. J Magn Magn Mat 22: 129–201
51. Williamson SJ, Romani GL, Kaufman L, Modena I (eds) (1983) Biomagnetism: an interdisciplinary approach. New York – London: Plenum Press

20. High resolution electrocardiography and magnetocardiography: clinical application

P. SILTANEN[1], T. KATILA[2], M. MÄKIJÄRVI[1], M. LEINIÖ[2],
J. NÉNONEN[2], J. MONTONEN[2], & S. MADEKIVI[2]

[1]Cardiovascular Laboratory, Helsinki University Central Hospital;[2] Department of Technical Physics, Helsinki University of Technology; Helsinki, Finland

Key words: high-resolution electrocardiography, high-resolution magneto-cadiography, late potentials, signal averaging

Abstract

A high-resolution (HR) surface ECG system is described, suitable for HR real-time (RT) recording and for signal averaging (SA). HR-ECG measurements were done in an electrically shielded room. The signal was amplified with a battery-driven 8-channel preamplifier, digitized with a 12(16)-bit A/D converter and stored in a microcomputer. The overall noise level of the system was below 1 μV_{p-p} in the band 0.05–300 Hz. RT- and SA-magnetocardiographic (MCG) measurements were done in a magnetically shielded room using a very sensitive (5 fT/$\sqrt{Hz}$) DC-SQUID magnetic gradiometer. The output signal was transferred to a minicomputer for analysis. Examples of ECG and MCG recordings of cardiac micropotentials are presented, using both RT- and SA-techniques with special reference to late potentials (LP). The MCG technique was also utilized for localizing the Kent bundle in 6 cases of WPW syndrome. The recovery rate of LP was 37% in patients with recent myocardial infarction (AMI), and 72% in patients with ventricular tachycardia (VT) or ventricular fibrillation (VF). The mean duration of LP in the VT/VF-group was 27 ms, and the mean amplitude 17 μV. The His-Purkinje signal was detected in 60% of cases examined. The RT-ECG proved to be superior to the SA-ECG in detecting intermittent or inconstantly timed signals. Preliminary base-line data of 2 prospective studies are presented (10 patients of which with VT, 10 with recent AMI without VT and 10 healthy controls) using both RT-ECG and SA-ECG, the latter with both time and frequency domain analysis. The initial and terminal QRS notches of the low-gain ECG were most frequent in the VT group, and probably belong to the same category of depolarization abnormalities as LPs.

V. Hombach, H. H. Hilger and H. L. Kennedy (eds), Electrocardiography and Cardiac Drug Therapy. ISBN 978-94-010-6976-2
© 1989, Kluwer Academic Publishers, Dordrecht –

Introduction and review

Sudden unexpected cardiac death is still today one of the big unsolved problems of medicine. It threatens particularly those populations among which the coronary morbidity is high. The findings from the Helsinki Coronary Register [1] revealed, that the annual incidence of sudden coronary death (SCD), for example in men of 50–60 years of age, is about 2%. This fact led the cardiologists to embark on a long series of investigations on detectable risk factors for SCD. It was already presumed at the very beginning of this research, that the final fatal event is determined mainly by basic electrophysiological abnormalities. Thus it was no surprise, that these studies did not reveal any other useful risk markers than poor myocardial function and poor coronary anatomy. Not even the thorough analysis of the 14 parameters of routine low-gain ECG recorded at discharge from hospital after Acute Myocardial Infarction (AMI) uncovered any other risk markers than enhanced P terminal force, implying left ventricular dsyfunction, and ischemic S-T segment changes [2]. On the other hand, it is a clinical fact that among the victims of SCD there is a considerable number of persons whose left ventricular function is nearly or fully normal, and whose coronary artery lesions are not necessarily extensive. Presuming that some discernible markers of the risk of SCD were hidden in the cardiac electrical events of these patients, the current routine ECG methods obviously failed to detect these factors. The predictive value of the exercise ECG was limited, and was based mainly on the same markers as that of the resting ECG. Holter monitoring technique was promising but cumbersome, and numerous reports about its predictive value were controversial.

It is known, that the myocardial scar may turn the physiological radially oriented ventricular activation into more or less circuitous and tangential spread in and around the affected myocardial segments. That was the reason why our research group resorted in 1973 to the newly launched magnetocardiography (MCG) technique as a parallel modality, with theoretically better spatial resolution than ECG, and with more sensitivity to tangential currents, contrasting again with the ECG, which is highly sensitive to radial currents. For a long time our group used exclusively the low gain technique because of unfavourable measuring circumstances and sensors too insensitive for high resolution recordings, and because of seeking after waveforms known from the ECG. Unfortunately we did not find any major novelty with the new technique as regards risk prediction.

First steps in the right direction were taken already 70 years ago by Oppenheimer [3], who found many small notches in the QRS complex in certain cases. This phenomenon, which he called 'arborization block' was followed over 20 years later by concepts of 'focal intraventricular block', 'peri-infarction block', 'parietal focal block', 'intrainfarction block', and 'post-excitation', as listed in Table 1. All workers hypothetized a principle of circuitous and more or less tangential local activation of the myocardium.

Initial QRS notches, similar to the intrainfarction block of Cabrera and terminal QRS notches, like the postexcitation of Zuckermann, which often were found in the ECG's of coronary patients, aroused the attention of some Finnish investigators in 1960's [12, 13, 14]. They were able to show by careful clinicopathological studies, that the occurrence of these notches in the vast majority of cases was associated with coronary artery disease and a previous (AMI), which in the cases of an initial notch usually was subendocardial and in cases of terminal notch usually an inferior lesion, as observed at postmortem examination. The initial and terminal notches were also recorded from 1600 men aged 35–65 in a cardiovascular study of the Helsinki police force, but no relationship was found between the notches and the prevalance of coronary morbidity, and only slight increase of notches was observed with age (Pyörälä, Siltanen and Punsar, unpublished data); a possible correlation between the appearance of QRS notches and coronary events in this material during the follow-up period are still under analysis. Recently two groups of researchers have demonstrated experimental and clinical evidence suggesting that terminal QRS notches 20–100 μV in amplitude, and thus often visible even in the low-gain ECG, represent one type of fragmented depolarization, separate from high-frequency low-amplitude delayed depolarization called 'late potentials' (LP) [31, 32].

Recent studies have demonstrated, that in ischaemic myocardial damage the initial QRS voltage, expressed as the RMS-value during the first 40 ms of filtered QRS complex is significantly lower in patients with previous myocardial infarction and sustained ventricular tachycardia (VT) than in patients without VT or in normals [33]. Using frequency-domain analysis it has been demonstrated, that ischaemic myocardial damage results in a reduction in the high-frequency content of initial and middle QRS complex [34, 35]. If the damaged muscle mass is great enough, initial QRS notching in the low-gain ECG is expected to appear.

After demonstration of fragmented delayed depolarization in the ischemic scar tissue of an isolated human heart [36], and experimentally in an ischemic canine heart [37, 38], the concept of the reentrant circuit as the main mechanism of VT in man, was introduced [39]. This idea was soon confirmed experimentally by demonstrating delayed fractionated activity in diastole during VT in an acutely ischaemic canine heart [40]. These fragmented late activities, called in clinical practice 'late potentials' (LP), were recognized and validated by endocardial and/or epicardial recordings

Table 1. Highlights in the development of external recording of cardial micropotentials

1917	Oppenheimer [3]	'Arborization block': Prolonged and highly notched QRS in surface ECG.
1940	Weinberg and Katz [4]	'Focal intraventricular block': One lead QRS prolongation.
1944	Wilson et al. [5]	Terminal slurring of QRS in myocardial infarction: Conduction defect.
1950	First et al. [6]	'Peri-infarction block': Circuitous tangential epicardial activation; terminal QRS notching.
1952	Langner [7]	High fidelity ECG: Concealed information in ECG.
1953	Alzamora-Castro et al. [8]	'Parietal focal block': Fiber block.
1959	Cabrera et al. [9]	'Intra-infarction block': initial QRS notching.
1960	Langner and Geselowitz [10]	High fidelity ECG in myocardial infarction: RMS voltage
1960	Zuckermann [11]	'Postexcitation': Terminal QRS notch in myocardial infarction.
1965	Raunio et al. [12]	Terminal QRS notch in myocardial infarction. First systematical clinicopathological study.
1967	Anttonen et al. [13]	Terminal QRS notch: Further clinicopathological studies.
1969	Raunio [14]	Initial QRS notch in myocardial infarction: First systematical clinicopathological study.
1969	Flowers et al. [15]	High frequency QRS notching associated with postmortem finding of myocardial scar.
1973	Stopczyk et al. [16] Flowers et al. [17] Berbari et al. [18]	First signal averaged surface ECG recording of His-Purkinje signal in man.
1974	Siltanen et al. [19]	The current magnetocardiographic lead system, i.e. the standard grid, and the normal MCG pattern.
1974	Saarinen et al. [20]	Recording of QRS notches by real time magnetocardiography in myocardial infarction.
1978	Farrell et al. [21]	Magnetocardiographic recording of His-Purkinje signal.
1978	Fontaine et al. [22]	Signal-averaged surface ECG recording of 'Late potentials' in man.
1980	Allor [23]	Real-time surface ECG recording of His-Purkinje signal.
1980	Walczak et al. [24]	Real-time surface ECG recording of His-Purkinje signal using spatial averaging.
1981	Wajszsuk et al. [25]	Signal-averaged and real-time surface ECG recording of sinus node activity.
1981	Simson [26]	Application of quantitative vectorcardiography to micropotential studies.
1983	Hombach et al. [27]	Real-time surface ECG recording of late potentials using spatial averaging.
1983	Erné et al. [28]	Signal averaged magnetocardiographic recording of late fields related to late potentials.
1984	Cain et al. [29]	Fast Fourier Transform analysis of the high-frequency content of QRS in myocardial infarction.
1985	Erné [30]	First three-dimensional localization of abnormal cardiac microfield using magnetocardiography.

and also by surface ECG recordings, first in an experimental animal [41] and then also in humans, by using high resolution (HR) measurements and sequential signal averaging (SA) [22, 31, 42, 43, 44].

High resolution (HR) magnetocardiography (MCG) became possible after the development of high-sensitivity SQUID sensors, which rendered it possible to record cardiac microcurrents. The first HR-MCG recording of late fields (LFs) corresponding to LPs occurred in a magnetically shielded room [28], but recording might also be possible in a hospital laboratory, where HR-MCG recording of the His-Purkinje signal (HPS) has been carried out, including validation with an intracardiac HPS ECG recording [45].

The SA technique was the earliest and still is the most commonly used means of enhancing the signal-to-noise ratio in recording weak signals. Good reviews of the use of this technique in cardiology have recently appeared [46, 47]. It is easy to use, and commercial devices for clinical use are available. On the other hand, it has some significant drawbacks; in particular, its failure to discern intermittent or inconsistently timed signals must be mentioned [27, 48, 49, 50], which renders it in many cases unfavourable for recordings of the HPS and LPs. However, the SA technique is at present the most usual means to record in the clinical setting the LP, the HPS, and even the preatrial signal, which probably is generated by the sinus node. The recovery rate of HPS using SA technique is about 60 percent according to various reports, which limits its use in clinical pracitice. The same applies in greater extent to recordings of the very weak preatrial signal.

In order to avoid the problems associated with the SA-ECG technique another ECG measurement technique has been developed, which is based on careful minimization of the external and instrumental noise, and when necessary by using spatial signal averaging, carried out with parallel composite electrodes, parallel low noise preamplifiers and appropriate filters [27, 48, 49, 50]. These arrangements render it possible to record cardiac micropotentials in real-time (RT) and examine them on a beat-to-beat basis.

Comparisons of SA-ECG and RT-ECG have revealed concordant findings in 74–78% of cases; the majority of the discordant findings are RT-ECG-positive cases, which indicates the superiority of the latter (RT-) technique [44, 51]. It has been pointed out, that a combination of sequential SA and HR-ECG, which is based on noise reduction including eventual spatial averaging to a 'double averaging', will reduce significantly the number of beats necessary for sequential SA [52]. As regards recording of LPs, both techniques are handicapped by the necessity of defining LPs, which has many problems [53]. Automated analysis of terminal low-voltage potentials of QRS complex has therefore utilized vectorcardiography either by computing the RMS vector of the terminal 40 ms of filtered QRS complex obtained using three orthogonal leads [26], or by measuring the relative high-frequency power of the terminal QRS plus S-T segment by applying Fast Fourier Transforms (FFT) [29]. The latter method is perhaps not as sensitive a discriminator for patients with and without VT as the former [54], but it may be less prone to interference by the presence of bundle branch block than the former method [55, 56]. Apparently the same problem is encountered in other SA-ECG rechniques too [57].

The association of LPs with the propensity to VT, particularly in patients with coronary heart disease, has been documented by several authors during the last ten years [26, 27, 31, 40, 44, 47, 53, 58, 59, 60, 61, 62, 63]. The association is loose in the early phase of AMI, but well developed at least at 8th week after AMI [64]. On the other hand, according to some subsequent reports, the SA-ECG at discharge from hospital after AMI presents all information as regards prediction of VT or SCD, the majority of which occurs during the first half year after AMI [63, 65, 66]. The relationship between VT and LP of other predictors of VT is important in this context, because observations on the mechanism of SCD occurring during Holter monitoring have revealed, that nearly always VT initiates the arrhythmic event finally leading to ventricular fibrillation (VF) and death [67, 68]. On the other hand, LPs have almost no relevance for primary VF and SCD at the very beginning of an ischaemic attack [31]. Programmed ventricular stimulation (PVS) studies have also made it evident, that in a great proportion of patients with LPs it is possible to induce a repetitive ventricular response, and that the combination of LP and positive PVS may be the best predictor of subsequent fatal arrhythmic events in AMI patients [69, 70, 71]. Sustained VT inducible by PVS predicts sudden death or non-fatal VT/VF with a high probability, in contrast to inducible VF, which lacks predictive value [65]. The predictive value of LPs have been compared by several investigators with other methods used for prediction of VT or SCD, namely Holter monitoring, left ventricular function and PVS [63, 64, 65, 69]. The predictive value for LPs varied between 21–26%, for Holter monitoring 15–18%, for PVS 22–24%, for left ventricular function 23%, for a combination of LP + PVS 27–30% and for LP + PVS + Holter 31%. The authors of one of the most recent studies, which is based on a material of 403 AMI patients [65], conclude that about one quarter of AMI survivors have a high risk of VT or SCD; patients who have either LP or inducible VT by PVS have a 27% probability to SCD or to non-fatal VT/VF during 2 subsequent years with highest incidence during first 6 months.

Studies reviewed above, as well as numerous other studies, have shown, that ischemic heart disease is prone to induce fragmentation of ventricular depolarization. The fragmentation can be detected by various techniques, and it seems to be very good marker for risk of VT or SCD. All the methods in question have special advantages and drawbacks, and for the present no unanimity exists about the most advantageous technique. In order to get personal experience of different ways of approaching these problems, our group started 1982 to develop instrumentation for HR-ECG studies and to put an effort in enhancing the resolution ability of our MCG-systems of that time. At various stages of the development of the instrumentation, the methods were tested and validated by recording cardiac microsignals like HPS and LP/LF in numerous sporadic cases. Our present HR-ECG instrumentation was installed in the hospital in 1985, a pilot series of recording LPs in consecutive patients with AMI was completed in spring 1986, and in November 1986 we began to collect HR-ECG recordings systematically (1) in patients with documented sustained VT, and (2) in patients with acute myocardial infarction before discharge from hospital. The data are stored for future analysis. They are to be reviewed later in the RT-mode (beat-to-beat) for intermittent or inconstantly timed LPs, and thereafter averaged and subjected to both time domain and frequency domain analysis. A small proportion of patients also are examined by HR-MCG. Some preliminary results of the base-line measurements are presented and the measurement methods are described in the following,

Methods

Electrical studies. The low signal amplitude (about 1–$20~\mu$V) of cardiac micropotentials requires extremely sensitive low noise equipment and preferably a low noise environment for recording. All our HR-ECG recordings were done in the electrically shielded room (Faraday cage) of the cardiovascular laboratory of the Helsinki University Central Hospital. A block diagram depicting the recording arrangements is presented in Figure 1. Data acquisition occurred using a laboratory-made microprocessor-based 8-channel ECG measurement system, which is suitable both for RT- and SA-measurements. The system was developed from the commercial KONE 620 ECG terminal. It uses battery-driven preamplifiers with a noise level of $0.5~\mu V_{p-p}$ in the frequency band 0.05–300 Hz, and with a 20 Mb Winchester unit allowing 10 minutes continuous recording. The device has 12- or 16-bit resolution and a noise level below $1~\mu V_{p-p}$ in the frequency band 0.05–300 Hz.

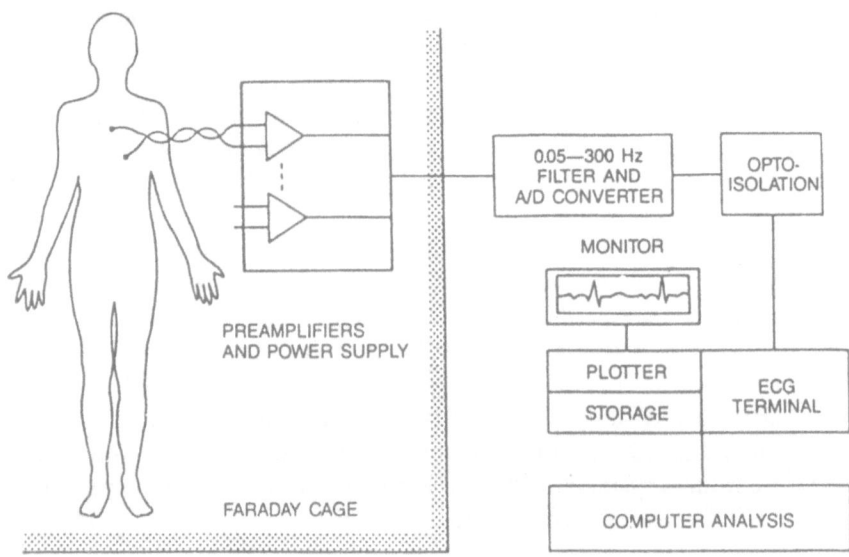

Figure 1. A block diagram depicting the high-resolution ECG recording and signal processing system used in the present study. The electrically shielded room and the ECG terminal are located at the cardiovascular laboratory of Helsinki University Central Hospital, and the computer at the Department of Technical Physics, Helsinki University of Technology.

The subsequent analysis of the retrieved HR-ECG data occurred using an HP-1000 minicomputer located at the Helsinki University of Technology. Before further processing the RT data were examined beat-to-beat for visual inspection of possible LPs. Any fractionated, polymorphic, low-amplitude signal is considered as an LP, if it follows the fundamental QRS complex after more than 10 ms, measured backwards from the point where it (RMS value) falls to a magnitude equal to twice the noise level. The complexes were averaged by the correlation method for accurate timing and classification of the complexes. Then the total duration of the QRS complex, including the possible LP, was measured. The signal processing continued either with time domain or frequency domain analysis.

For time domain analysis the signal was first filtered using an 80 Hz low-pass filter (-60 dB/oct at 25 Hz), and the sampling frequency was reduced from 2000 to 250 Hz in order to minimize filter ringing. This was followed by filtering with a 25 Hz high-pass FIR filter (-60 dB/oct), constructing the RMS complex obtained from three modified orthogonal leads and determining the Low Amplitude (<40 μV) Signal (LAS) duration and the RMS value of the last 40 ms of QRS (V_{40}); the RMS complex was considered abnormal, if LAS was >40 ms and/or V_{40} was <25 μV.

The frequency domain analysis of QRS complexes from three modified orthogonal leads was carried out with the aid of a 512 point Fast Fourier Transform (FFT) using a Hamming-window. The discriminating power was evaluated by comparing the amount of high frequency energy (40–100 Hz) of each lead to the respective amount of low frequency energy (<40 Hz) both visually and by calculating area ratios for the terminal 40 ms of the QRS complex and also for the whole QRS complex.

We used low noise disposable silver/silver chloride electrodes with no spatial averaging. The lead system is depicted in Figure 2. The total noise level varied between 3 and 10 μV, the mean being 6.0 μV.

The low-gain standard 12-lead ECG's were visually examined for initial and terminal QRS notches. Criteria for notches are [12, 14]: A positive or negative notch appearing in two or more of the 12 standard leads during the initial or terminal 40 ms of QRS complex, provided that its duration is 20 ms or more in at least one lead; the initial notch of duration mentioned above is significant if it appears at least in one of the precordial leads.

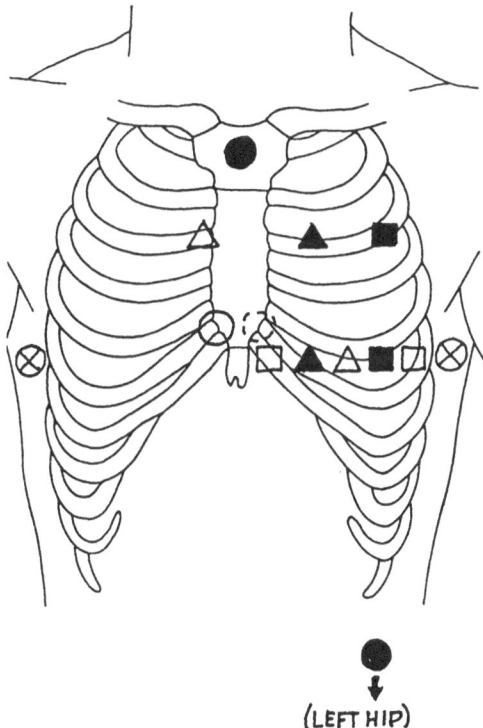

(LEFT HIP)

Figure 2. The system of bipolar ECG leads used in the high resolution measurements of the present study. The modified orthogonal leads are signed as follows: $x = \otimes$, $y = \bullet$, $z = \bigcirc\!\bigcirc$.

Magnetic studies. The magnetic microfields generated by the cardiac conduction system and by LPs are very weak, usually about 0.1–0.5 pT in amplitude. Therefore, HR-MCG-studies require very sensitive measurement devices. The general arrangements of the measuring facility is described in the block diagram of Figure 3. All our measurements were done in the magnetically shielded room of Helsinki University of Technology. A very sensitive DC-SQUID magnetic gradiometer was constructed for this purpose. The superconducting flux transformer forms a first-order asymmetric gradiometer. The diameter of the main sensing coil is 3.7 cm, and the base length of the gradiometer 8 cm. The equivalent flux noise at the input coil of the DC-SQUID used (S.H.E. Corp., U.S.A.) is 1.5×10^{-5} $\Phi_0/\sqrt{\text{Hz}}$, and the current noise 1.5 pA/$\sqrt{\text{Hz}}$. The device is coupled to a commercial electronics unit. The field sensitivity of the gradiometer is better than 5 fT/$\sqrt{\text{Hz}}$, to our knowledge the highest sensitivity reported so far. Reaching such noise levels also requires careful minimizing of the dewar noise.

The output signal is transferred via an optical line to an HP-1000 minicomputer and additionally stored on magnetic tape. The data analysis is performed both by examining the RT recording beat-to-beat and by using the SA technique with correlation methods and digital filtering. The

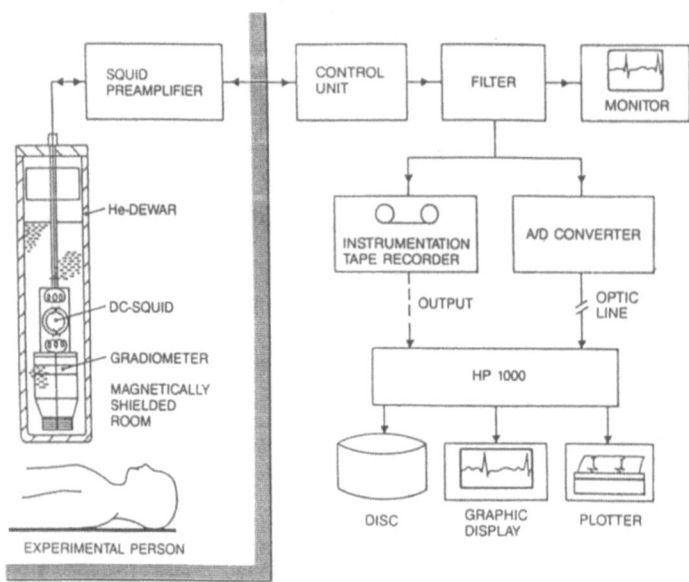

Figure 3. A block diagram of the MCG recording and signal processing system used at the Department of Technical Physics, Helsinki University of Technology.

recording positions on the anterior chest wall are determined by the standard 36-position grid developed in our laboratory and applied internationally [19, 72, 73], as modified by adding an extra (7th) vertical row of positions to the left. In studies dealing with localization of the cardiac microcurrent sources we have applied the current multipole model with dipole and quadrupole terms [74].

Patients

During the running-in period, 1984–1986, numerous sporadic representative cases were examined electrically and magnetically both by RT- and SA-ECG. Measurements consisted mostly of recording the HPS, preexcitation signal in WPW syndrome, and LPs. Because our main clinical interest is in the electrophysiological background of SCD, our present activity is focused to the minor abnormalities of the ECG including possible changes in the high frequency content of the QRS complex. Two types of patient have been recruited:

(1) Consecutive patients aged less than 65 years and suffering from their first AMI, for a prospective study. All patients were examined with HR-ECG on the 10th day after onset of symptoms. Standard 12-lead discharge ECGs were examined for initial and terminal QRS notches. Other examinations before discharge consist of routine clinical examination, a low-grade exercise test, a 24-hours ambulatory ECG and radionuclide ventriculography. The follow-up covers a period of 6 months and includes clinical examination, both low-gain and HR-ECG at 3 and 6 months, and recording of all SCDs, total mortality and all tachyarrhythmic episodes possible to trace anamnestically, or from hospital or health centre documents.

(2) Patients with documented sustained VT, for investigation of the behaviour of LPs during atrial pacing and administration of antiarrhythmic drugs. Most of these patients had suffered from more than one AMI. All patients were examined with HR-ECG with and without transosophageal atrial pacing. The standard 12-lead low-gain ECGs were examined for initial and terminal QRS notches. Other investigations were a 24-hour ambulatory ECG, a standard bicycle exercise test, radionuclide ventriculography PVS and introduction of antiarrhythmic treatment according to a free protocol. The effect of drug therapy is monitored with repeated electrical studies including PVS if necessary. All patients are under clinical follow-up.

In the present study, thirty subjects have been examined using RT-ECG, time-domain analysis and frequency domain analysis techniques in order to investigate high-frequency, low-amplitude signals throughout the QRS complex including possible LPs. The group consists of three subgroups: group (A) 10 patients from the above patient series (1), who have passed the 3rd month postinfarction follow-up without arrhythmic events; group (B) 10 patients from the above patient series (2) with sustained VT; group (C) 10 healthy control subjects under 35 years of age. Thus, these data represent a part of the baseline data of the two prospective studies.

Additionally, some selected patients were examined magnetically for demonstrating LFs and HPS, and in order to localize the break-through site of preexcitation or the source of the LP current.

Results

His-Purkinje signal. A typical example of a RT-ECG recording of HPS is demonstrated in Figure 4. In Figure 5 both RT- and SA-ECG recordings (59 beats) of HPS are presented. HPS has been recovered by HR-ECG in 21/35 cases (60%) in our laboratory. Both RT- and SA-MCG recordings (123 beats) of HPs are presented in Figure 6 showing in the upper (SA-) curve a small bump which probably represents the H-spike. A ramp pattern has been seen in most cases examined with MCG, often with a superposed bump timed simultaneously with the H-spike of an intracardial HPS-recording obtained in advance, and in some cases additional small deflections in the H-V segment can be surmised. No attempt has been done to localize the conductive tissue.

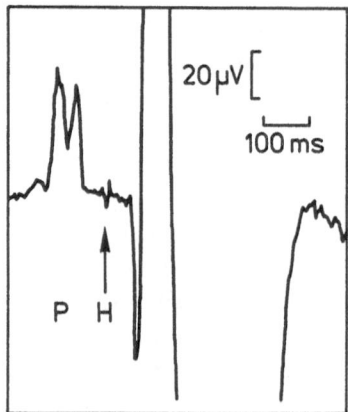

Figure 4. Real-time high-resolution surface ECG recording of HPS, done in the hospital laboratory. The HPS was seen regularly beat-to-beat with an identical timing.

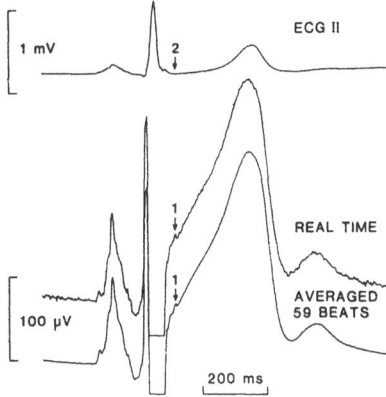

Figure 5. Electrical recordings in a case of sustained ventricular tachycardia. Upper curve: low gain ECG (lead II) recording of one beat. Middle curve: Real time high resolution recording of one beat. Lower curve: an average of 62 beats; note the LP deflection (2) in the RT- and SA-ECG, not visible in the low gain ECG (1). The frequency band is 0.05–300 Hz. The measurements were done using the hospital ECG terminal and the magnetically shielded room of the Helsinki University of Technology.

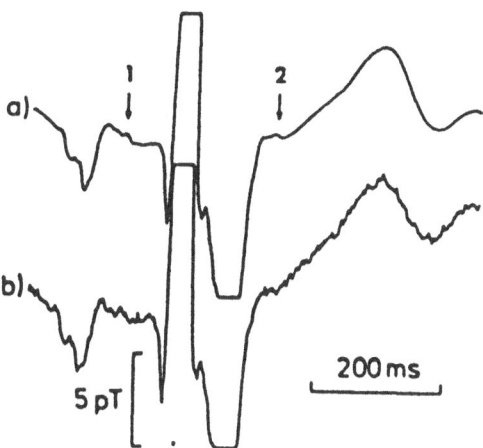

Figure 6. High-resolution MCG recordings in the same case as in Figure 5. a) average of 123 beats, b) real time signal. The frequency band is 0.05–300 Hz, and the measurement location is D3-4 of the standard grid. The HPS and LF magnitudes (1 and 2, respectively) are relatively small in this case, only about 0.2 pT.

272

Preexcitation. In 6 cases of WPW syndrome we have carried out computations based on HR-MCG data in order to localize the site of the Kent bundle on the strength of the break-through site of the preexcitation. In Figure 7 an example of a case is presented, in which the localization was validated by invasive electrophysiological investigation, and further also by surgery.

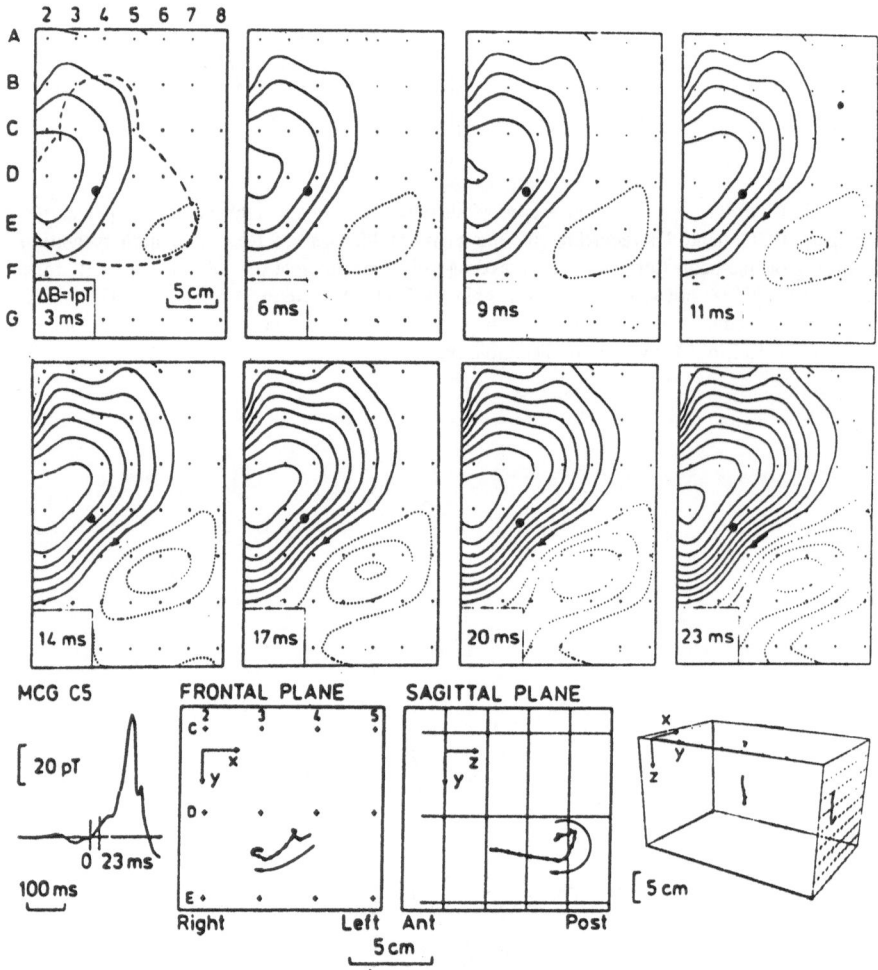

Figure 7. Magnetocardiographic localization of the break-through site of preexcitation in a case of WPW syndrome. The eight panels in the upper part of the figure present the isofield maps at different time instants beginning from the earliest upstroke of the delta wave. The heavy circuitous lines provided with dots in the two lower panels are constructed by computing from the map data, and present the projections of the pathway of the equivalent current dipole generated by the preexcitation on the frontal and sagittal plane. The letters (A–G) and the numbers (1–8) refer to the rows of the modified MCG standard grid.

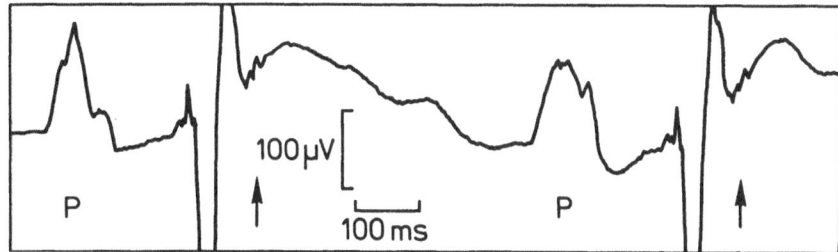

Figure 8. A real-time high-resolution ECG recording, done in the hospital laboratory in a case of sustained ventricular tachycardia. Late potentials (arrows) can be seen following both QRS complexes.

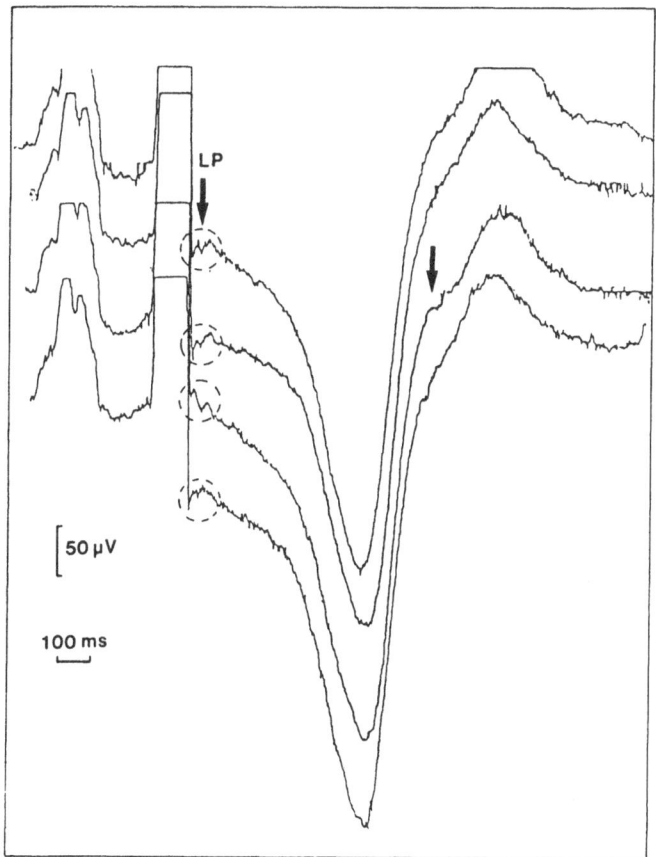

Figure 9. Real-time high-resolution recordings in a case of sustained ventricular tachycardia, done in the hospital laboratory. Late potentials (arrows) appear after each of the four consecutive QRS complexes, and also intermittently on the terminal ascending slope of the T wave.

Late potentials. Examples of LP recordings are presented in Figures 5, 6, 8 and 9. Figure 5 shows LPs recorded with HR-ECG both using RT- and SA-ECG (59 beats). The LFs in Figure 6 were recorded with HR-MCG using both the RT- and SA-technique (123 beats). An example of RT-ECG recording of LP in two consecutive beats can be seen in Figure 8, and in four consecutive beats in Figure 9. Notice the small fluctuations in the LP wave-forms on the early S-T segment in Figure 9, and also the variability of the very delayed LP on the ascending slope of the negative T wave. Intermittent and moving late potentials were often found, many of them (>20%) disappeared after averaging. LPs were found from RT-ECG recordings in 13/35 patients with recent AMI without VT/VF (37%), and in 72% of patients with documented VT/VF during hospital care. No-one of the healthy controls had LP in the HR-ECG. The duration of LPs in the VT/VF-group varied between 20 and 40 ms (mean 27 ms), and their amplitude between 10 and 30 μV (mean 17 μV). The LPs were clearly smaller and shorter in patients with AMI. LP findings in the present study group of 30 subjects are given in Table 2. The better sensitivity of the RT-ECG in detecting LPs can also be seen from these observations as compared to SA-ECG.

In a case of previous AMI and sustained VT with a clearcut LP in the

Table 2. Fragmented ventricular depolarization: low-gain and high-resolution ECG findings in 10 patients with sustained ventricular tachycardia after previous myocardial infarction, 10 patients with recent myocardial infarction and without tachycardia, and 10 healthy subjects

	VT		no VT		Controls	
Initial QRS notch in low-gain ECG	7/10	(70%)	5/10	(50%)	2/10	(20%)
Terminal QRS notch in low-gain ECG	8/10	(80%)	2/10	(20%)	2/10	(20%)
Late potentials in real-time ECG	7/10	(70%)	3/10	(30%)	–	–
Late potentials in signal-averaged ECG	6/10	(60%)	1/10	(10%)	–	–
QRS duration (MS) in signal-averaged ECG	164 ± 38		136 ± 29		104 ± 10	
Abnormal RMS-complex (LAS, V$_{40}$)	6/10	(60%)	1/10	(10%)	1/10	(10%)
FFT: relative energy at 40–100 Hz in the terminal 40 MS of QRS-complex increased	7/10	(70%)	5/10	(50%)	7/10	(70%)
FFT: relative energy at 40–100 Hz in the total QRS-complex decreased	7/10	(70%)	1/10	(10%)	–	–

ECG and LF in the MCG, the MCG isofield maps were utilized for efforts to localize the origin of the LF. However, subtraction of the background signals for computing the origin of the LF encountered problems, which have not yet been overcome.

Time domain analysis of QRS complex. Thirty persons (Groups A–C) were subjected to time domain analysis of QRS comlex. The number of findings of abnormal RMS complexes in each group is indicated in Table 2. An example of a typical finding in the group B (patients with VT) is shown in Figure 10, and an example of a normal finding in Figure 11. The amplitudes of the RMS complex were markedly lower in the VT-group than in

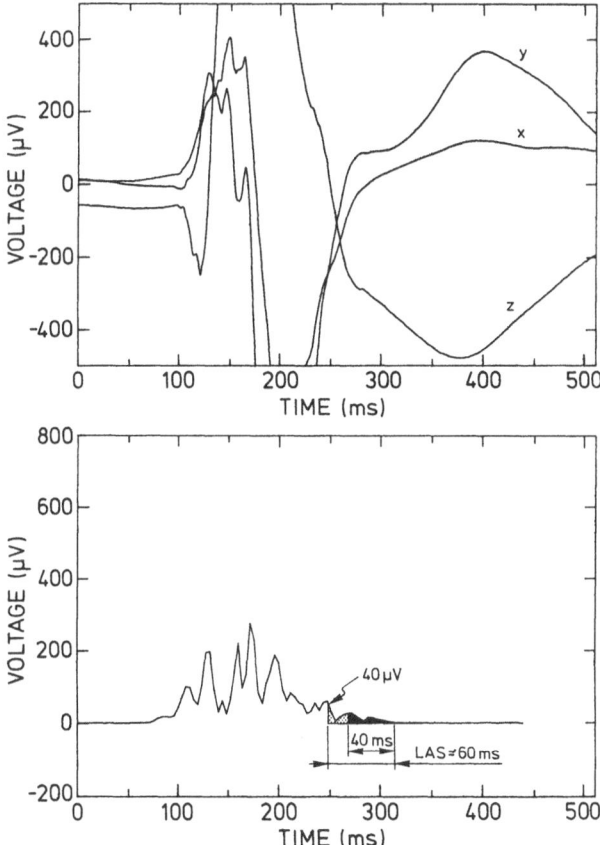

Figure 10. Signal averaged high-resolution ECG recording in a case of sustained ventricular tachycardia after myocardial infarction. The RMS complex at the bottom panel is computed from the QRS complex data obtained using the orthogonal leads *x*, *y* and *z*, and shown in the upper panel. The black area indicates the terminal 40 ms of QRS, and the black and shaded areas together the LAS (see text).

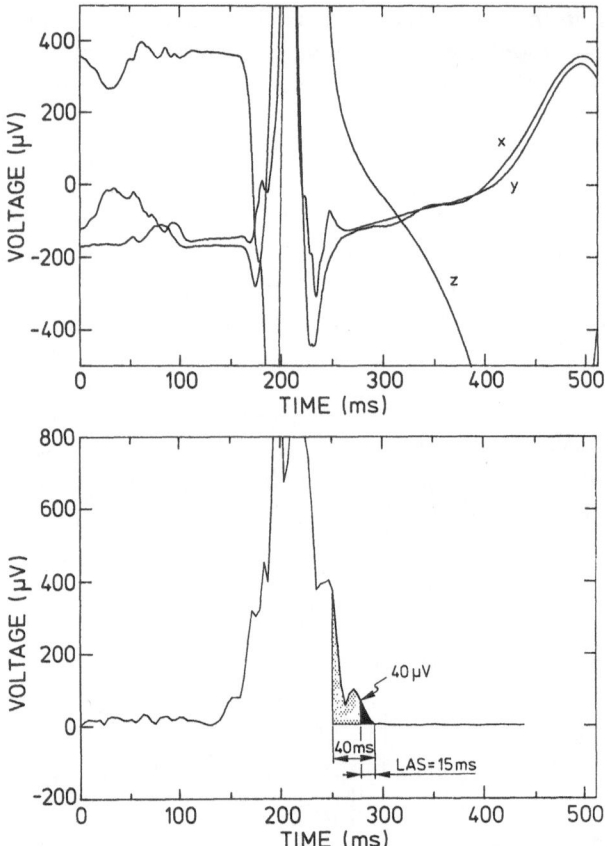

Figure 11. Signal averaged high-resolution ECG recording and an RMS complex of a healthy young man. The RMS complex at the bottom panel is computed from the QRS complex data obtained using orthogonal leads *x*, *y* and *z*, and shown in the upper panel. The shaded plus black areas together indicate the terminal 40 ms of QRS, and the black area the LAS (see text).

the control subjects, and were also diminished to some extent in the AMI-group.

Frequency domain analysis of QRS complex. In thirty persons (Groups A–C) FFT was used. The results are given in Table 2. In all three groups there was relatively much energy in the terminal 40 ms of the QRS complex between frequencies 40 and 100 Hz. The mean area ratios were close to each other, overlapping with a large S.D. and possessed no discriminating power. However, the VT-patient group showed a clear lack of high frequency energy of the whole QRS complex as compared with the AMI- and control groups.

Initial and terminal QRS notches. The prevalence of initial and terminal notches in groups A–C are given in Table 2. The prevalence is greatest in patients with VT, actually 3 times that in normal subjects, among whom the notches were in all cases associated with a duration of the filtered averaged QRS of less than 120 ms. The prevalence of notches in the AMI-group was between that of the VT- and control groups. The appearance of both initial and terminal notches in the VT- and AMI-groups was always associated with a prolongation of the filtered averaged QRS complex.

Discussion

The SA techniques are very important both in clinical practice and in medical research [46]. Electrocardiology has probably most profited from this technique, which being originally adopted by medical researchers, was introduced to clinical use for discriminating the foetal ECG from the ECG of the mother [75]. Actually, our experience on the averaging of cardiac signals also derives from foetal monitoring [76]. Its great advantages are the improved signal-to-noise ratio, and the relatively rapid procedure which may largely be automated. Drawbacks are its failure to detect moving signals, and the complexity of the devices, particularly if automation is desired.

Our observations (e.g. Figure 8) support the view of previous authors [27, 49, 50], that the sensitivity of RT-HR-ECG in detecting LPs is markedly better than that of SA-ECG. The retrieval of LPs in a recent study [51] was over 29% better using RT-ECG than using SA-ECG, which is consistent with our observations. In our series over 20% of LPs discerned in the RT-ECG disappeared during sequential signal averaging, although we did not use spatial averaging. Unfortunately, RT recording requires the best possible signal-to-noise ratio and preferably a shielded environment, is often more time consuming, and necessitates an experienced ECG reader for interpretation of tracings.

Recording of HPS using the HR-ECG is without any doubt a useful diagnostic tool in diseases of A-V conductive tissue and e.g. in monitoring certain drug effects on A-V conduction. Computer model experiments suggest, that the ramp-like pattern of the His-Purkinje recordings obtained using HR-MCG, or HR-ECG without filtering may tell more comprehensively about the function of the conductive tissue, beginning from the A-V node down to the bundle branches [77, 78]. However, today only HR-ECG is applicable as a diagnostic tool in hospital environment, where it offers the possibility to measure A-H and H-V intervals noninvasively in about

2/3 of cases. Generally, the signal is high-pass filtered in order to reveal a distinct H-spike.

Localization of the electric source in the His-Purkinje system has challenged several investigators. It would be tempting to selectively 'image' noninvasively the diseased His-Purkinje system. However, from the clinical point of view it does not seem realistic to expect much contribution to decisions from this rather laborous technique in clinical practice. On the other hand, localization of the Kent bundle and sources of currents associated with LPs by using the HR-MCG technique may be of clinical importance, when surgical treatment or catheter ablation is aimed. In these settings, which occur rather infrequently, the laboriousness of the technique is no big problem.

The prevalence of LPs in this study was of the same magnitude as in previous reports on cases of recent AMI. According to various reports the incidence of LP during the early hours of AMI varies between 16–33% [27, 31, 66], but its appearance is rather inconsistent during the first six weeks [66]. It is possible, that this inconsistency is related to a beat-to-beat variability of the appearance of LP in this period. Later on, the incidence decreases down from 33–55% during the first half year to 20–36% during the second half year after AMI [53, 65].

Time-domain analysis revealed a general reduction of high frequency amplitudes throughout the QRS complex, which was often associated with a prolongation of the total QRS duration including the possible LP, or 'ventricular activation time' [79]. Since the original report of Simson [26] over twenty different reports have appeared presenting consistent evidence of the high predictive power of RMS voltage of terminal 40 ms of QRS complex, and/or of duration of low-amplitude ($<40 \mu$V) terminal QRS signal, and/or prolongation of QRS duration over 120 ms, as measured at discharge from hospital after AMI, in differentiating between patients with and without VT. The predictive values reported in various papers have already been referred to above. A careful study [80] analyzed the power of SA-ECG, Holter monitoring and cardiac catheterization to distinguish between two groups of patients with recent AMI, with and without sustained VT. In that study 81% of patients were categorized correctly on the strength of LP or duration of the filtered QRS complex. Combination with Holter monitoring and/or left ventricular function data actually slightly worsened the categorization. Presence or absence of LP, and duration of the filtered QRS complex independently differentiated the two patient groups in a multivariate logistic regression analysis. It is certainly possible to combine more variables of HR-ECG into an appropriate risk index in order to augment the predictive power.

The results of frequency domain analysis of the SA-ECG using FFT of the last 40 ms of the QRS are not consistent with the previous reports of its differentiation power [81]. The observations of the present study on this issue are very limited, but they support the results of another more recent study demonstrating a low sensitivity and specificity of this method [54]. Contrary to some earlier observations [29], the high-frequency spectrum of the whole QRS complex seems to have some differentiating power between patients with VT, and with AMI or normal subjects.

The present data do not allow an evaluation of this method and further investigation is needed to elucidate the importance of the high-frequency analysis of the QRS complex and maybe also of the S-T segment [81]. Presently, we have not yet evaluated the various alternatives, e.g. the 'area ratios' or other indexes of the frequency distribution of energy. Further, high-frequency QRS analysis on the band 150–250 Hz using envelope curves [34] has to be evaluated for possible predictive value. Frequency domain analysis of the single beat HR-ECG has recently been presented [82]. The rapid processing and printout ability of this system are great advantages from the clinical point of view.

The initial and terminal notches were very frequent among patients with VT. This is consistent with a previous study [31], in which terminal notches were found in 90% of patients with sustained VT, in 43% of patients with recent AMI, and in only 25% of patients with VF. In the present study, initial and terminal notches we found in 20–30% of controls, but always associated with normal duration of the filtered QRS complex in contrast to patients of the VT-group, in which QRS duration was always prolonged over 120 ms. The frequency of the notches diminishes with time after AMI, i.e. from the initial frequency of about 30% to almost 10% during the first year past AMI [83]. The corresponding reduction of the frequency of LPs after AMI is 15–20% [53, 65]. Apparently the initial and terminal notches belong to the same category of depolarization abnormalities as LPs, and may contribute to prediction of the risk of VT and SCD. Actually, in the only prospective study in the literature [83], of 7 patients with their first AMI dying during the year of follow-up, 4 (57%) had had an initial and/or terminal QRS notch at admission; this is almost twice the frequency of notches in the whole series at admission.

Conclusions

(1) RT-ECG seems to be a superior technique to SA-ECG for detecting micropotentials like His-Purkinje signals and LPs. The method is, however, time consuming, sensitive to subjective bias, and cannot easily be

automated. The same is not true as regards the sensitivity of RT-MCG versus SA-MCG, because for the present the instrument at its best still is often too noisy to detect the smallest cardiac microsignals discernible by HR-ECG.

(2) SA-ECG and maybe also SA-MCG are useful tools for large scale prognostication in spite of imperfect retrieval of intermittent or inconstantly timed microsignals.

(3) The MCG technique has proved to be useful in localizing, in three dimensions, sources of certain weak signals, such as preexcitation and probably also LPs.

(4) More elaborate time-domain and frequency-domain analyses of ventricular depolarization will be needed to discover more sensitive and more specific markers for risk of life-threatening arrhythmias and SCD, especially after AMI.

(5) The value of initial and terminal notches as adjuncts to the other noninvasive electrophysiological means for predicting the risk of VT and SCD should be evaluated, because of their easy availability from the routine 12-lead low-gain ECG.

Acknowledgements

The authors thank O. Mela, M.S. Nieminen, S. Nieminen, J. Puurtinen, M. Raivio. A. Salli and L. Toivonen for their assistance at various stages of this work, and for useful discussions. The economic aid of the Academy of Finland and SITRA foundation are acknowledged. The authors thank the Instrument Division of Kone Inc. for the positive attitude to the project.

References

1. Siltanen P (1972) The ischaemic heart disease register as a frame for preventive measures. Adv Cardiol 8:214–225
2. Siltanen P, Pohjola-Sintonen S, Haapakoski J, Mäkijärvi M, Pajari R (1985) The mortality predictive power of discharge electrocardiogram after first acute myocardial infarction. Am Heart J 109:1231–1237
3. Oppenheimer BS, Rothschild MA (1917) Electrocardiographic changes associated with myocardial involvement. JAMA 69:429–431
4. Weinberg HB, Katz LN (1940) Two unusual types of electrocardiograms. Am Heart J 19:519–528
5. Wilson FN, Johnston FD, Rosenbaum FF, Erlanger H, Kossmann CE, Hecht H, Cotrim M, de Oliveira RM, Scarsi R, Barker PS (1944) The precordial electrocardiogram. Am Heart J 27:19–85

281

6. First SR, Bayley RH, Bedford DR (1950) Peri-infarction block: Electrocardiographic abnormality occasionally resembling bundle branch block and local ventricular block of other types. Circulation 2:31–36
7. Langner PH Jr (1952) Value of high fidelity electrocardiography using cathode ray oscilloscope and expanded time scale. Circulation 5:249–256
8. Alzamora-Castro V, Abugattas R, Rubio C, Bouroncle J, Zapata C, Santa-María E, Paredes D (1953) Parietal focal block: an experimental and electrocardiographic study. Circulation 7:108–115
9. Cabrera E, Rocha JC, Flores G (1959) El vectorcardiograma de los infartos miocardicos co tras tornos en la conducción intraventricular. Arc Inst Cardiol Méx 29:625–646
10. Langner PH Jr, Geselowitz DB (1960) Characteristics of the frequency spectrum in the normal electrocardiogram and in subject following myocardial infarction. Circ Res 8:577–584
11. Zuckermann R (1960) Postexcitation. Z Kreislauff 4:654–658
12. Raunio H, Anttonen V-M, Meurman L (1965) Terminal QRS forces in posterior myocardial infarction. Ann Med Int Fenn 54:157–168
13. Anttonen V-M, Raunio H, Krogerus J, Meurman L (1967) The significance of a notch during the terminal 0.04 second of the QRS complex in an electrocardiogram. Ann Med Int Fenn 56:1–7
14. Raunio H (1969) Significance of a notch during the initial 0.04 sec of the QRS complex in the electrocardiogram. Ann Clin Res 1:Suppl 3
15. Flowers NC, Horan LG, Tolleson WJ, Thomas JR (1969) Circulation 40:927–933
16. Stopczyk MJ, Kopeć, J. Żochowski RJ, Pieniak M (1973) Surface recording of electrical heart activity during the P-R segment in man by computer averaging technique. Int Res Com Syst (73-8):11, 21, 2
17. Flowers NC, Horan LG (1973) His bundle and bundle branch recordings from the body surface. Circulation 48:Suppl 4:102 (abstr)
18. Berbari EJ, Lazzara R, Samet P, Scherlag BJ (1973) Noninvasive technique for detection of electrical activity during the PR segment. Circulation 48:1005–1013
19. Siltanen P, Saarinen M, Katila T, Ahopelto J (1974) Magnetocardiogram in healthy men and women. Proc VIII World Congr Cardiol, Buenos Aires (abstr)
20. Saarinen M, Karp PJ, Katila TE, Siltanen P (1974) The magnetocardiogram in cardiac disorders. Cardiovasc Res 8:820–834
21. Farrell DE, Tripp JH, Norgren R (1978) Non-invasive information on the PR segment of the cardiac cycle: an assessment of the clinical potential of the electric and magnetic methods. Proc SPIE 167:173–177
22. Fontaine G, Frank R, Gallais-Hamonno F, Allali I, Phan-Thuc H, Grosgogeat Y (1978) Electrocardiographie des potentials tardifs du syndrome de post-excitation. Arch Mal Coeur 71:854–864
23. A noninvasive method of recording a serial His-Purkinje Study in man. CVP April/May:16–19 (1980)
24. Walczak F, Kepski R, Pluciński Z, Piatkowski A (1980) Noninvasive method of HPS system activity measurements without averaging. Preliminary report. Kardiologia Polska 23:625–679
25. Wajszczuk WL, Palko T, Przybylski J, Stopczyk MJ, Bauld ThJ, Rubenfire M (1981) External recording of sinus node region activity in anomals and in man. In: Hombach V, Hilger HH (eds) Signal averaging technique in clinical cardiology. Stuttgart – New York: F.K. Schattauer Verlag, pp 65–79
26. Simson MB (1981) Use of signals in the terminal QRS complex to identify patients with ventricular tachycardia after myocardial infarction. Circulation 64:235–242

27. Hombach V, Kebbel U, Höpp H-W, Winter U-J, Braun V, Deutsch H, Hirche H, Hilger HH (1982) Fortlaufende Registrierung von Mikropotentialen de meschlichen Herzens. Erste Erfahrungen mit einem neuen hochauflösenden EKG-Verstärkersystem. D Med Wchschr 107:1951–1956

28. Erné SN, Fenici RR, Hahlbohm H-D, Jaszczuk W, Lehman HD, Masselli M (1983) High-resolution isofield mapping in magnetocardiography. Il Nuovo Cimento 2D:291–300

29. Cain ME, Ambos HD, Witkowski FX, Sobel BE (1984) Fast Fourier Transform analysis of signal-averaged electrocardiograms for identification of patients prone to sustained ventricular tachycardia. Circulation 69:711–720

30. Erné SN (1985) High resolution magnetocardiography: modeling and sources localization. Med Biol Eng Comp 23:suppl:1447–1450

31. Kertes PJ, Glabus M, Murray A, Julian DG, Campbell WF (1984) Delayed ventricular depolarization—correlation with ventricular activation and relevance to ventricular fibrillation in acute myocardial infarction. Eur Heart J 5:974–983

32. Scherlag BJ, Chesterfield GG, Berbari EJ, Lazzara R (1985) Peri-infarction block (1950)—late potentials (1980): Their relationship, significance and diagnostic implications (Editorial). Am J Cardiol 55:839–841

33. Kienzle MG, Falcone RA, Josephson ME, Simson MB (1984) High frequency signal amplitude in the early and middle QRS in patients with and without ventricular tachycardia. JACC 3:623 (abstr)

34. Abboud S, Belhassen B, Miller HI, Sadeh D (1986) High frequency electrocardiography using an advanced method of signal averaging for non-invasive detection of coronary artery disease in patients with normal conventional electrocardiogram. J Electrocardiol 19:371–380

35. DeCaro M, Volosin KJ, Greenspan AJ (1987) Optimal interval to predict ventricular tachycardia based on frequency analysis of the signal averaged electrocardiogram. JACC 9:suppl:208 (abstr)

36. Durrer D, VanLier A, Buller J (1964) Epicardial and intramural excitation in chronic myocardial infarction. Am Heart J 68:765–776

37. Boineau JP, Cox JL (1973) Slow ventricular activation in acute myocardial infarction. A source of reentrant premature ventricular contractions. Circulation 48:702–713

38. Waldo AL, Kaiser GA (1973) A study of ventricular arrhythmias associated with acute myocardial infarction in the canine heart. Circulation 47:1222–1228

39. Wellens HJ, Durrer DR, Lie KI (1976) Observations on mechanisms of ventricular tachycardia in man. Circulation 54:237–244

40. El-Sherif N, Scherlag BJ, Lazzara R, Hope RR (1977) Reentrant ventricular arrhythmias in late myocardial period. 1. Conduction characteristics in the infarction zone. Circulation 55:686–702

41. Berbari EJ, Scherlag BJ, Hope RR, Lazzara R (1978) Recording from the body surface of arrhythmogenic ventricular activity during ST segment. Am J Cardiol 41:697–702

42. Abdollah H, Brugada B, Richards DA, van der Dool A, Green M, Wehr M, Wellens HJJ (1983) Late potentials detected with signal averaged ECG and left ventricular endocardial mapping in patients with ventricular tachycardia. Circulation 68:suppl 3:174 (abstr)

43. Vassallo JA, Cassidy DM, Simson MB, Marchlinski FE, Buxton AE, Waxman HL, Dresden C, Falcone RA, Josephson ME (1983) Relationship of signal averaged late potentials, endocardial late activity, and origin of ventricular tachycardia. Circulation 68:suppl 3:174 (abstr)

44. El-Sherif N, Gomes JAC, Restivo M, Mehra R (1985) Late potentials and arrhythmogenesis. PACE 8:440–462

45. Fenici RR, Masselli M, Erné SN, Hahlbohm HD (1985) Magnetocardiographic mapping

of the P-R interval phenomena in an unshielded hospital laboratory. In: Weinberg H, Stroink G, Katila T (eds) Biomagnetism, application and theory. Oxford – New York: Pergamon Press Inc., pp 137–141

46. Hombach V, Barun V, Höpp H-W, Gil-Sanchez D, Scholl H, Behrenbeck DW, Tauchert M, Hilger HH (1982) The applicability of the signal averaging technique in clinical cardiology. Clin Cardiol 5:107–124

47. Hombach V, Höpp HV, Kebbel U, Eggeling T, Osterspey A, Hirche H, Hilger HH (1985) Signal averaged and high resolution beat-to-beat ECG technique for recovery of cardiac microvolt potentials. Med Biol Eng Comp 23:suppl:1451–1452

48. Flowers NC, Shvartsman V, Sohi GS, Horan LG (1981) Signal averaged versus beat-to-beat recording of surface His-Purkinje potentials. In: Hombach V, Hilger HH (eds): Signal averaging technique in clinical cardiology. Stuttgart: FK Schattauer Verlag, pp 329–349

49. Stopczyk MJ, Walczak F, Kepski R, Plucinski Z, Peczalski K (1981) The history of non-invasive His-Bundle recording: From averaging to continuous record. In: Hombach V, Hilger HH (eds): Signal averaging technique in clinical cardiology. Stuttgart: FK Schattauer Verlag, pp 283–289

50. El-Sherif N, Mehra R, Gomes JAC (1983) Appraisal of a low noise electrocardiogram. JACC 1:456–467

51. Hombach V, Höpp HV, Kebbel U, Treis I, Osterspey A, Eggeling T, Winter U, Hirche H, Hilger HH (1986) Recovery of ventricular late potentials from body surface using the signal averaging and high resolution ECG techniques. Clin Cardiol 9:361–368

52. Stopczyk MJ (1985) Studies on His-Purkinje activity from the body surface. From digital-time to Spatial-time (4-dimensional, analog-digital) averaging. Med Biol Eng Comp 23:suppl:1453–1454

53. Breithardt G, Borggrefe M (1986) Pathophysiological mechanisms and clinical significance of ventricular late potentials. Eur Heart J 7:364–385

54. Machac J, Weiss A, Winters SL, Barecca P, Gomes JA (1987) A comparative study of frequency- and time-domain analysis of signal averaged ECG's in ventricular tachycardia. JACC 9:suppl:208 (abstr)

55. Gomes JA, Stewart D, Winters SL, Barreca P (1987) The signal averaged electrocardiogram in patients with ventricular tachycardia and bundle branch block. JACC 9:suppl:208 (abstr)

56. Lindsay BD, Ambos HD, Markham J, Casin ME (1987) Identification by frequency-domain analysis of patients with bundle branch block at risk for sustained ventricular tachycardia. JACC 9:suppl:207 (abstr)

57. Oeff M, von Leitner ER, Schwarz W, Schröder R (1986) Nichtinvasive Registrierung ventrikulärer Spätpotentiale bei Herzgesunden und bei patienten mit intraventrikulären Reitzleitungstörungen. Methode und Ergebnisse der Signalmittelungstechnik. Z Kardiol 7:666–672

58. Hombach V, Höpp H-V, Braun V, Behrenbeck DW, Tauchert M, Hilger HH (1980) Die Bedeutung von Nachpotentialen innerhalb des ST-Segmentes im Oberflächen-EKG bei Patienten mit koronarer Herzkrankheit. Dtsch med Wschr 105:1457–1462

59. Breithardt G, Schwarzmaier J, Abendroth RR, Borggrefe M, Seipel L (1981) Prospective study on the incidence of late potentials in post-myocardial infarction patients. Circulation 64:suppl 4:328 (abstr)

60. Denes P, Santarelli P, Hauser RG, Uretz EF (1983) Quantitative analysis of the high-frequency components of the terminal portion of the body surface QRS in normal subjects and in patients with ventricular tachycardia. Circulation 67:1129–1138

61. Denes P, Uretz E, Santarelli P (1984) Determinants of arrhythmogenic ventricular

activity detected on the body surface QRS in patients with coronary artery disease. Am J Cardiol 53:1519–1523

62. Denniss AR, Richards DA, Cody DV, Russell PA, Young AA, Cooper MJ, Ross DL, Uther JB (1986) Prognostic significance of ventricular tachycardia and fibrillation induced at programmed stimulation and delayed potentials detected on the signal-averaged electrocardiograms of survivors of acute myocardial infarction. Circulation 74:731–745

63. Kuchar DL, Thorburn CW, Sammel NL (1986) Late potentials detected after myocardial infarction: natural history and prognostic significance. Circulation 74:1280–1289

64. Osterspey A, Höpp H-W, Hombach V, Deutsch H-J, Winter U, Behrenbeck DW, Tauchert M, Hilger HH (1983) Diagnostic and prognostic significance of ventricular late potentials in patients with coronary heart disease. In: Steinbach K (ed.) Cardiac pacing. Proceedings of the 7th World Symposium on Cardiac Pacing, Vienna 1983. Darmstatt: Steinkopff, pp 283–290

65. Denniss AR, Ross DL, Richards DA, Uther JB (1985) Changes in incidence of delayed potentials after myocardial infarction. Circulation 72:suppl 3:164 (abstr)

66. Lewis SJ, Lander OT, Taylor PA, Chamberlain DA, Vincent R (1987) The natural history of ventricular late potential activity in acute myocardial infarction. JACC 9:suppl:151 (abstr)

67. Panidis J, Morganroth J (1983) Sudden death in hospitalized patients: cardiac rhythm disturbances detected by ambulatory electrocardiographic monitoirng. JACC 2:798–805

68. Pratt GM, Francis MJ, Luck JC, Wyndham CR, Miller RR, Quinones MA (1983) Analysis of ambulatory electrocardiograms in 15 patients during spontaneous ventricular fibrillation with special reference to preceding arrhythmic events. JACC 2:789–797

69. Höpp H-W, Hombach V, Deutsch H-H, Osterspey A, Winter U, Hilger HH (1983) Assessment of ventricular vulnerability by Holter ECG, programmed ventricular stimulation and recording of ventricular late potentials. In: Steinbach K (ed.): Cardiac pacing, proceedings of the 7th World Symposium on Cardiac Pacing, Vienna 1983. Darmstadt: Steinkopff, pp 283–290

70. Haerten K, Borggrefe M, Breithardt G (1983) Repetitive ventricular response and late potentials in patients early after myocardial infarction. Circulation 68:suppl 3:174 (abstr)

71. Breithardt G, Borggrefe M, Karbenn U, Abendroth R-R, Seipel L (1983) Ventricular vulnerability and presence of late potentials in patients without documented ventricular tachycardia. PACE 6:suppl:108 (abstr)

72. Saarinen M, Siltanen P, Karp PJ, Katila T (1978) The normal magnetocardiogram. I. Morphology. Ann Clin Res 10:suppl 21

73. Siltanen P (1987) Magnetocardiography. In: Macfarlane PW, Lawrie TDW (eds) Electrocardiology, Ch 37. London: Baillière & Tindall

74. Katila T, Maniewski R, Mäkijärvi M, Nenonen J, Siltanen P (1987) On the accuracy of source localization in cardiac measurements. Phys Med Biol 32:125–131

75. Docker MF (1971) Computing in the study of the fetal electrocardiogram. In: Computer for analysis and control in medical and biological research. IEEE Conference Publication 79:17

76. Kariniemi V, Ahopelto J, Karp PJ, Katila TE (1974) The fetal magnetocardiogram. J Perinat Med 2:214–216

77. Leoni R, Romani GL (1982) Computer simulation of magnetic field patterns from the human cardiac conduction system. Il Nuovo Cimento 1D:737–750

78. Berbari EJ, Collins SM, Salu, Y, Arzbaecher R (1983) Orthogonal surface lead recordings of His-Purkinje activity: comparison of actual and simulated waveforms. IEEE Trans Biomed Eng BME-30:160–167

79. Denniss AR, Ross DL, Uther JB (1986) Reproducibility of measurements of ventricular

activation time using the signal-averaged Frank vector-cardiogram. Am J Cardiol 57:156–160

80. Kanowsky MS, Falcone RA, Dresden CA, Josephson ME, Simson MB (1984) Identification of patients with ventricular tachycardia after myocardial infarction: signal-averaged electrocardiogram, Holter monitoring and cardiac catheterization. Circulation 70:264–270

81. Cain ME, Ambos HD, Markham J, Fisher A, Sobel BE (1985) Quantification of differences in frequency content of signal-averaged electrocardiograms in patients with compared to those without sustained ventricular tachycardia. Am J Cardiol 55:1500–1505

82. Haberl R, Hengstenberg E, Pulter R, Steinbeck G (1986) Frequenzanalyse des Einzelschlag-Elektrokardiogrammes zur Diagnostik von Kammer-tachykardien. Z Kardiol 75:659–665

83. Pyörälä K, Raunio H, Kentala E (1975) Occurrence and regression of initial and terminal notching of the QRS complex in the electrocardiograms of patients with acute myocardial infarction. Ann Clin Res 7:426–432

Part IV: Drug Therapy

21. Diuretics – water depriving measures

H.G. SIEBERTH

Dept. of Internal Medicine, Technical University of Aachen, F.R.G.

Introduction

Even after the Second World War, dropsy as it was then called was one of the most frequent diseases found on internal medical wards. A large proportion of these patients died from this no longer controllable hyperhydration.

In industrialised countries, the leading cause of oedemas is cardiac disease. Oedemas of renal and hepatic origin follow, but are much less frequent. At the turn of the century therapy still consisted largely of the same remedies known since ancient times:

The organic mercury compounds used as diuretics between 1920 and 1950 derived from the observation, during the treatment of syphilis, that inorganic mercury compounds increased diuresis. Numerous very effective organic mercury diuretics were developed—all of which were extremely nephrotoxic and could therefore only be used at infrequent intervals [9]. From about 1950 onwards a large number of highly effective saluretic drugs of wide therapeutic range were developed, so that today there remain only a few situations in which saluretic drugs can not be effectively used. In these situations, extracorporeal haemofiltration now allows us quickly to withdraw any desired amount of water from the body.

In 1987 it is thus possible without exaggeration to state that depriving the body of water can be achieved in every clinical situation. The rate of fluid withdrawal can also be well controlled.

I would like to divide the remainder of my remarks into three sections:

1. factors causing oedemas to form, particularly in cardiac insufficiency;
2. diuretic drugs and water depriving measures—primarily haemofiltration, and
3. clinical strategy for using diuretics and haemofiltration.

V. Hombach, H. H. Hilger and H. L. Kennedy (eds), Electrocardiography and Cardiac Drug Therapy. ISBN 978-94-010-6976-2
© 1989, Kluwer Academic Publishers, Dordrecht –

1. *Factors causing oedemas particularly in heart failure*

There are many varied factors which can cause fluid retention or oedemas. Haemodynamic factors, disorders of renal function, humoral factors, stimulation of the autonomic nervous system and reduced lymph transport and reduced protein synthesis in inanition or cirrhosis of the liver are some of them. Each of these groups subdivides into further individual factors which play a role. And of course the individual organs also interact with one another to further complicate the picture.

With a simplified picture one should briefly recapitulate of how cardiac insufficiency causes fluid retention. Cardiac insufficiency reduces the effective circulating blood volume. This stimulates the controlling receptors located in both venous and arterial branches. These receptors in turn stimulate the sympathetic system with increased production of catecholamines, followed by raised vascular resistance and reduced renal blood flow. This results in increased release of renin and angiotensin. The release

Table 1. Factors mediating edema

Factors Mediating Edema

1. Haemodynamic Factors
   Heart
   Venous Pressure
   Effective Circulatory Blood Volume
   Blood Pressure
   Capillary Filtration

2. Kidney Function
   Renal Vascular Resistance
   Clearance, Filtration Fraction
   Hormone Release
   Protein Loss → Nephrotic Syndrome
   Kidney Insufficiency

3. Hormonal Factors
   Increased Renin-Angiotensin Activity
   Stimulated Aldosterone Release
   Increased Anti-Diuretic Hormonon Secretion
   Decreased Natriuretic Activity (Hormone?)
   Augmented Catecholamine Release

4. Stimulated Sympathetic Nervous System
5. Diminished Lymphtransport

of angiotensin increases the secretion of aldosterone, which in turn raises the re-absorption of sodium and water, thus increasing plasma volume [10]. The aim of this initially natural compensation mechanism is to raise the left ventricular end-systolic filling pressure to increase cardiac output especially under load. This mechanism finally results in increased capillary filtration with increased interstitial fluid retention causing peripheral and pulmonary oedemas.

Oedemas from kidney and liver disease arise in a completely different way [13]. It is essential to understand the genesis of the oedema to decide on suitable diuretic therapy.

In patients of average weight, peripheral oedemas are only found once about 5 litres of fluid have been retained. Extensive cardiac oedemas usually develop only slowly. The blood pressure may remain within normal range, or may be elevated or depressed.

The situation is different in hypertensive crisis, which occurs in 80% of patients with already impaired renal function. Retained fluid raises the afterload with excessively elevated blood pressure. In such situations the central venous pressure is not necessarily elevated. The extent of the hyperhydration is low in comparison with the conditions described above. Often no peripheral oedemas are found.

Finally I should mention hyperhydration in cardiac shock. The hyperhydration arises because cardiac output is so severely reduced that blood pressure falls below the minimum glomerular filtration pressure [6], so that fluid can no longer be excreted via the kidneys even under saluretic therapy. The fluid administered—often wrongly, as 'treatment for shock'—causes hyperhydration with excessive increase of the preload, i.e. a rise of the central venous pressure and substantial deposits of water in the lungs. In these cases peripheral oedemas are often only slight or not present at all.

2. *Diuretic drugs and water depriving measures—primarily hemofiltration*

The therapies for each of the three conditions described above are extensive oedemas which differ widely. Clinical and laboratory parameters for differential indication between diuretic therapy and haemofiltration are given in Table 2. The laboratory parameters listed here are also suitable for monitoring the therapy and detecting side effects.

It would not be appropriate to try to outline here the chemistry and mechanism of action of all saluretic drugs. I would however like to mention those groups of diuretics which are in current clinical use. The basic drugs used in cardiac insufficiency with unimpaired renal function are sulphonamide derivatives, especially thiazide, for example hydrochlorthiazide.

Table 2. Parmeters for differential indications in diuretic therapy

Parameters for differential indications in diuretic therapy

I. Clinical Parameters
   Peripheral Edema
   Blood Pressure
   Venous Pressure (CVP)
   Heart Examination!
   Pulmonary Edema
   Consciousness/Brain Edema
   Diuresis

II. Chest X-ray
    ECG
    UCG
    Sonography of the Kidneys

III. Laboratory Results
     Na, K, Creatinine, Urea, Clearance
     pH, apO_2, $apCO_2$. O_2Sat, % Haemoglob.
     CK, CKmB

IV. CVP
    Cardiac Output, Pulm. Art. Pressure,
    Wedge pressure
    Peripheral Resistance

This acts primarily on the proximal tubulus and to a slight extent also on the distal tubulus. The effect commences 1 to 2 hours after administration and lasts for 6 to 24 hours. Sodium and potassium excretion are increased. This increased potassium excretion is the main disadvantage of most of the saluretic drugs. For this reason, combination with potassium sparing diuretics is indicated for most patients and especially for those with unstable cardiac rhythm. This point will be discussed later.

The high ceiling diuretics, of which the most important is furosemide, act on the entire tubulus. The decisive site of action is however the loop of Henle. The action starts rapidly, within a few minutes of administration, and lasts only 2 to 3 hours for an individual dose. The drug has a wide therapeutic range—from 20 to 2000 mg/day and is also effective in advanced renal insufficiency [5].

Two problems important in diuretic therapy, should be stress more in detail:

A) Indications for different potassium sparing diuretics;

B) Management of the so called resistance for diuretic therapy.

Table 3. Election of diuretic sufficient for clinical use

Saluretics

Sulfonamides → Thiazides
Furosemide   ⎫ High
Etacrynic Acid ⎬ Ceiling
Muzolimine   ⎭ Diuretics
Potassium Sparing Diuretics
Aldosterone Antagonists
Amiloride
Triamterene

A) *Indications for different potassium sparing diuretics*

With a few exceptions, potassium sparing diuretics should only be used in combination with other diuretics [15]. Amylorid and triamteren act in the distal tubulus to inhibit sodium-potassium exchange. Their action is independent of aldosterone. Even with moderate renal insufficiency (creatinine levels above 1.5 mg/dl), life-threatening hyperkalaemia can arise, especially if the diet is rich in potassium. Amylorid and triamterene are just as effective at potassium saving as spironolactone, but much cheaper. If restricted renal function compels the use of potassium saving diuretics, then it is advisable for safety reasons to use spironolactones. At higher plasma potassium concentrations, increased amounts of aldosterone are secreted, and thus again more potassium is exchanged for sodium in the distal tubulus. Spironolactone does not block completely but competitively inhibits the aldosterone action.

B) *Management of the so called resistance to diuretic therapy*

a) *Complete resistance to diuretics is rare.* As the glomerular filtration rate falls, the dose of diuretics acting in the proportional tubules has to be increased [2]. At glomerular filtration rates below 30 ml/min, thiazides are completely ineffective. In healthy subjects the fractional sodium excretion is less than 1%. That means more than 99% are reabsorbed, therefrom 60–65% in the proximal tubule. With diminished glomerulumfiltrate, for instance creatinine clearance 30 ml/min, fractional sodium excretion rises to 4%. Under this situation the saluretic effect of thiazides is completely eliminated by the sodium reabsorption in the loop of Henle. When sodium reabsorption in the loop of Henle is diminished by high ceiling diuretics, one can demonstrate that chlorothiazide is still effective even in renal insufficiency. High ceiling diuretics act as already mentioned in kidney insufficiency even in dialysis patients. Hyponatriaemia can substantially reduce or completely block the efficacy of furosemide. Substitution of sodium chloride or sodium bicarbonate can restore saluretic efficacy very soon. If furosemide is ineffective and serum electrolytes are normal, it can be used in combination with ethacrynic acid to increase effectiveness. In contrast to furosemide and ethacrynic acid, muzolimine acts from the contraluminal side [14]. This appears to be relevant for its action in advanced renal insufficiency. It could be shown that muzolimine further increases diuresis over that produced by furosemide [7].

b) *Haemofiltration*. In cases where saluretic drugs are not effective or do not act quickly enough, haemofiltration is indicated. This is the case in shock, in cases where blood pressure falls below the glomerular filtration pressure, in acute and chronic renal insufficiency, in excessive hypernatraemia, and in postrenal obstructive renal failure if the cause of the blockage cannot immediately be removed. The principle of action is simple: plasma water is filtered by convection through a membrane [12]. The necessary pressure across the membrane can in veno-venous filtration be provided by a pump or in arterio-venous filtration by the arterial pressure. Although veno-venous haemofiltration is technically somewhat complicated since a pump and an air trap are needed, we prefer this method to arterio-venous filtration for the following reasons. Even in the most severe cases of shock, with arterial pressure no longer sufficient to perform filtration, veno-venous filtration is still able to remove the desired amount of fluid in the desired time [3, 4]. The maximum rate we ever aim at is 20 to 30 ml/min. Technically it is possible to achieve higher rates. We regard as a further advantage the fact that a venous puncture is easier to make than an arterial puncture. An arterial puncture also prevents any thrombolysis therapy from being given.

3. *Clinical strategy for using diuretics and haemofiltration*

Oedemas of cardiac origin can usually be removed by thiazide diuretics alone. The fluid removal is often sufficient to achieve recompensation of the heart. The rate of fluid withdrawal should be slow, particularly in older patients, to avoid hypovolaemia with cardiac, cerebral and renal complications. The net withdrawal rate should not exceed 2 litres/day. Prophylaxis against thrombosis and accurate electrolyte balancing are indicated. Especially in digitalised patients, arrythmia can occur or be accentuated even when serum potassium is reduced to low normal range.

Combinations with potassium sparing diuretics should therefore be used, provided there are no renal contraindications.

Initial use of high ceiling diuretics in these patients is only indicated in two situations:

a) threatening clinical symptoms, for the benefit of quicker action, and

b) where thiazides are no longer effective because of concomitant renal insufficiency.

In patients with minimal-range cardiac performance, we adjust the body weight to be optimum. These patients receive a basic therapy with thiazide diuretics. Fluctuations in body weight can be compensated with furosemide, administered by the patient himself. Hypertensive crisis is in most cases due to hyperhydration with renal damage. The critical volume of fluid is often relatively small. The initial therapy, consisting of lowering the blood pressure and redistributing the blood, increasing the venous pooling, will be discussed in detail in the following papers. High ceiling diuretics are always used in this situation to remove the water from the body.

If these substances are not effective, which is for instance the case in

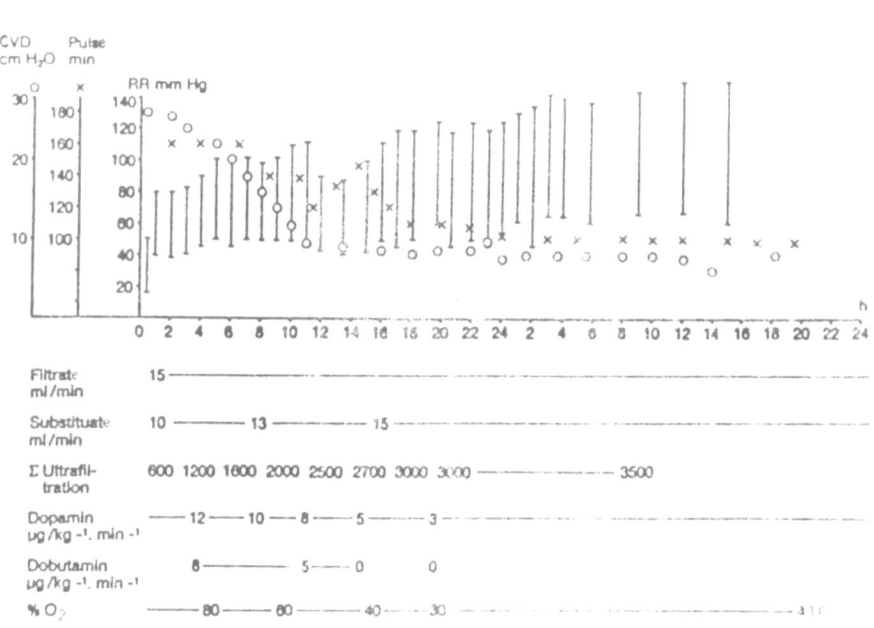

Figure 1. 64 years old patient with myocardial infarction and cardiogenic shock. The high central venous pressure could be reduced by continuous hemofiltration, followed by a diminished pulse rate and rising blood pressure. The amount of catecholamines could be reduced consecutively.

dialysis patients, then haemofiltration or dialysis with ultrafiltration is indicated.

In patients with severe shock, particularly cardiogenic shock, it is often not possible even with maximum doses of catecholamines to raise the blood pressure above the glomerular filtration pressure. An additional volume increase causes a further rise in the already severely elevated central venous pressure and only worsens the patient's condition. Saluretic drugs are not effective here. In such cases the only way of depriving the body of water is by arterio-venous or veno-venous haemofiltration. Often this succeeds in lowering the central venous pressure to a level optimum for the heart and in raising cardiac output. Frequently the blood pressure then rises, with falling catecholamine demand. If acute renal failure has not yet occurred, then once the blood pressure exceeds the glomerular filtration pressure high ceiling diuretics can be used to reinstate adequate diuresis. An example, is shown in Figure 1.

References

1. Baer JE, Fotz EL (1969) Availability of amiloride at distal site of action. Int Congr of Nephrol 4:204
2. Beermann B, Groschinsky-Grind M (1977) Pharmacokinetics of hydrochlorothiazide in mans. Europ J Clin Pharmacol 12:297–303
3. Coraim F, Wolner E (1985) Management of Cardiac Surgery Patients with Continuous Arteriovenous Hemofiltration. In: Sieberth HG, Mann H (eds) Continuous Arteriovenous Hemofiltration (CAVH), München – Paris – London – New York: Karger Verlag, Basel, p 103
4. Coraim F, Fasol R, Stellwag F, Wolner E (1985) Continuous Arteriovenous Hemofiltration (CAVH) after Cardiac Surgery. In Sieberth HG, Mann H (eds) Continuous Arteriovenous Hemofiltration (CAVH), München – Paris – London – New York: Karger Verlag, Basel, p 116
5. Cutler RE, Blair AD (1979) Clinical pharmacokinetics of furosemide. Clin Pharm 4:279–296
6. Deetjen J, Boylan JW, Kramer K (1976) Niere und Wasserhaushalt. In: Gauer, Kramer, Jung (eds) Physiologie des Menschen, 7. München – Berlin – Wien: Verlag Urban & Schwarzenberg
7. Garthoff B, Hanisch M (1984) Muzolimine. Cardiovascular Drugs 2:51–70
8. Greither A, Goldman S, Edelen JS, Benet LZ, Cohn K (1979) Pharmacokinetics of furosemide in patients with congestive heart failure. Pharmacology 19:121–131
9. Herken H (1969) Handbuch der experimentellen Pharmakologie. Bd. XXIV Diuretika. Heidelberg – New York: Springer Verlag Berlin
10. Kaloyamide GJ (1983), Textbook of Nephrology. Massry SG, Glassock RJ (eds) Baltimore – London: Williams and Wilkings, pp 430–441
11. Knauf H, Mutschler E (1980) Pharmakokinetik von Diuretika bei eingeschränkter Nierenfunktion. In: Rosenthal J, Knauf H (eds) Diuretika, Weinheim

12. Kramer P, Wigger W, Rieger J, Matthai D, Scheler F (1977) Arterio-venous hemofiltration. A new and simple method for treatment of over-hydrated patients resistant to diuretics. Klin Wschr 55:1121
13. Lange H (1982) Wasserhaushalt: Oedeme und Überwässerung. Internist 23:710–717
14. Loew D, Ritterm W, Dycka J (1977) Comparison of the pharmacodynamic effects of furosemide and Bay g 2821 and correlation of the pharmacodynamics and pharmacokinetics of Bay g 2821 (Muzolimine). Europ J Clin Pharmacol 12:341–344
15. Truniger B (1978) Diuretika – Kaliumverluste – Kaliummangel und Kaliumsubstitution. Schweiz Med Wschr 108:1009–1912

22. Beta adrenoceptor blocking drugs

BRIAN N.C. PRICHARD

Department of Clinical Pharmacology, University College London and The Middlesex Hospital Medical School, London WC1, U.K.

Pharmacodynamics

The variation in properties of beta adrenoceptor blocking drugs can be used as a basis for classification. There are those which are non-selective, those which have a selective action on the $beta_1$ receptors, and then those drugs which in addition possess vasodilator or alpha receptor blocking properties. They may be further sub-divided into various groups according to the presence or absence of intrinsic sympathomimetic activity (I.S.A) or partial agonist activity and membrane stabilising activity (M.S.A) [1, 2, 3] (Table 1). $Beta_1$ selective drugs have been previously termed 'cardioselective' reflecting their preferential effect on the heart in contrast to certain other tissues, such as bronchial smooth muscle, however as $beta_1$ and $beta_2$ receptors are found in the heart the term 'cardioselective' is inaccurate.

The property of M.S.A. does not appear to be important. The *d*-isomer of proparanolol, for instance, which has the same membrane stabilising action but not the beta blocking effect of racaemic i.e. ordinary proparanolol, lacks anti-hypertensive effect [4, 5], or anti-anginal [6].

Competitive inhibition

Beta adrenoceptor blocking drugs are competitive antagonists, and thus the receptor occupancy is dependent on the ratio of the concentration of agonist and antagonist. It is possible to construct a series of dose response curves to isoprenaline in the presence of increasing doses of beta adrenoceptor antagonist. The dose response curves demonstrate a parallel shift to the right, with the same maximum response being obtained after the various doses of antagonist by increasing the dose of the agonist, isoprenaline [7]. As an increase in agonist overcomes the blockade, there is

V. Hombach, H. H. Hilger and H. L. Kennedy (eds), Electrocardiography and Cardiac Drug Therapy. ISBN 978-94-010-6976-2
© 1989. Kluwer Academic Publishers, Dordrecht –

Table 1. Classification of beta-adrenoceptor blocking drugs

		Partial Agonist Effect (Intrinsic sympathomimetic effect)	Membrane Stabilising Effect (Quinidine like effect)
DIVISION I: NON-SELECTIVE (beta$_1$ + beta$_2$) BLOCK			
Group I	Oxprenolol Alprenolol Penbutolol	+	+
Group II	Propranolol	–	+
Group III	Pindolol Carteolol	+	–
Group IV	Sotalol Timolol Nadolol	–	–
DIVISION II: CARDIOSELECTIVE BLOCK (beta$_1$)			
Group I	Acebutolol	+	+
Group III	Practolol	+	–
Group IV	Atenolol Bisoprolol Metropolol	–	–
DIVISION III: NON-SELECTIVE BLOCK + ALPHA BLOCK/VASODILATOR			
Group II	Labetalol	–	+
DIVISION IV: CARDIOVASCULAR BLOCK + ALPHA BLOCK No example yet available			

therefore no completely beta blocking dose in terms of an exogenous stimulus.

Beta$_1$ selectivity

The ability of beta blocking drugs to inhibit the effect of isoprenaline on the heart shows considerable variation. For equivalent inhibition of exercise tachycardia far less antagonism of the cardiac effects of isoprenaline is seen with the beta$_1$-selective drugs than the non selective agents with or without I.S.A. [8, 9, 10, 11, 12]. The reason for this discrepancy appears to be the presence of β_2 receptors in the atria in addition to β_1 receptors [11, 13, 14]. It does not appear to be due to unopposed β_2 vasodilator activity from isoprenaline following cardioselective blockade. Such a fall in blood pressure could indeed produce vagal de-inhibition, thus cardiac acceleration, minimising any cardiac blockade of isoprenaline. However, the difference is not affected by angiotensin to maintain blood pressure [1], or by prior administration of atropine [15].

A pressor reaction, involving the liberation of adrenaline, e.g. smoking [16], insulin hypoglycaemia [17] tends to be aggrevated when the dilator action of adrenaline is antagonised. The antagonism of the dilator component of adrenaline by non-selective blockade in effect converts the action of adrenaline into that of nonradrenaline [18]. As might be expected therefore pressor responses involving the liberation of adrenaline are differently affected by beta$_1$-selective blockade, for instance the pressor responses to a combination of coffee and cigarettes has been reported to be atenuated by atenolol whereas neither oxprenolol or propranolol had any effect [19]. There is less increase in airways resistance with beta$_1$ blockade than with non-selective blockade and this is the most important difference of the beta$_1$ selective agents [20, 21, 22]. However even the beta$_1$-selective drugs must be regarded as a potential risk in asthmatic subjects [22].

It also appears that beta$_1$-selective drugs result in less of an increase in LDL, less of a fall in HDL than non-selective agents [3]. Also beta$_1$-selective agents do not appear to prolong insulin hypoglycaemia whereas there is some prolongation with non-selective drugs [3, 23]. Lastly beta$_1$ selective agents do not impair the metabolic changes in muscles associated with exercise to the degree seen with other beta blocking drugs [3].

Intrinsic Sympathomimetic Activity (ISA)

Of the various effects of ISA [24], the most marked are the central haemodynamic effects. A drug with a significant degree of ISA results in less of a reduction in resting heart rate [25, 26] and cardiac output [27, 28] and, at least partly because of this, less of a reduction in peripheral blood flow [29, 30, 31]. If prevailing sympathetic tone is low enough (e.g. sleep) and the degree of ISA is sufficient, even an increase in heart rate may be seen from an ISA possessing drug. If the drug possesses beta$_2$ ISA then a peripheral vasodilation action from stimulation of beta$_2$ vasodilator receptors may also be relevant [32]. Provided high levels of exercise are used and full doses of the drugs, a beta blocking drug with ISA gives less of a reduction in heart rate [12, 22]. In asthmatic subjects the modest beta stimulant action on bronchial smooth muscle is not important in this context as these patients are potentially sensitive to any receptor blockade [33]. A drug with ISA down regulates beta receptors and thus when the drug is stopped there is no post beta blocking drug hypersensitivity in contrast to non-ISA agents [24, 34, 35]. Finally there is evidence that the possession of ISA results in less of a disturbance in certain metabolic processes, particularly lipid metabolism, i.e. less increase in VDL or decrease in HDL [3] and also the metabolism of liver metabolised drugs [36].

The combination of beta and alpha blockade or vasodilator activity

Labetalol is the only drug with beta and alpha receptor blocking properties that is widely available at present [7]; it has been extensively evaluated in hypertension [37, 38]. Medroxalol also possesses both beta- and alpha-blocking properties, but probably additional vasodilator effect mediated by beta$_2$ adrenergic stimulation [39, 40]. Its beta- and alpha-blocking properties have been confirmed in man [41] and it is an effective drug in hypertension [42]. Celiprilol has beta$_1$ blocking properties and also a vasodilator action which seems to be a combination of some beta$_2$ stimulatory action besides a direct vasodilator action [43]. It has been shown to be effective in hypertension [44, 45].

Laterly several drugs have been evaluated that possess beta-blocking plus vasodilator activity. Prizidolol [46] after considerable investigation has been withdrawn because of animal toxicity. Bucindolol [47, 48] and carvedilol [49, 50, 51, 52, 53, 54, 55, 56] and other similar drugs are at present in an early stage of evaluation.

Pharmacokinetic properties

There are two broad groups of beta blocking drugs in terms of their pharmacokinetic properties. There are those drugs which are lipid soluble, they undergo extensive first pass metabolism in the liver and readily penetrate the brain, and secondly those that are hydrophilic, excreted unchanged in the urine and have low brain penetration. As the liver metabolism, of the lipid soluble beta blocking drugs, e.g. alprenolol, metoprolol, labetalol, oxprenolol, propranolol, shows variability these compounds exhibit considerable variation in plasma concentration between individuals after the same oral dose [57, 58, 59]. Additionally the relationship between the dose and the area under the plasma concentration curve (AUC) varies at low doses. For example at doses of less than 200 mg of alprenolol [60] or 40 mg propranolol [61], changes in AUC are non linear and smaller incremental increases are seen than at greater dose levels. However, oxprenolol, which undergoes hepatic metabolism, appears to produce a dose related linear increase in plasma concentration from the lowest doses [62]. Although the first pass effect becomes saturated at high doses, even with larger doses of propranolol systemic bioavailability does not exceed 50% [63]. Hepatic metabolism and therefore steady state plasma concentrations depend on hepatic blood flow [58, 64], and thus conditions which reduce liver blood flow, e.g. congestive heart failure, cirrhosis will reduce hepatic clearance and prolong half life. Also those drugs, such as propranolol, which reduce cardiac output and hepatic blood flow will slow their own metablism and that of any other drug metabolised by the liver. Whereas single doses have a plasma elimination half life of two to three hours, it may extend to six hours with chronic administration.

The Lipid solubility of pindolol is also high, however only about 50% of pindolol is metabolised in the liver and therefore first pass effects are less important [65]. Pindolol is less dependent on hepatic blood flow for plasma clearance, as it is also eliminated by renal excretion. The intrinsic sympathomimetic activity of pindolol and oxprenolol means that they have less effect on cardiac output at rest, and thus it would be expected that plasma half lives would be similar after acute and chronic administration [66].

Those compounds which are water soluble are eliminated in the urine as parent drugs or active metabolites. Hydrophilic atenolol and sotalol are excreted unchanged in the urine. Renal insufficiency results in an increase in half life. Atenolol has been reported to have an increase of three to four times in renal insufficiency [67, 68], with sotalol an eight fold increase has been found in end stage renal failure. The water soluble beta blockers reach more predictable plasma concentrations as they are independent of variable liver metabolism. Atenolol, for instance, shows a variation of two to five fold in plasma concentrations between individuals [69, 70], much less than is seen with, for example, propranolol.

The amount of lipid solubility affects the volume of distribution which may vary about eight fold, (0.7–5.6 l/kg for atenolol and propranolol respectively, and mostly exceeds the physiological space [71]. There is a slight reduction of volume of distribution in renal failure or in the elderly, e.g. with sotalol [72]. When the volume of distribution is greater than total body water it is indicative of concentration into certain tissues (particularly lung, liver and heart) as has been confirmed in animal tissues [73, 74]. High liposolubility is associated with rapid penetration across the blood brain barrier, e.g. alprenolol and propranolol [71]. The concentration of propranolol in the brain is about twenty times higher than the concentration of atenolol. The lung is a major organ of deposition for propranolol [73]. Although the lipophilic substances have the larger volumes of distribution, they have shorter plasma elimination half lives, as drug clearance by the liver rather than the kidneys represents a greater capacity for elimination from the body [71].

Uses of beta adrenoceptor blocking drugs in cardiovascular disease

Beta adrenoceptor blocking drugs have become a very widely used group of drugs in cardiovascular medicine, in many indications markedly changing therapeutic practice [75].

Ischaemic heart disease

There is a reduction in oxygen demand of the heart particularly on exercise and under other forms of sympathetic stress, with beta blocking drugs. They reduce heart rate, systolic blood pressure and ventricular contractility, though ventricular size increases which is a factor increasing oxygen consumption, but this only partly offsets the benefit. Overall coronary flow diminishes, presumably due to an autoregulatory effect. There is, however, a redistribution of flow in ischaemia, into the vulnerable areas as the relatively well perfused myocardium uses less oxygen. Besides these haemodynamic effects, beta blockers lower free fatty acid concentration and this improves myocardial utilisation of carbohydrates. Angina pectoris was one of the original indications for beta adrenoceptor blocking drugs, and they have become established as a highly effective prophylactic [38].

There has lately been considerable interest in the phenomenon of silent ischaemia [76]. The majority of episodes of S-T segment depression over 24 hours are not associated with pain. These episodes of 'silent ischaemia' are often haemodynamically indistinguishable from overt ischaemic events. They may, or may not, be preceded by an increase in heart rate. Beta blockade has been shown to be effective in reducing the episodes not preceded by an increase in heart rate.

Beta blocking drugs have been found useful in myocardial infarction. When beta-blockers are administered intravenously infarct size is reduced by about 25%. $Beta_1$ blockade appears to be the necessary component. The pyrexial response which accompanies infarction is also significantly diminished. The number of patients with threatened infarction who go on to develop frank infarction is probably significantly reduced, though this has not been the finding in all studies [77, 78]. The effects on mortality have been less impressive than in late intervention studies. Results of large studies indicated a significant reduction in vascular mortality in the beta-blockers group of about 15% at one week as shown with metoprolol [79] and atenolol [80]. The benefits from i.v. followed by oral beta-blockade are probably most likely to be observed if the i.v. administration occurs within 12 hours of the onset of pain. At one year a significant reduction in mortality is still apparent [80, 81]. The results of studies related to a low risk group of patients cannot be extrapolated to all patients entering a coronary care unit. Pooled data from 28 randomised trials suggest that the incidence of reinfarction and cardiac arrest are significantly decreased (15–18%) by early beta-blockade involving the intravenous route. Few problems have arisen concerning morbidity or adverse reactions with early-entry studies. Bradycardia and hypotension can occur but rarely require active intervention. Cardiogenic shock and heart failure, even in high risk patients, are uncommon [79, 80]: in the case of i.v. beta-blocker given in the very early hours after onset of chest pain, this might reflect salvaged myocardium. The excess usage of inotropic agents occurs mainly on days 0–1, a time coincident with maximal beta-blocker benefit in terms of mortality reduction. Heart block is also uncommmon in the treated groups and is not associated with excess mortality.

The long term administration of beta blockers post infarction, secondary prevention studies, when analysed on an 'intent to treat' basis indicated that beta-blockers decrease total mortality by about 25%. This benefit derives from $beta_1$-blockade; thus both $beta_1$-selective and non-selective agents may be expected to render equal benefit. The pooled results in 'late intervention' trials are highly significant ($P < 0.0001$) [78]. Some have suggested that the possession of ISA reduces benefit. It was found from various studies that when they were pooled there was an approximate 10% decrease in mortality with beta-blockers possessing ISA, significantly less than the approximate 30% with beta-blockers with no ISA [78]. A positive relationship between the decrease in resting heart rate on beta-blocker treatment and the decrease in mortality exists: beta-blockers with moderate-high ISA have little effect on resting heart rate [82].

Hypertension

The beta-adrenoceptor blocking drugs are often used as first choice drugs for hypertension [83]. Although they have been in use for over 20 years their anti-hypertensive mode of action remained a matter for debate. There is a fall of blood pressure regardless of the presence or absence of the associated properties, $beta_1$ selectivity, intrinsic sympathomimetic activity and membrane activity, except perhaps a high level of pure $beta_1$ stimulation. The membrane active non-beta- blocking isomers are without anti-hypertensive effect [5, 84], it therefore seems clear that beta-adrenoceptor blocking drugs lower the blood pressure as a result of their beta-receptor blocking action. A number of attempts have been made to explain the hypotensive effect of beta-adrenergic blocking drugs, including a direct action on the central nervous system, adrenergic neurone blocking perhaps via pre-synaptic beta$_2$ receptors, anti-renin activity, an increase of vasodilator prostaglandins, effects secondary to reduced cardiac output, and resetting of baroreceptors secondary to reduced pressor peaks to various pressor stimuli from the reduction in cardiac activity consequent to beta-blockade. However, the exact mode of action remains unclear [83]. It may be that in some patients one of the many effects may be of overriding importance.

Most attention has been given to a possible correlation to the effect of beta adrenoceptor blocking drugs on the blood pressure and renin levels. Buhler et al. 1975 [85] found patients with high renin levels responded best to propranolol, normal renin patients less well and low renin patients had a poor response. Others have found a good correlation between renin levels and response of blood pressure with a variety of beta adrenoceptor blocking drugs [85, 86]. Hollifield et al. [87] also found propranolol at a relatively low dose of 160 mg a day readily lowered the blood pressure in high renin patients, while higher doses of propranolol, 320–960 mg a day, lowered the blood pressure in low renin patients, independent of effects on renin levels.

On the other hand investigators have not found a correlation between renin levels and response to beta adrenoceptor blocking drugs, with propranolol [88, 89, 90, 91], alprenolol [92], oxprenolol [93], pindolol [91, 94], sotalol [95], timolol [96] or metoprolol [97, 98]. Leonetti et al. [99] for instance found a relatively small dose of propranolol gave full suppression of renin but only a minor lowering of blood pressure whereas only a larger dose above 40 mg a day gave a significant fall in diastolic blood pressure. Similar findings were obtained when propranolol was given to patients already on chlorthalidone [100, 101].

It was demonstrated by Man in't Veld and Schalekamp [29] that while beta adrenoceptor blocking drugs with no intrinsic sympathomimetic activity (ISA) lowered blood pressure and renin levels, those with ISA, like pindolol, lowered blood pressure also but had little effect on renin activity. Lastly it has been found in patients not fully responding to the converting enzyme inhibitor, captopril, that suppressing the renin system the addition of propranolol gave a lowering of blood pressure [102].

Beta blockers compared with other drugs

In a comparison of propranolol up to 640 mg/d with hydrochlorothiazide up to 200 mg/d in a between patient study it was found that hydrochlorothiazide lowered blood pressure by 17.5/13.1 (66% achieving a diastolic blood pressure less than 90 mmHg) and propranolol lowered it by 8.3/11.3 mmHg (53% achieving a diastolic blood pressure less than 90 mmHg). The response to thiazides was best in blacks and the response to propranolol was best in whites [103, 104]. In the MRC study [105], propranolol (up to 240 mg/d) and bendrofluazide (10 mg/d) were equieffective in hypertensives aged 35–44 but propranolol was less effective in older patients. Other non selective beta blocking drugs without ISA, sotalol [106], nadolol [107, 108] and timolol [109] appear similar to thiazide diuretics in their antihypertensive effect. The same is true for non selective agents with ISA, oxprenolol [110, 111], pindolol [112]. There is some evidence that beta$_1$ selective drugs may be more effective than diuretics, as shown by studies with atenolol [113, 114], and metoprolol [115]. Diuretics have been found by others to be similar with metoprolol [116] or acebutolol [117]. Studies in the elderly have found atenolol similar to diuretics in their effect [118]. Spironolactone (100 mg/d) has been found to be similar to 160 mg/d [119] or 320 mg/d propranolol [120] and 1–2 Moduretic was observed to have an equivalent effect to 80–320 mg nadolol [121].

The calcium antagonist verapramil and beta blockers are probably equally effective in lowering blood pressure though verapamil appears more effective in older patients and beta blockers more effective in younger subjects [122, 123]. Nitrendipine 40 mg/d has been shown to be similar to 240–280 mg propranolol [124, 125] while atenolol (100 g) was similar to nitrendepine (20 mg/day) [126]. Nifedipine has also been found to have a similar anti-hypertensive effect to metoprolol [127] and to atenolol in black patients [128].

Propranolol up to 360 mg a day has been found to be equivalent to up to 450 mg/d captopril in various races, Caucasian [129, 130] Indian and Negros [131]. In the presence of a diuretic then 60–120 mg/d propranolol has been found to be as effective as 37.5–75 mg/d captopril [132]. Patients with systolic hypertension had a similar effect from 120 mg/d propranolol and 25–50 mg/d captopril [133]. Atenolol has also been found to be overall similar in its antihypertensive efficacy to captopril [134]. Enalapril in doses of 20–80 mg/d has been shown to be similar to propranolol 160–480 mg/d [135, 136, 137]. Others have found 10–40 mg/d enalapril to produce a greater effect than 80–240 mg/d propranolol [138]. Several investigators have reported atenolol and enalapril similar in effect [139, 140, 141], but others have found a greater effect from enalapril [142], others vice versa [143].

It has been observed that prazosin 2–24 mg produced the same effect on the supine blood pressure but much more on the standing levels than propranolol 80–480 mg/d [144]. Similar reductions of supine and standing blood pressure were obtained by up to 100 mg hydrochlorthiazide, up to

320 mg/d propranolol, and to up to 20 mg/d prazosin, but the greatest effect on exercise blood pressure was obtained with propranolol [145]. Clonidine (0.15 to 0.30 mg/d) is as effective as 120–240 mg propranolol [146].

Orthostatic hypotension

Some attempt has been made to treat orthostatic hypotension with beta receptor blocking drugs. The rationale has been the expectation the $beta_2$ blockade would allow the unopposed alpha constrictor activity of circulating adrenaline to improve the blood pressure. Some reports show good results with pindolol (moderate ISA) [147] or propranolol, but others have not found either drug effective [148]. Some promising results have been obtained with agents with ISA such as prenalterol or xamaterol [149], which may also give additional benefit by maintaining or increasing cardiac output.

Valvular disease

Postural hypotension accompanied by faintness and syncope has been described with mitral valve prolapse [150]. It was found in 7 patients that falls of mean systolic blood pressure from 114 to 78 mmHg on standing and accompanying symptoms were abolished by oral propranolol (80–160 mg/day) given for 4–6 weeks.

Beta blockade reduces the pressure gradient across the mitral valve in mitral stenosis by allowing longer for diastolic filling. This has been shown in pure mitral stenosis after intravenous propranolol and after chronic oral administration [75].

There have been few studies in aortic stenosis. Stockins et al. 1985 found one weeks atenolol (100 mg) improved exercise tolerance and reduced exercise induced angina and dyspnoea.

Arrhythmias

The efficacy of beta blocking drugs varies considerably according to the type of arrhythmia. Catecholamines increase the rate of diastolic depolarisation of automatic pacemaker cells and thus increase the rate of impulse formation, speed the conduction process through the A-V node and shorten the refractory period. They also produce a shortening of the refractory period of ventricular cells and so predispose to extrasystoles by re-entry and the threshold to ventricular fibrillation is lowered [151]. Beta blocking drugs act in arrhythmias to inhibit these influences [152] but also they may act indirectly to modify the process which predisposes to arrhythmias e.g. myocardial ischaemia, thryotoxicosis, anaesthesia etc. [75].

All the evidence suggests that the direct antiarrhythmic property of beta-blockers is via $beta_1$-blockade [75]. Although they have less effect on stress induced hypokalaemia, it appears that they and non-selective agents are equally effective in inhibiting stress-induced arrhythmias. In conditions of high sympathetic tone beta-blockers with and without ISA have similar antiarrhythmic effects. In experimental animals or with catecholamine depletion with reserpine beta-blockers with high ISA e.g. pindolol, can increase heart rate and lower the threshold to ventricular fibrillation. The membrane stabilising activity is manifest only at very high dosages [153] e.g. propranolol over 640 mg/day, where a quinidine-like antiarrhythmic effect might be observed [75]. Sotalol differs from the other beta-blockers in possessing a class III effect [154, 155] when administered acutely, i.e. involving a lengthening of the monophasic action potential duration, increasing the Q-T interval, prolonging atrial and ventricular effective refractory periods and also prolonging the refractoriness of accessory pathways.

Supraventricular tachycardias

The ectopic atrial tachycardias are often associated with increased sympathetic activity and may respond well to a beta-blocker [156] but multifocal atrial tachycardia occurring in association with pulmonary disease is usually unresponsive.

Paroxysmal supraventricular tachycardias not due to pre-excitation often respond to intravenous beta blockade with a return to sinus rhythm and vagal manoeuvres are often more successful in the presence of a beta-blocker [157]. Oral beta blockers are often successful in preventing the onset of these arrhytmias, particularly if the arrhythmia is precipitated by emotion or exercise [151]. Sotalol, with its additional class III properties, is probably superior to other beta-blockers in benefitting patients with SVT [158]. The effective refractory period of accessory pathways involved in supra-ventricular tachycardias arising from pre-excitation e.g. Wolff-Parkinson-White Syndrome, are unaffected by beta-blockers other than sotalol with its Class III properties. However, by modifying conduction and refractoriness in the A-V node or supressing initiating premature beats, intravenous [159] or oral propranolol can be very effective in supressing or preventing these arrhythmias, particularly in children or if combined with quinidine [159]. Atrial flutter and fibrillation complicating the WPW syndrome should not be treated with beta-blockade.

Atrial fibrillation may be converted to sinus rhythm by beta blockade if the precipitating cause involves a high sympathetic tone e.g. exercise [157]. Longstanding cases rarely convert to sinus rhythm [160] but a useful slowing of the heart rate at rest and with exercise may be achieved if higher dosage of digoxin is contraindicated [157]. Atrial flutter, like fibrillation, rarely converts to sinus rhythm with beta-blockers, but a slowing of the heart rate by increasing the A-V block can be useful [157, 161].

Ventricular arrhythmias

Ventricular premature beats which occur in the presence of ischaemic heart disease, or that are induced by exercise, stress or emotion, may respond to beta blockade [162]. Sustained ventricular tachycardia often does not respond to beta-blockers and there is the additional risk of precipitating heart failure in the presence of severe heart disease. Paroxysmal ventricular tachycardia, particularly if induced by high sympathetic activity, responds to either non-selective or beta$_1$ selective beta blockade [157]. Ventricular tachycardia is a medical emergency and cardioversion should be employed. A beta blocker can sometimes be helpful in this process. Recurrent ventricular tachycardia induced by stress or exercise, particularly in children, responds well to beta-blockade [75].

Ventricular arrhythmias arising from digitalis toxicity often show a response to beta-blockers. However beta-blockers cannot be regarded as the drugs of choice in view of the risk of heart block which can sometimes be fatal [157].

Beta-blockers are the drugs of choice in the prevention of ventricular premature beats, ventricular tachycardia and fibrillation associated with a prolapsing mitral valve. This has been found with lethal ventricular arrhythmia prevention in the long Q-T syndrome so that a 73% mortality rate in the hereditary (but not idiopathic) variety has been reduced to 6% by propranolol [75].

Outflow tract obstruction

Fallot's tetralogy patients may experience attacks of severe cyanosis and syncope, often precipitated by effort, crying or stress. These attacks are associated with shut-down of the right ventricular outflow tract with disappearance of the systolic murmur, and are thought to be due to stimulation of the hypertrophied right ventricular outflow tract by catecholamines. This has been the rationale for the use of beta blocking drugs. The intravenous administration of propranolol improves pulmonary artery flow and arterial oxygen saturation in most cases [163]. The use of long term oral propranolol, given in suitable dosage (as high as 6 mg/kg/day or more) is highly effective in abolishing syncopal attacks and improving effort tolerance [164]. Side effects are uncommon, but break-through syncopal attacks occasionally occur. Oral propranolol is probably preferable to palliative shunt surgery in buying time before corrective surgery. This applies also to some patients with unpromising cardiac anatomy e.g. pulmonary atresia. The mortality of corrective surgery is high in the first 18 months of life and propranolol can normally be given for a time so that safer surgery can be performed when the child is older [164].

Patients who have hypertrophic obstructive cardiomyopathy have an outflow tract gradient which may appear only with sympathetic stimulation such as isoprenaline infusion or exercise. The intravenous administration of beta-blockers usually diminishes such a gradient and usually improves left ventricular compliance or distensibility. Sudden death is often effort-related [165]. There is thus a good rationale for the long-term use of beta blockers. Provided an optimal beta-blocking dose is given, e.g. propranolol 320–460 mg/day, symptoms may be abolished or diminished and there may be a decrease in sudden death [166].

Congestive cardiomyopathy

The aetiology of congestive cardiomyopathy (COCM) is unknown [165]. However catecholamines are known to have toxic myocardial effects and patients with COCM may be hypersensitive as there is a down-regulation of cardiac $beta_1$-receptors. It is possible that beta-blockers diminish the effect of catecholamines, decreasing heart rate. This results in a decreased myocardial oxygen requirement and an up-regulation of cardiac $beta_1$ receptors [75]. Beta-blockers given initially in low dosage can benefit patients with COCM-improved effort tolerance, decrease in heart size, improved diastolic function and an increase in ejection fraction, mortality may also be improved [167]. The beneficial effects may not be seen for weeks or months, but improvement can occur up to 2 years or more [168]. Not all patients benefit and some are precipitated into heart failure and shock, even with initial very low dosage.

Phaeochromocytoma

A phaeochromocytoma is characterised by the secretion of high levels of noradrenaline and adrenaline. Severe hypertension and arrhythmias can thus occur, providing the reasons for using alpha- and beta-blockade. Phenoxybenzamine is the alpha-blocker most often used for the treatment of hypertension. A beta-blocker is often needed to counteract increased beta activity after phenoxybenzamine—propranolol has been most often employed. Such a combination provides good preparation for the removal of the tumour and diminishes problems of hypertension and arrhythmias, and reverses hypovolaemia associated with peripheral vasoconstriction [169, 170]. Labetalol combining alpha and beta blocking activity has also been employed [38]. A beta blocker given alone can give rise to unopposed alpha activity and an excessive rise in blood pressure [18].

Anxiety

Anxiety patients may experience predominantly cardiovascular symptoms such as palpitations, excessive effort dyspnoea, fatigue, precordial discomfort and sometimes tremor and sweating. The symptoms are like those of sympathetic overstimulation and this is the rationale for treatment with beta-blockers; Beta-blockers, in low dosage, are effective in mitigating or abolishing cardiovascular symptoms and signs [171, 172].

Portal hypertension

There is a reduction in portal venous pressure from beta blockade because cardiac output falls, and possibly also because of $beta_2$-blockade resulting in unopposed alpha-induced vasoconstriction in the hepatic artery. The non-selective drugs, giving a fall of 20–25% in portal pressure, are probably more effective than $beta_1$-selective agents [173]. Labetalol, with alpha- and beta-blocking properties, is relatively ineffective in lowering portal venous pressure [174]. There is evidence to suggest that oral propranolol (40–360 mg/day) markedly diminished the incidence of haematemesis and possibly death, in cirrhotic patients who had a history of gastrointestinal bleeding [175]. However, not all studies have confirmed these results. Patient selection may explain these differences.

312

Dissection of the aorta

Dissection of the aorta is a highly lethal condition and without treatment 90% of patients will be dead within 3 months of the event [176]. Hypertension is commonly present. Medical treatment is aimed at lowering the blood pressure, but also it is desirable to reduce left ventricular ejection velocity. Thus, whether high blood pressure is present or not, i.v. beta-blockade should be administered, propranolol 0.15 mg/kg or its equivalent with other agents. Blood pressure if high may be acutely lowered with, for instance, nitroprusside [177]. For distal dissections long-term medical therapy, rather than surgery, may be desirable, the goal being good antihypertensive control and a decrease in left ventricular ejection velocity [177]. As beta$_1$-blockade is desirable the choice of beta-blocker is unimportant, unless there is a contraindication to beta$_2$-blockade e.g. asthma, in which case a beta$_1$-selective agent should be cautiously tried. Late survival can be expected to be reduced from 90% untreated to about 40–50% treated by medical or surgical means [177, 178].

Subarachnoid haemorrhage

This extremely stressful occurrence is associated with high levels of catecholamines. There are bizarre ECG abnormalities and focal myocardial necrosis in those patients with particularly high catecholamine levels and are associated with a poor prognosis. Many of the ECG abnormalities can be abolished by the administration of propranolol and prophylactic beta-blockade which prevents catecholamine-induced myocardial necrosis [179]. The administration of propranolol (80 mg tds) started within 48 hours of the SAH and continued for 3 weeks has been found to lead to a significantly lower incidence of CNS complications. At 1 year follow-up there were significantly fewer deaths and disabled patients in the treated group [180].

Head injury

Cardiovascular and metabolic signs of marked sympathetic overactivity occur with the severe trauma associated with head injury. Continuous ECG monitoring indicated that ischaemics and arrhythmics occur. Myocardial damage, presumably catecholamine-induced, is indicated by raised serum CKMB (cardiac isoenzyme) and necropsy findings. The administration of intravenous atenolol for 3 days followed by oral for 4 days significantly decreased the incidence of supraventricular arrhythmias, diminished the plasma concentration of CKMB and prevented catecholamine-induced myocardial necrosis [181].

Conclusion

The beta adrenoceptor blocking drugs 25 years after their first introduction remain an area of continuing investigation with new compounds still being developed. Likewise all the many indications of beta blocking drugs have yet to be fully exploited.

References

1. Fitzgerald JD (1972) Beta adrenergic blocking drugs. Present position and future developments. Acta Cardiol (Brux) 15 Suppl XV:199–216
2. Prichard BNC (1978) β-adrenergic receptor blockade in hypertension, past, present and future. Br J Clin Pharmacol 5:379–399
3. Prichard BNC, Tomlinson B (1986) The additional properties of beta adrenoceptor blocking drugs. J Cardiovasc Pharmacol 8 (Suppl 4):S1–S15
4. Waal-Manning HJ (1970) Comparative studies on the hypotensive effects of beta-adrenergic receptor blockade. In: Simpson FO (ed.) Symposium on beta-adrenergic receptor blocking drugs. Ciba, Auckland p 64
5. Prichard BNC, Boakes AJ (1977) The use of beta-adrenergic blocking drugs in hypertension: A review. Curr Med Res Opin 4 (Suppl 5):51–76
6. Wilson AG, Brooke OG, Lloyd HJ, Robinson BF (1969) Mechanism of action of beta-adrenergic receptor blocking agents in angina pectoris: comparison of action of propranolol with dexpropranolol and practolol. Br Med J 4:399–401
7. Richards DA, Prichard BNC, Boaks AJ, Tuckman J, Knight EJ (1977) Pharmacological basis for antihypersensitive effects of intravenous labetalol. Br Heart J 39:99–106
8. Briant RH, Dollery CT, Fenyvesi T, George CF (1973) Assessment of selective beta-adrenoceptor blockade in man. Br J Pharmacol 49:106–114
9. Graham BR, Littlejohns DW, Prichard BNC, Scales B, Southorn P (1973) Preliminary observations on the human pharmacology of ICI 66082 in normal volunteers. Br J Pharmacol 49:154P–155P
10. Walden RJ, Bhattacharjee P, Tomlinson B, Cashin J, Graham BR, Prichard BNC (1982) The effect of intrisic sympathomimetic activity on beta receptor responsiveness after beta adrenoceptor blockade withdrawal. Br J Clin Pharmacol 13:359S–364S
11. McGibney D, Singleton W, Silke B, Taylor SH (1983) Observations on the mechanism underlying the differences in exercise and isoprenaline tachycardia after cardioselective and non-selective β-adrenoceptor antagonists. Br J Clin Pharmacol 15:15–19
12. Tomlinson B, Bhattacharjee P, Graham BR, Hill JM, Raeburn J, Prichard, BNC (1984) A comparison of penbutolol with atenolol and long-acting propranolol. Br J Clin Pharmacol 17:117–182
13. Andersson K-E (1982) Drugs blocking adrenoceptors. Acta Med Scand (Suppl) 665:9–17

314

14. Zerkowski H-R, Ikezono K, Rohm N, Reidemeister J Chr, Brodde O-E (1986) Human myocardial beta-adrenoceptors: demonstration of both beta$_1$ and beta$_2$-adrenoceptors mediating contractile responses to beta-agonists on the isolated right atrium. Naunyn-Schmiedeberg's Arch Pharmacol 322:142–147

15. Arnold JMO, McDevitt DG (1982) Interpretation of isoprenaline dose-response curves in the presence of selective and non-selective β-adrenoceptor blocking drugs. Br J Clin Pharmacol 13:585p

16. Trap-Jensen J, Carlsen JE, Svendsen TL, Christensen NJ (1979) Cardiovascular and adrenergic effects of cigarette smoking during immediate non-selective and selective beta adrenoceptor blockade in humans. Eur J Clin Invest 9:181–183

17. Davidson NMcD, Corrall RJM, Shaw TRD, French EB (1977) Observations in man of hypoglycaemia during selective and non-selective beta blockade. Scott Med J 22:69–72

18. Prichard BNC, Ross EJ (1966) Use of propranolol in conjunction with alpha-receptor blocking drugs in phaeochromocytoma. Am J Cardiol 18:394–398

19. Freestone S, Ramsay LE (1983) Effect of beta-blockade on the pressor response to coffee plus smoking in patients with mild hypertension. Drugs 25 Suppl 2:141–145

20. Tattersfield AE, Harrison RN (1983) Effect of β-blocker therapy on airway function. Drugs 25 (Suppl 2) 227–231

21 Decalmer PBS, Chattarjee SS, Cruickshank JM, Benson MK, Sterling GM (1978) Beta-blockers and asthma. Br Heart J 40:184–189

22. McDevitt DG (1987) Pharmacologic aspects of cardioselectivity in a beta-blocking drug. Am J Cardiol 59:10F–12F

23. Kendall MJ (1987) Impact of beta$_1$ selectivity and intrinsic sympathomimetic activity on potential unwanted noncardiovascular effects of beta blockers. Am J Cardiol 59:44F–47F

24. Prichard BNC (1987) Pharmacologic aspects of intrinsic sympathomimetic activity in beta-blocking drugs. Am J Cardiol 59:13F–17F

25 Prichard BNC, Aellig WH, Richardson GA (1970a) The action of intravenous oxprenolol, practolol, propranolol and sotalol on acute exercise tolerance in angina pectoris: The effect on heart rate and the electrocardiogram. Postgrad Med J 46 (Suppl Nov):77–85

26. Kostis JB, Frishman W, Hosler MH, Thorsen NL, Gonasun L, Weinstein J (1982) Treatment of angina pectoris with pindolol: the significance of intrinsic sympathomimetic activity of beta blockers. Am Heart J 104:495–504

27. Svendsen TL, Hartling O, Trap-Jensen J (1979) Immediate haemodynamic effects of propranolol, practolol, pindolol, atenolol and ICI 89406 in healthy volunteers. Eur J Clin Pharmacol 15:223–228

28. Taylor SH, Silke B, Lee PS, Hilal A (1982) Haemodynamic dose-response effects of intravenous beta-blocking drugs with different ancillary properties in patients with coronary heart disease. Eur Heart J 3:564–569

29. Man In 't Veld AJ, Schalekamp MADH (1982) How intrinsic sympathomimetic activity modulates the haemodynamic responses to beta-adrenoceptor antagonists. A clue to the nature of their antihypertensive mechanism. Br J Clin Pharmacol 13 (Suppl 2):245S–257S

30. Svensson A, Gudbrandsson T, Sivertsson R, Hansson L (1982) Haemodynamic effects of metoprolol and pindolol: a comparison in hypertensive patients. Br J Clin Pharmacol 13: 259S–267S

31. Man in't Veld AJ (1987) Effect of beta blockers on vascular resistanin ce systemic hypertension. Am J Cardiol 50:21F–25F

32. Chang PC, Blauw GJ, Van Brummelen P (1983) Pindolol: a beta-blocker with vasodilating properties due to stimulation of vascular β_2 adrenoceptors. Journal of Hypertension 1 Suppl 2:338–339

33. McDevitt DG (1978) β-adrenoceptor antagonists and respiratory function. Br J Clin Pharmacol 5:97–99

34. Prichard BNC, Tomlinson B, Walden RJ, Bhattacharjee P (1983) The β-adrenergic blockade withdrawal phenomenon. J Cardiovasc Pharmacol 5:S56–S62

35. Frishman WH (1987) Clinical significance of beta$_1$ selectivity and intrinsic sympathomimetic activity in a beta-adrenergic blocking drug. Am J Cardiol 59:33F–37F

36. Lysbo Svendsen T, Tango M, Waldorff S, Steiness E, Trap-Jensen J (1982) Effects of propranolol and pindolol on plasma lignocaine clearance in, man. Br J Clin Pharmacol 13:223S–226S

37. Lund-Johansen P, Omvik P (1984) Long-term haemodynamic effects of enalapril (alone and in combination with hydrochlorothiazide) at rest and during exercise in essential hypertension. J Hypertension 2 (Suppl 2):49–56

38. Prichard BNC (1984) Combined a- and b-receptor inhibition in the treatment of hypertension. Drugs 28 (Suppl 2):51–68

39. Dage RC, Cheng HC, Woodward JK (1981) Cardiovascular properties of medroxalol, a new anti-hypertensive drug. J Cardiovasc Pharmacol 3:299–315

40. Dage RC, Hsieh CP, Spedding M (1983) Vasodilation by medroxalol mediated by beta-2 adrenergic receptor stimulation. J Cardiovasc Pharmacol 5:143–150

41. Jaillon P, Weissenburger J, Biour M, Cheymol G, Haegele K, Schechter PJ, Koch-Wester J (1982) Beta- and alpha-adrenoceptor antagonism by medraxolol in healthy volunteers: relationship to dose and plasma concentration. J Cardiovasc Pharmacol 4:705–713

42. Schechter PJ, Tanskanen A, Tuomilehto J, Koch-Weser J (1982) Treatment of mild and moderate hypertension with medroxalol, and alpha- and beta-adrenergic antagonist. J Cardiovasc Pharmacol 4:955–959

43. Pruss TP, Khandwala A, Wolf PS, Grebow P, Wong L (1986) Celiprolol: A new beta adrenoceptor antagonist with novel ancillary properties. J Cardiovasc Pharmacol 8 (Suppl 4):S29–S32

44. Capone P, Mayol R (1986) A placebo-controlled double-blind multicenter study of celiprolol in the treatment of mild and moderate hypertension. J Cardiovasc Pharmacol 8 (Suppl 4):S119–S121

45. Silke B, Verma SP, Frais MA, Reynolds G, Taylor SH (1986) Differential actions of atenolol and celiprolol on cardiac performance in ischemic heart disease. J Cardiovasc Pharmacol 8 (Suppl 4):S138–S144

46. Lund-Johansen P, Omvik P (1982) Prizidilol in essential hypertension: Long-term effects on plasma volume, extracellular fluid volume and central haemodynamics at rest and during exercise. J Cardiovasc Pharmacol 4:1012–1017

47. Dietchman D, LaBudde JA, Seidehamel RJ (1983) Bucindolol New Drugs Annual: Cardiovascular Drugs Scriabine, A (ed.) New York, Raven Press, 1983 pp 1–18

48. Malini PL, Strocchi E, Ambrosioni E (1983) Comparison of the anti-hypertensive efficacy of bucindolol and propranolol. J Hypertension 1 (Suppl. 2):348–350

49. Schnurr E, Widmann L, Glocke M (1987) Efficacy and safety of carvedilol in the treatment of hypertension. J Cardiovasc Pharmacol (In Press)

50. Eggertsen R, Sivertsson R, Andrén L, Hansson L (1987) Acute and long-term hemodynamic effects of carvedilol, a combined beta-adrenoceptor blocking and precapillary vasodilating agent, in hypertensive patients. J Cardiovasc Pharmacol (In Press)

51. Dupont AG, Van der Niepen P, Taeymans Y, Ingels M, Piepsz A, Bossuyt AM, Block P, Six RO, Jonckheer MH, Vanhaelst L (1987) Effect of carvedilol on ambulatory blood pressure, renal hemodynamics and cardiac function in essential hypertension. J Cardiovasc Pharmacol (In Press)

52. Morgan T, Snowden R, Butcher L (1987) Effect of carvedilol and metoprolol on blood pressure, blood flow and vascular resistance. J Cardiovasc Pharmacol (In Press)

53. Meyer-Sabellek W, Schulte K-L, Distler A, Gotzen R (1987) Circadian antihypertensive profile of carvedilol (BM14190). J Cardiovasc Pharmacol (In Press)

54. Ogihara T, Ikeda M, Goto Y, Yoshinaga K, Kumahara Y, Iimura O, Ishi M, Murakami E, Takeda T, Kokubu T, Arakawa K (1987) The effect of low dose carvedilol on circadian variation of blood pressure in patients with essential hypertension. J Cardiovasc Pharmacol (In Press)

55. Tanaka M, Masumura H, Tanaka S, Akashi A (1987) Studies on antihypertensive properties of carvedilol, a compound with beta-blocking and vasodilating effects. J Cardiovasc Pharmacol (In Press)

56. Abshagen U (1987) A new molecule with vasodilating and β-adrenoceptor blocking properties. J Cardiovasc Pharmacol (In Press)

57. Shand DG (1974) Pharmacokinetic properties of β-adrenergic receptor blocking drugs. Drugs 7:39–47

58. Routledge PA, Shand DG (1979) Clinical pharmacokinetics of propranolol. Clin Pharmacokinet 4:73–90

59. Melander A, Danielson K, Schersten B, Wahlin E (1977) Enhancement of the bioavailability of propranolol and metoprolol by food. Clin Pharmacol Ther 22:108–112

60. Ablad B, Ervik M, Hallgren J, Johnsson G, Solvell L (1972) Pharmacological effects and serum levels of orally administered alprenolol in man. Eur J Clin Pharmacol 5:44–52

61. Shand DG, Rangno RE (1972) The disposition of propranolol. I. Elimination during oral absorption in man. Pharmacol 7:159–168

62. Riess W, Brechbuhler S, Brunner L, Imhof PR, Jack DB (1974) The metabolism of β-blockers in relation to their pharmacokinetic and pharmacodynamic behaviour. In: Schweizer W (ed.) Beta blockers – present status and future prospects. Ciba, Horsham: UK pp 276–289

63. Nies AS, Shand DG (1975) Clinical pharmacology of propranolol. Circulation 52: 6–15

64. Shand DG, Branch RA, Evans GH, Nies AS, Wilkinson GR (1973) The disposition of propranolol. VII. The effects of saturable hepatic tissue uptake on drug clearance by the perfused rat liver. Drug Metab Dispos 1:679–686

65. Gugler R, Herold W, Dengler HJ (1974) Pharmacokinetics of pindolol in man. Eur J Clin Pharmacol 7:17–24

66. Gugler R, Bodem G (1978) Single and multiple does pharmacokinetics of pindolol. Eur J Clin Pharmacol 13:13–16

67 Sassard J, Pozet N, McAinsh J, Legheand J, Zech P (1977) Pharmacokinetics of atenolol in patients with renal impairment. Eur J Clin Pharmacol 12:175–180

68. Wan SH, Koda RT, Maronde RF (1979) Pharmacokinetics, pharmacology or atenolol and effect of renal disease. Br J Clin Pharmacol 7:569–574

69. Brown HC, Carruthers SG, Johnston GD, Kelly JG, McAinsh J, McDevitt DG, Shanks RG (1976) Clinical pharmacologic observations on atenolol, a β-adrenoceptor blocker. Clin Pharmacol Ther 20:524–534

70. Fitzgerald JD, Ruffin R, Smedstad R, Roberts R, McAinsh J (1978) Studies on the pharmacokinetics and pharmacodynamics of atenolol in man. Eur J Clin Pharmacol 13:81–89

71. Johnsson G, Regardh C-G (1976) Clinical pharmacokinetics of β-adrenoceptor blocking drugs. Clin Pharmacokinet 1:233–263

72. Ishizaki T, Hirayama H, Tawara K, Nakaya H, Sato M, Sato K (1980) Pharmacokinetics and pharmacodynamics in young normal and elderly hypertensive subjects: a study using sotalol as a model drug. J Pharmacol Exp Ther 212:173–181

73. Dollery CT, Junod AF (1976) Concentration of (+) – propranolol in isolated, perfused lungs of rat. Br J Pharmacol 57:67–71

74. Bodin N-O, Borg, K-O, Johansson R, Obianwu H, Svensson R (1974) Absorption, distribution and excretion of alprenolol in man, dog and rat. Acta Pharmacol Toxicol 35:261–269

75. Cruickshank JM, Prichard BNC (1988) Beta-Blockers in Clinical Practice. Churchill Livingstone (In Press)

76. Pepine CJ, Lambert CR, Hill JA, Imperi G, Norvell N (1987) Silent myocardial ischemia: rationale for management

77. Yusuf S, Sleight P (1983) Limitation of myocardial infarct size. Drugs 25:441–450

78. Yusuf S, Peto R, Lewis J, Collins R, Sleight P (1985) Beta-blockade during and after myocardial infarction: an overview of the randomised trials. Prog Cardiovasc Dis XXVII(5):335–371

79. MIAMI Trial Research Group (1985) Metoprolol in acute myocardial infarction (MIAMI). A randomised placebo-controlled international trial. Eur Heart J 6:199–226

80. ISIS-I (First International Study of Infarct Survival) Collaborative Group (1986) Randomised trial of intravenous atenolol among 16 027 cases of suspected acute myocardial infarction: ISIS-I. Lancet 2:57–66

81. Herlitz J, Hjalmarson A, Swedberg K, Vedin A, Waagstein F, Waldenstrom A, Wilhelmsson C (1986) The influence of early intervention in acute myocardial infarction on long-term mortality and morbidity as assessed in the Goteborg metoprolol trial. Int J Cardiol 10:291–301

82 Kjekshus J (1985) Comments—beta-blockers: heart rate reduction a mechanism of benefit. Eur Heart J 6 (Suppl A):29–30

83. Prichard BNC, Owens CWI (1984) Clinical Pharmacology of Beta-Adrenoceptor Blocking Drugs. In: Kostis JB, De Felice EA (eds) Beta Blockers in the Treatment of Cardiovascular Disease Raven Press New York: pp. 1–56

84. Waal-Manning HJ (1970) Comparative studies on the hypotensive effects of beta-adrenergic receptor blockade. In: Simpson FO (ed.) Symposium on beta-adrenergic receptor blocking drugs. 1970 Auckland: Ciba p. 64

85. Buhler FR, Burkart F, Lutold BE, Kung M, Marbet G, Pfisterer M (1975) Anti-hypertensive beta blocking action as related to renin and age: a pharmacologic tool to identify pathogenic mechanisms in essential hypertension. Am J Cardiol 36:653–669

86. Castenfors H (1977) Long term effects of timolol and hydrochlorthiazide or hydro-chlorthiazide and amiloride in essential hypertension. Eur J Clin Pharmacol 12:97–103

87. Hollifield JW, Sherman K, Vander Zwaag R, Shand DG (1976) Proposed mechanisms of propranolol's anti-hypertensive effect in essential hypertension. New Engl J Med 295–73

88. Bravo EL, Tarazi RC, Dustan HP, Lewis JW (1975) Dissociation between renin and arterial pressure responses to beta-adrenergic blockade in human essential hypertension. Circ Res Supp I:36–37

89. Hansson L (1973) Beta-adrenergic blockade in essential hypertension. Effects of pro-pranolol on haemodynamic parameters and plasma renin activity. Acta Med Scand 55 (Suppl 1):1–40

90. Leonetti G, Mayer G, Morganti A, Terzoli L, Zanchetti A, Bianchetti G, DiSalle E, Morselli PL, Chidsey CA (1975) Hypotensive and renin supressing activities of pro-pranolol in hypertensive patients. Clin Sci Mol Med 48:491–499

91. Morgan TO, Roberts R, Carney SI, Louis WJ, Doyle AF (1975) Beta adrenergic receptor blocking drugs, hypertension and plasma renin. Br J Clin Pharmacol 2:159–164

318

92. Pedersen EB, Kornerup HJ (1977) Plasma renin concentration in essential hypertension during beta-adrenergic blockade and vasodilator therapy. Eur J Clin Pharmacol 12:93–96

93. Gavras I, Gavras H, Sullivan PC, Tifft CP, Chobanian AV, Brunner HR (1979) A comparative study of the effects of oxprenolol versus propranolol in essential hypertension. J Clin Pharmacol 19:8–14

94. Anavekar SN, Louis WJ, Morgan TO, Doyle AE, Johnston CI (1975) The relationship of plasma levels of pindolol in hypertensive patients to effect on blood pressure, plasma-renin and plasma noradrenaline levels. Clin Exper Pharmacol and Physiol 2:203–212

95. Verniory A, Staroukine M, Telerman M, Delwiche F (1974) Effect of sotalol on arterial pressure and renin-angiotensin system in hypertensive patients. In: Sotalol E. Smart (ed.) Clinical Advances in beta-blocking therapy. Amsterdam: Excerpta Medica IV:36–45

96. Simon G, Kiowski W, Julius S (1978) Anti-hypertensive and beta-adrenoceptor antagonist action of timolol. J Clin Pharmacol Ther 23:152–157

97. Genest J, Dornier A, Boucher R, Nowaczynski W, Rojo-Ortega JM, Kuchel O (1976) β-adrenergic blocking agents and renin spectrum. In: Scriabine A, Sweet CS (eds) New Anti-Hypertensive Drugs. New York: Spectrum, pp 215–226

98, Hansson BG, Dymling JF, Hedeland H, Hulthen UL (1977) Long-term teratment of moderate hypertension with the beta$_1$-receptor blocking agent metoprolol. Eur J Clin Pharmacol 11:239–245

99. Leonetti G, Mayer G, Morganti A, Terzoli L, Zanchetti A, Bianchetti G, DiSalle E, Morselli PL, Chidsey CA (1975) Hypotensive and renin supressing activities of propranolol in hypertensive patients. Clin Sci Mol Med 48:491–499

100. Morganti AA, Terzoli L, Sala C, Bianchini C, Leonetti G, Zanchetti AS (1979b) Interactions between diuretics and propranolol in treatment of arterial hypertension. Cardiovascular Medicine 4:43–52

101 Zanchetti A, Leonetti G, Terzoli L, Sala C (1983) Beta-blockers and renin. Drugs (Symposium on beta-blockers in the 1980's) 25 (Suppl 2):58–63

102 Staessen J, Fagard R, Lijnen P, Verschueren LJ, Amery A (1983) Double-blind comparison between propranolol and bendroflumethiazide in captopril-treated resistant hypertensive patients. Am Heart J 106(2):321–328

103 Veterans Administration Cooperative Study Group (1982a) Comparison of propranolol and hydrochlorothiazide for the initial treatment of hypertension. I. Results of short-term titration with emphasis on racial differences in response. JAMA 248:1996–2003

104. Veterans Administration Cooperative Study Group on Antihypertensive Agents (1982b). Racial differences in response to low dose captopril. Br J Clin Pharmacol 14: p 975

105. Greenberg G, Brennan PJ, Miall WE (1984) Effects of diuretic and beta-blocker therapy in the Medical Research Council trial. Am J Med 76: 45–51

106 Tuomilehto J, Arstila M, Savilahti R, Sundquist H (1977) Sotalol and a combination of hydrochlorothiazide and spironolactone in the treatment of hypertension with a single daily dose. Curr Ther Res 21:668–675

107 Finnerty FA (1980) Initial therapy of essential hypertension: diuretic or beta-blocker? J Fam Practice 11:199–205

108 Heel RC, Brogden GE, Pakes GE, Speight TM, Avery GS (1980) Nadolol: A review of its pharmacological properties and therapeutic efficacy in hypertension and angina pectoris. Drugs 20:1–23

109 Wilcox RG (1978) Randomised study of six beta-blockers and a thiazide diuretic in essential hypertension. Br Med J 2:383–385

110 Taylor SH, Watt SJ, Goldstraw PW (1978b) Effects of treatment on pressor responses to exertion in hypertensive patients. Br Heart J 40: p 431

111. Friedman B, Gray JM, Gross S, Levit SA (1983) United States experience with oxprenolol in hypertension. Am J Cardiol 52:43D–48D

112. Davidov M, Green AM (1980) Effect of pindolol on arterial pressure in patients with essential hypertension. Curr Ther Res 27:507–515

113. Fagard R, Amery A, Deplaen JF, Lijnen P, Missotten A (1976) Plasma renin concentration and the hypotensive effect of bendrofluazide and of atenolol. Clinical Science and Molecular Medicine 51:215s–217s

114. Petrie JC, Jeffers TA, Robb OJ, Scott AK, Webster J (1980) Atenolol, sustained-release oxprenolol, and long-acting propranolol in hypertension. Br Med J 280:1573–1574

115. Stokkeland OM, Sangvik K, Lindseth Ditlefsen E-M (1975) A comparative study of metoprolol and trichlormethiazide in hypertension. Curr Ther Res 18:755–768

116. Pedersen OL, Mikkelsen E, Nielsen JL, Christensen NJ (1979) Abrupt withdrawal of beta-blocking agents in patients with arterial hypertension. Effect on blood pressure, heart rate and plasma catecholamines and prolactin. Eur J Clin Pharmacol 15:215–217

117. Leary WP, Morris M, Asmal AC (1979) Effect of beta-blocking agents on renal function. S African Med J 56: p.745

118. Andersen GS (1985) Atenolol versus bendroflumethiazide in middle-aged and elderly hypertensives. Acta Med Scand 218:165–172

119. Lawrie TDV, Lorimer AR, Jones RW, Kidner PH, James IM, Cummin P, Joy MD, Kubik MM, Bennett PN, Lewis LD (1984) Spironolactone and propranolol in the management of idiopathic hypertension. Acta Ther 10:257–272

120. Karlberg BE, Kagedal B, Tegler L, Tolagen K, Bergman B (1976) Controlled treatment of primary hypertension with propranolol and spironolactone. Am J Cardiol 37:642–649

121. Furberg B, Kjellmert A, Nisell J, Olofsson B-O (1981) Nadolol in hypertension. In: Gross, F (ed.) Royal Society of Medicine Congress Symposium Series No 37, International experience with nadolol: a long-acting beta-blocking agent, proceedings of a symposium, Paris, 1980. London: Academic Press, pp 169–174

122. Buhler FR, Hulthen UL, Kiowski W, Bolli P (1983) Beta-blockers and calcium antagonists. Drugs (Symposium on beta-blockers in the 1980's) 25 (Suppl 2):50–57

123. Hornung RS, Jones RI, Gould BA, Sonecha T, Raftery FB (1984) Propranolol versus verapamil for the treatment of essential hypertension. Am Heart J 108:554–560

124. Johnson BF, Romero L, Marwaha R (1983) Comparative effects of the calcium channel blocker nitrendipine and propranolol on BP, renin and metabolism. Clin Pharmacol Ther 32(2):84th Ann Mtg Am Soc Clin Pharmacol Therap San Diego, March 9–12, 1983 (abstr)

125. Fritschka E, Distler A, Gotzen R, Thiede H-M, Philipp T (1984) Crossover comparison of nitrendipine with propranolol in patients with essential hypertension. J Cardiovasc Pharmacol 6:S1100–S1104

126. de Divitiis O, Petitto M, Di Somma S, Galderisi M, Villari B, Santomauro M, Fazio S (1985) Nitrendipine and atenolol: comparison and combination in the treatment of arterial hypertension. Arznzneim Forsch 35:727–729

127. Ekelund L-G, Ekelund C, Rossner S (1982) Antihypertensive effects at rest and during exercise of a calcium blocker, nifedipine, alone and in combination with metoprolol. Acta Med Scand 212:71–75

128. Isles CG, Johnson AOC, Milne FJ (1986) Slow release nifedipine and atenolol initial treatment in blacks with malignant hypertension. Br J Clin Pharmacol 21:377–383

129. Friedlander DH (1979) Captopril and propranolol in mild and moderate essential hypertension: preliminary report. NZ Med J 90:146–148

130. Huang CM, Salomon J, Molteni A, Quintanilla A, Del Greco F (1980) Antihypertensive effect of captopril and propranolol. Clin Pharmacol Ther 27:258–259 (Abst)
131. Seedat YK (1979a) Comparison of captopril with propranolol in the treatment of mild and moderate essential hypertension. S Afr med J 56:983–986
132. Ofen A, Rotmensch HH, Vlasses PH, Riley LJ, Tadros SS, Koplin JR, Ferguson RK (1985) Crossover comparison of captopril and propranolol as step 2 agents in hypertension. Am Heart J 109:554–557
133. Niarchos AP, Laragh JH (1981) Renin dependency of isolated systolic hypertension. 8th Scientific Meeting of the International Society of Hypertension, Milan 31 May–3 June, 1981, 314 (abstr)
134. Andren L, Karlberg B, Ohman P, Svensson A, Asplund J, Hansson L (1982) Catopril and atenolol combined with hydrochlorothiazide in essential hypertension. Br J Clin Pharmacol 14:107S–111S
135. Amabile G, Ceraulo C, Serradimigni A (1984) A comparison of propranolol and enalapril (MK 421) in the treatment of mild to moderate essential hypertension. J Hypertension 2:427 (abstr)
136. Boer P, Geyskes GG (1984) Plasma renin substrate concentration during chronic propranolol therapy. Hypertension 6:132–133
137. Simon A Ch, Levenson JA, Bouthier JD, Benetos A, Achimastos A, Fouchard M, Maarek BC, Safar ME (1984) Comparison of Oral MK 421 and propranolol in mild to moderate essential hypertension and their effects on arterial and venous vessels of the forearm. Am J Cardiol 53:781–785
138. Enalapril in Hypertension Study Group (1984) Enalapril in essential hypertension: a comparative study with propranolol. Br J Clin Pharmacol 18:51–56
139. Webster J, Petrie JC, Robb OJ, Trafford J, Burgess J, Richardson PJ, Davidson C, Fairhurst G, Vandenberg MJ, Cooper WD, Arr SM, Kimber G (1986) Enalapril in moderate to severe hypertension: a comparison with atenolol. Br J Clin Pharmacol 21:489–495
140. Ohman KP, Karlberg BE (1984) Enalapril and atenolol in primary hypertension—a comparative study of blood pressure lowering and hormonal effects. Scand J Urol Nephrol 579:93–97
141. Silas JH, McGourty JC (1986) Comparison of enalapril and atenolol in hypertension. X World Congress of Cardiology, September 14–19, 1986 Washington DC (abstr)1118
142. Helgeland A, Hagelund CHJ, Strommen R, Tretli S (1986) Enalapril, atenolol, and hydrochlorothiazide in mild to moderate hypertension. Lancet
143. Franz I-W, Ketehut R, Behr U, Agrawal B (1986) A comparison of the antihypertensive efficacy at rest and during exercise of atenolol, enalapril and their combination. 11th Scientific Meeting of the International Society of Hypertension, August 31–September 7, 1986, Heidelberg, (abstr)
144. Wood DA (1981) A double-blind cross-over study in hypertension to compare prazosin and propranolol using a twice daily dosage regime. In: Royal Society of Medicine Congress Symposium Series No 41: Prazosin: Pharmacology, hypertension and congestive heart failure (Proc Symp Pfizer, London 16–17 November, 1980) London: Academic Press, pp 61–65
145. Inouye I, Massie B, Benowitz N, Simpson P, Loge D, Topic N (1984) Monotherapy in mild to moderate hypertension: comparison of hydrochlorothiazide, propranolol and prazosin. Am J Cardiol 53:24A–28A
146. Wilkinson PR, Raftery EB (1977) A comparative trial of clonidine propranolol and placebo in the treatment of moderate hypertension. Br J Clin Pharmacol 4:289–294
147. Man in't Veld AJ, Schalekamp MADH (1981) Pindolol acts as beta-adrenoceptor agonist in orthostatic hypotension: therapeutic implications. Br Med J 282:929–931

148. Davies B, Bannister R, Mathias C, Sever P (1981) Pindolol in postural hypotension, the case for caution. Lancet 2:982–983

149. Melsen J, Trap-Jensen J (1986) Xamtouol, a new selective beta$_1$-adrenoceptor partial agonist, in the treatment of postural hypotension. Acta Med scand 219:173–177

150. Santos AD, Mathew PK, Hilal A, Wallace WA (1981) Orthostatic hypotension: a commonly unrecognized cause of symptoms in mitral valve prolapse. Am J Med 71:746–750

151. Gibson D, Sowton E (1969) The use of beta-adrenergic receptor blocking drugs in dysrhythmias. Prog Cardiovasc Dis 12:16–39

152. Hombach V, Braun V, Hopp HW, Gil-Sanchez D, Behrenbeck DW, Tauchert M, Hilger HH (1982) Electrophysiological effects of cardioselective and non-cardioselective beta-adrenoceptor blockers with and without ISA at rest and during exercise. Br J Clin Pharmacol 13:285S–293S

153. Coltart DJ, Gibson DG, Shand DG (1971) Plasma propranolol levels associated with suppression of ventricular ectopic beats. Br Med J 1:490–491

154. Echt DS, Berte LE, Clusin WT, Samuelsson RG, Harrison DC, Mason JW (1982) Prolongation of the human cardiac monophasic action potential by sotalol. Am J Cardiol 50:1082–1086

155. Creamer JE, Nathan AW, Shennan A, Camm AJ (1986) Acute and chronic effects of sotalol and propranolol on ventricular repolarization using constant-rate pacing. Am J Cardiol 57:1092–1096

156. Singh BN (1973) Clinical aspects of the antiarrhythmic actions of beta-receptor blocking drugs: Part 1 Pattern of response of common arrhythmias. N Z Med J 78:482–486

157. Singh BN, Jewitt DE (1977) Beta-adrenoreceptor blocking drugs in cardiac arrhythmias. Cardiovasc Drugs 2:119–159

158. Schofield PM, Reid F, Bennett DH (1987) A comparison of atenolol and sotalol in the treatment of patients with paroxysmal supraventricular tachycardia. Br Heart J 57: Proceedings of the British Cardiac Society, London, 25–27 Nov 1986 (abstr)

159. Gallagher JJ, Pritchett ELC, Sealy WC, Kasell J, Wallace AG (1978) The preexcitation syndromes. Prog Cardiovasc Dis 20:285–327

160. Frishman W, Davis R, Strom J et al (1979) Clinical pharmacology of the new beta-adrenergic blocking drugs. Part 5: Pindolal (LB-46) therapy for supraventricular arrhythmia: a viable alternative to propranolol in patients with bronchospasm. Am Heart J 98:393–398

161. Rehnqvist N (1981) Clinical experience with intravenous metoprolol in supraventricular tachyarrhythmias. A multicentre study. Ann Clin Res 13 (Suppl 30):68–72

162. Pratt CM, Yepsin SC, Bloom MGK, Taylor AA, Young JB, Quinones MA (1983) Evaluation of metoprolol in suppressing complex ventricular arrhythmias. Am J Cardiol 52:73–78

163. Lue HC, Su WJ, Wang NK, Shen CT (1978) Right ventricular outflow tract obstruction and its response to propranolol in tetralogy of Fallot. VIII World Congress of Cardiology, Tokyo, 17–23 September 1978 (Abstr)

164. Garson A, Gillette PC, McNamara DG (1981) Propranolol: the preferred palliation for tetralogy of Fallot. Am J Cardiol 47:1098–1104

165. Goodwin JF (1973) Hypertrophic diseases of the myocardium. Prog Cardiovasc Dis 16:199–238

166. Frank MJ, Abdulla AM, Canedo MI, Saylors RE (1978) Long-term medical management of hypertrophic obstructive cardiomyopathy. Am J Cardiol 42:993–1001

167. Anderson JL (1987) Treatment of cardiac myopathies with beta-blockers: What do we know, where do we go from here?

168. Swedberg K, Hjalmarson A, Waagstein F, Wallentin I (1980) Beneficial effects of

long-term beta-blockade in congestive cardiomyopathy. Br Heart J 44:117–133

169. Ross EJ, Prichard BNC, Kaufman L, Robertson AIG, Harris BJ (1967) Pre-operative and operative management of patients with phaeochromocytoma. Br Med J 1:191–198

170. Delarue NC, Morrow JD, Kerr JH, Colapinto RF (1978) Phaeochromocytoma in the modern context. Can J Surg 21:387–394

171. Rimon R, Kampman R, Viukari M (1979) Propranolol in the treatment of neurocirculatory asthenia—an open pilot study. Isr Ann Psychiatry Relat Discip 17:144–148

172. Hanak T (1978). Efficacy of alprenolol and diazepam in the treatment of functional sympathicotonic cardiovascular disorders: a double-blind crossover study. Curr Ther Res 774–785

173. Hillon P, Lebrec D, Munoz C et al (1982) Comparison of the effects of a cardioselective and a non-selective beta-blocker on portal hypertension in patients with cirrhosis. Hepatology 2:528–531

174. Freeman JG, Barton JR, Record CO (1983) Effects of vasodilators on portal pressure in patients with portal hypertension. Gut 24:A971

175. Lebrec D, Poynard T, Bernuau J, Bercoff E, Nouel O, Capron J-P Poupon R, Bouvry M, Rueff B, Benhamou J-P (1984) A randomized controlled study of propranolol for prevention of recurrent gastrointestinal bleeding in patients with cirrhosis: a final report. Hepatology 4:355–358

176. Wheat MW (1973) Treatment of dissecting aneurysms of the aorta: current status. Prog Cardiovasc Dis XVI:87–101

177. Doroghazi R, Slater EE, DeSanctis RW (1981) Medical therapy for aortic dissections. J Cardiovasc Med 6:187–197

178. McFarland J, Willerson JT, Dinsmore RE, Austen WG, Buckley MJ, Sanders CA, DeSanctis RW (1972) The medical treatment of dissecting aortic aneurysms. New Engl J Med 286:115–119

179. Neil-Swyer G, Walter P, Cruickshank JM, Doshi B, O'Gorman P (1978) Effect of propranolol and phentolamine on myocardial necrosis after subarachnoid haemorrhage. Br Med J 2:990–992

180. Neil-Dwyer G, Walter P, Cruickshank J, Stratton C (1983) Beta-blockade in subarachnoid haemorrhage. Drugs (Symposium on beta-blockers in the 1980s) 25 (Suppl 2):273–277

181. Cruickshank JM, Neil-Dwyer G, Hayes Y, Degaute JP, Kuurne T, Kytta J, Vincent JL, Carruthers ME, Patel S (1987) Reduction of stress/catecholamine-induced cardiac necrosis by β_1-selective blockade. New Engl J Med (In press)

23. Antiarrhythmic agents – 1987

A. JOHN CAMM & NICHOLAS J. LINKER

Department of Cardiological Sciences, St George's Hospital Medical School, Cranmer Terrace, London SW17 0RE, U.K.

Introduction

The drug therapy of arrhythmias has developed rapidly over the last 25 years. During this period, the number of available antiarrhythmic agents has increased dramatically and many more compounds are in development. In the United Kingdom there are more than ·forty antiarrhythmic drugs (including beta adrenergic blocking agents) currently listed in the pharmacopoeia. This chapter will describe some aspects of newly introduced antiarrhythmic agents and methods of assessing the efficacy of drug therapy, with particular reference to the arrhythmogenic effects of drugs.

Antiarrhythmic drug therapy is only one means of treating tachyarrhythmias. In many patients an arrhythmia (for example, ventricular premature contractions) may not cause troublesome symptoms nor have any prognostic importance. In such cases, no therapy is warranted. Some patients have symptomatic, sustained tachyarrhythmias which are very responsive to vagal manoeuvres such as carotid sinus massage or the Valsalva manoeuvre and the patient may be able to terminate attacks in this way without the need for additional treatment, and drug treatment may not be necessary. Antiarrhythmic agents constitute the most popular therapy for those patients with symptomatic arrhythmias, but disappointingly achieve control in only a minority of patients. For other patients refractory to these treatments, a more aggressive approach needs to be taken with recourse to implantable electronic devices, such as anti-tachycardia pacemakers or defibrillators, and electrical or surgical ablation techniques.

Antiarrhythmic agents

Antiarrhythmic drug therapy is the mainstay of treatment for the majority of patients with troublesome tachyarrhythmias. Many of the agents in use at

V. Hombach, H. H. Hilger and H. L. Kennedy (eds). Electrocardiography and Cardiac Drug Therapy. ISBN 978-94-010-6976-2
© 1989, Kluwer Academic Publishers, Dordrecht –

324

present have been widely studied in the past, although there have been some recent studies on established medications. For example, an evaluation has been made of the effectiveness of intravenous lignocaine in preventing ventricular fibrillation in association with acute myocardial infarction [1]. This study was a randomised, placebo-controlled, double-blind, prospective trial of the administration of lignocaine by paramedics to patients suspected of having suffered an acute myocardial infarction. The results of this important study showed that only 2 cases of ventricular fibrillation occurred in the treated group compared to 12 in the control group ($p < 0.01$), and that ventricular tachycardia terminated a mean of ten minutes after injection in six out of nine lignocaine-treated patients but in none of five control patients ($p < 0.02$).

Advances in new antiarrhythmic agents

New agents that have been undergoing clinical trial recently include drugs that have an action which can be described by a single Vaughan Williams class, and agents that combine the actions of two or more classes (Table 1). For example, d-Sotalol and Penticainide have actions that can be classified as class III and Ib respectively, whereas bepridil and propafenone have multiple actions (classes III + IV and Ic + II + III respectively). Other agents such as somatostatin and adenosine cannot be fitted into the Vaughan Williams classification.

Table 1. Classification of new antiarrhythmic agents

Drug	VW Class
Cibenzoline	I and III
Bepridil	I and IV
Penticainide	Ib
Pirmenol	Ic
Recainam	Ic
Propafenone	Ic, II and III
Esmolol	II
Flestolol	II
d-Sotolol	III

Others: Adenosine, Somatostatin

Table 2. Treatment of supraventricular tachyarrhythmias

Drug	Response
Adenosine	Termination of AVRT/AVNRT in 80–100% of cases
Esmolol and	Reduction of ventricular rate of AF/flutter in 72–100% of cases;
Flestolol	conversion of AF/flutter to sinus rhythm in 6–45% of cases
Somatostatin	Termination of AVRT/AVNRT in 85% of cases

Drug therapy of supraventricular tachyarrhythmias

Drugs that have been studied particularly in the context of supraventricular arrhythmias include adenosine, esmolol, flestolol and somatostatin (Table 2). Adenosine, an endogenous purine nucleoside, is a potent AV nodal blocking agent, producing prolongation of the AH interval and increasing the AVERP [2]. It increases sinus cycle length but has no effect on the HV interval. Studies to date have shown that given in doses of 0.05–0.25 mg/kg it is effective in terminating 80–100% of atrioventricular reentry tachycardias and atrioventricular nodal reentry tachycardias [2, 3, 4]. It is a valuable research tool in view of the fact that it has a very short half-life, in the order of 30 secs and is relatively free of side effects with the exception of transient tachypnoea.

Esmolol and flestolol are two recently introduced beta-blockers. They both share a major pharmacological difference from other beta-blockers in that their halflives are very short (9.2 mins and 6.9 mins respectively) [5, 6]. There have been a number of reports on the use of these agents for the control of ventricular rate in supraventricular tachyarrhythmias; and also of their efficacy in converting spontaneously occurring supraventricular arrhythmias [5–11]. Esmolol was shown to produce a 15% or greater reduction in the ventricular rate of atrial fibrillation or flutter in 72–100% of patients. The ability of this agent to convert atrial fibrillation and flutter to sinus rhythm was variable, having success rates from 6 to 45%.

Somatostatin is, like adenosine, a naturally occurring compound. It is a peptide, and has many actions, one of which is to act as a neurotransmitter. It is found in high concentrations in the sinus and atrioventricular nodes. It slows sinus cycle length and prolongs the AH interval and the AVERP. A recent study has shown that, given intravenously, it is as effective as verapamil in terminating atrioventricular reentry and atrioventricular nodal reentry tachycardias [12].

Drug therapy of ventricular tachyarrhythmias

A number of the newer pharmacological agents have been developed for the treatment of ventricular tachyarrhythmias (Table 3). These drugs include pirmenol, cibenzoline, bepridil, recainam and penticainide.

Pirmenol is a class Ic agent and has been extensively investigated particularly in Finland [13, 14]. Oral pirmenol has been shown to be effective in causing a mean reduction of >80% of VPCs and a >95% reduction in repetitive VPCs in 11 out of 16 patients. The agent was well tolerated but was found to cause aggravation of the arrhythmia in one patient secondary to prolongation of the QT interval [13].

A predominantly class Ia antiarrhythmic agent, cibenzoline also has a weak class III action [15, 16]. In comparison with quinidine, it is equally effective in suppressing VPCs (60% vs 50%) but would appear to have fewer side effects. It is negatively inotropic and has a similar proarrhythmic propensity to quinidine.

Another class Ic drug recainam, is one of the newest antiarrhythmic agents undergoing clinical trial, and at present little information is available. In the one reported study, the effect of an infusion of recainam was monitored in patients who had frequent complex ventricular ectopic beats [18]. It was shown to be effective in suppressing more than 90% of total VPCs in 9 out of 10 patients. There was no evidence of a proarrhythmic effect nor was any depression of myocardial function noted. The drug did produce lengthening of the PR and QRS intervals, with a normal JT interval, consistent with a class Ic action.

Penticainide is a class Ib antiarrhythmic agent. It decreases sinus cycle length and increases the AH and HV intervals; it also effects the conduction properties of accessory pathways [19]. Given intravenously, it was found to be effective in terminating spontaneously occurring ventricular tachycardia in 5 out of 8 patients, and prevented the induction of ventricular tachycardia in 3 out of 6 patients [20].

Table 3. Treatment of ventricular tachyarrhythmias

Drug	Response
Pirmenol	Reduction of >80% of VPCs in 11/16 cases [13]
Cibenzoline	Suppression of VPCs in 60% of cases [15]
Bepridil	Prevented induction of VT in 46% of cases [17]
Recainam	Reduction of >90% fVPCs in 9/10 cases [18]
Penticainide	Terminated spontaneously occurring VT in 5/8 patients; prevented Vt induction in 3/6 cases [20]
d-sotalol	Prevention of ischaemia-induced VF in 8/8 dogs [22]

Calcium antagonists have been developed mainly for the treatment of angina and hypertension. A new agent bepridil, was originally introduced as an antianginal agent, however it was found to increase the QT interval secondary to a prolongation of repolarisation and was consequently investigated for use as an antiarrhythmic agent [17]. Bepridil prevented the re-induction of ventricular tachycardia in 46% of patients who had inducible sustained or non-sustained VT. Unfortunately, the proarrhythmic effect of this agent necessitates caution in its use, particularly in patients who may have QT interval prolongation.

d-Sotalol is the dextrorotatory isomer of sotalol. The commercially available sotalol is a racemic mixture of the dextro- and laevorotatory isomers of the drug. Work has shown that it is the laevorotatory isomer that possesses beta-blocking activity, in addition to a class III action, whilst the dextrorotatory isomer possesses class III activity without a significant beta-blocking effect [21]. Whilst studies in humans are not yet available, preliminary animal studies have shown that *d*-sotalol is effective in suppressing the induction of ventricular tachyarrhythmias, whilst having no appreciable beta-blocking effect [21, 22].

Developments in the use of antiarrhythmic drugs

There are at present a number of trials which are attempting to devise ways of determining drug efficacy in the management of arrhythmias; these include the Cardiac Arrhythmia Pilot Study (CAPS) [23, 24], the Cardiac Arrhythmia Suppression Trial (CAST), the Electrophysiologic Study Vs Electrocardiographic Monitoring trial (ESVEM) [25] and the 'Maastricht experiment' [26].

The CAPS investigation included an assessment of the efficacy and incidence of proarrhythmic effects between four class I antiarrhythmic agents (encainide, flecainide, imipramine and moricizine) and a placebo-controlled group in patients who have ventricular arrhythmias on 24-hour tape recordings following myocardial infarction. The preliminary reports have been based on a dose-titration study, which has demonstrated that a proarrhythmic effect is uncommon in post-infarct patients with non-sustained ventricular arrhythmias when dose increases are made at greater than 5 day intervals and that drug washout is a helpful manoeuvre in documenting a proarrhythmic response to class I agents [23]. Five hundred and two patients were randomised into the various treatment groups, the results showing that a reduction of >70% of VPCs and >90% decrease in episodes of non-sustained ventricular tachycardia occurred in 53 to 80% of patients in the treatment groups compared with 36% in the placebo group, with adverse reactions occurring in 7 to 31% of the treatment groups and 15% of the placebo group [24].

In the ESVEM trial, patients with recurrent, sustained ventricular tachycardia or a cardiac arrest are screened for inclusion. Patients who have sustained monomorphic ventricular tachycardia in response to programmed ventricular stimulation and average at least 10 VPCs per hour during a 48-hour tape recording are randomised to have serial drug evaluation by either non-invasive methods or programmed ventricular stimulation [25].

The 'Maastricht experiment' is proposed to test the validity of programmed ventricular stimulation as a method for selecting drug therapy of malignant ventricular arrhythmias [26]. A baseline ventricular stimulation protocol is performed to establish if a patient has inducible ventricular tachycardia. Whether or not patients are inducible, they are tested on an antiarrhythmic drug, which whether it is effective or not, is continued until a clinical recurrence of ventricular tachycardia occurs. Should the ventricular tachycardia recur, a second drug is assessed in the same way.

Proarrhythmic effects of drugs

The arrhythmogenic effects of antiarrhythmic drugs are a particular cause for concern, as often antiarrhythmic effects can be difficult to separate from proarrhythmic effects. All antiarrhythmic agents have the potential for arrhythmogenesis, some more so than others.

There have been two methods used to assess arrhythmogenic effects; firstly ambulatory monitoring in combination with exercise testing [27], and secondly electrophysiological studies [28]. The former involves a washout period, after which baseline exercise testing and Holter monitoring were carried out. A series of acute drug tests were then carried out to assess drug efficacy, following which an agent found to be effective in the first phase was administered for 48 hours during which the exercise test and Holter monitoring was repeated. The electrophysiological study consisted of a washout period, followed by attempted induction of VT by a stimulation protocol that involved one, two and three extrastimuli being delivered at the right ventricular apex during sinus rhythm and following ventricular pacing. The study was repeated two hours after a single large oral dose of the selected antiarrhythmic agent, and again after 48–96 hours of oral therapy with the same agent.

Table 4. Proarrhythmic effects of antiarrhythmic agents

Class Ia, III, ?Ib	Class Ic
QT(JT) prolongation	?JT prolongation
Polymorphic VT	Monomorphic VT
(Non-sustained VT)	(Sustained VT)

The results of these studies showed the average incidence of arrhythmogenic effects with antiarrhythmic agents to be 12%. There was broad agreement between the outcome of both types of study and from the data supplied, certain drugs, particularly quinidine and encainide showed a high incidence of proarrhythmic effects.

The arrhythmogenic effect of quinidine has been known for many years [29]. The drug produces a polymorphic ventricular tachycardia associated with marked QT interval prolongation (Table 4). This effect occurs with other members of class Ia such as disopyramide [30], and also amiodarone [31].

The class Ic agents flecainide and encainide have a similar high incidence of arrhythmogenic effects [27, 28], although the mechanism of this action is as yet undefined. These agents produce widening of the QRS with a variable effect on the QT interval [32, 33]. However the JT interval is usually unaffected, and the width of the QRS alone does not distinguish those patients at risk of an arrhythmogenic effect [34]. Proarrhythmic effects observed with these agents include an increased frequency of VPCs and spontaneous polymorphic ventricular tachycardia [34].

Conclusion

Of the recently developed antiarrhythmic drugs, few seem to offer any significant advantage over established agents. The exception to this is adenosine, which has great potential for the effective and safe treatment of supraventricular arrhythmias.

The investigation of the mechanisms of drug arrhythmogenesis is an important and challenging field for research, yet there is still need for a generally accepted definition of the criteria for arrhythmogenic effects. Present evidence suggests many of the present antiarrhythmic drugs have a significant proarrhythmic effect and cautious prescribing of these agents is required.

References

1. Koster RW, Dunning AJ (1985) Intramuscular lidocaine for prevention of lethal arrhythmias in the prehospitalization phase of acute myocardial infarction. N Engl J Med 313:1105–1110
2. DiMarco JP, Sellers TD, Berne RM, West GA, Belardinelli L (1983) Adenosine: electrophysiologic effects and therapeutic use for terminating paroxysmal supraventricular tachycardia. Circulation 68:1254–1263
3. Munoz A, Leenhardt A, Sassine A, Galley P, Puech P (1984) Therapeutic use of adenosine for terminating spontaneous paroxysmal supraventricular tachycardia. Eur Heart J. 5:735–738
4. Clarke B, Till J, Rowland E, Ward DE, Barnes PJ, Shinebourne EA (1987) Rapid and safe termination of supraventricular tachycardia in children by adenosine. Lancet i:299–301
5. Sum CY, Yacobi A, Kartzinel R, Stampfli H, Davis CS, Lai CM (1983) Kinetics of esmolol, an ultra-short-acting beta-blocker, and of its major metabolite. Clin Pharmacol Ther 34:427–434
6. Steinberg JS, Katz RJ, Somberg JC, Keefe D, Laddu AR, Burge J (1986) Safety and efficacy of flestolol, a new ultrashort-acting beta-adrenergic blocking agent, for supraventricular tachyarrhythmias. Am J Cardiol 58:1005–1008
7. Gray RJ, Bateman TM, Czer LSC, Conklin CM, Matloff JM (1985) Esmolol: a new ultrashort-acting beta-adrenergic blocking agent for rapid control of heart rate in postoperative supraventricular tachyarrhythmias. J Am Coll Cardiol 5:1451–1456
8. Esmolol vs Placebo Multicenter Study Group, 1986. Comparison of the efficacy and safety of esmolol, a short-acting beta blocker, with placebo in the treatment of supraventricular tachyarrhythmias. Am Heart J 111:42–48
9. Byrd RC, Sung RJ, Marks J, Parmley WW (1984) Safety and efficacy of esmolol (ASL-8052: an ultrashort-acting beta-adrenergic blocking agent) for control of ventricular rate in supraventricular tachycardias. J Am Coll Cardiol 3:394–399
10. Esmolol Research Group (1986) Intravenous esmolol for the treatment of supraventricular tachyarrhythmia: results of a multicenter, base-line controlled safety and efficacy study in 160 patients. Am Heart J 112:498–505
11. Esmolol Multicenter Study Research Group (1985) Efficacy and safety of esmolol vs propranolol in the treatment of supraventricular tachyarrhythmias: a multicenter double-blind clinical trial. Am Heart J 110:913–922
12. Webb SC, Hendry WG, Bloom SR, Krikler DM (1986) Somatostatin: a neuroregulatory peptide with electrophysiological activity. Brit Heart J 55:513
13. Toivonen LK, Nieminen MS, Manninen V, Frick MH (1985) Antiarrhythmic efficacy of pirmenol in the treatment of premature ventricular complexes. Eur Heart J 6:737–744
14. Toivonen LK, Nieminen MS, Manninen V, Frick MH (1986) Pirmenol in the long-term treatment of chronic ventricular arrhythmias: a placebo-controlled study. J Cardiovasc Pharmacol 8:156–160
15. Wasty N, Saksena S, Barr MJ (1985) Comparative efficacy and safety of oral cibenzoline and quinidine in ventricular arrhythmias: a randomized crossover study. Am Heart J 110:1181–1188
16. Touboul P (1985) Cibenzoline. Arch Mal Coeur 78:91–94.
17. Somberg J, Torres V, Flowers D, Miura D, Butler B, Gottlieb S (1985) Prolongation of QT interval and antiarrhythmic action of bepridil. Am Heart J 109:19–27
18. Anastasiou-Nana MI, Anderson JL, Hampton EM, Nanas JN, Heath BM (1986) Recainam, a potent new antiarrhythmic agent: effects on complex ventricular arrhythmias. J Am Coll Cardiol 8:427–435.

19. Munoz A, Aliot E, Prestat MP, Toussain P, Gagnol JP, Gilgenkrantz JM (1986) Cardiac electrophysiologic and antiarrhythmic effects of penticainide (CM 7857). Proceedings of X World Congress of Cardiology, p 179

20. Alio: E, Khalife K, Munoz A, Zannad F, Gagnol JP, Gilgenkrantz JM (1986) Efficacy of intravenous penticainide on spontaneous and induced sustained ventricular tachycardias. Proceedings of X World Congress of Cardiology, p 114

21. Lynch JJ, Wilber DJ, Montgomery DG, Hsieh TM, Patterson E, Lucchesi BR (1984) Antiarrhythmic and antifibrillatory actions of the levo- and dextrorotatory isomers of sotalol. J Cardiovasc Pharmacol 6:1132–1141

22. Taggart P, Sutton P, Donaldson R (1985) d-Sotalol: a new potent class III anti-arrhythmic agent. Clinical Science 69:631–636

23. Bigger JT, Woosley RL, Roden DM, Hallstrom A, Echt D, Greene L, Butler L, and CAPS investigators (1987) A placebo-controlled study of the proarrhythmic effects of class I antiarrhythmic drugs. J Am Coll Cardiol 9:245A

24. Woosley RL, Giardina E-G, Roden DM, Henthorn RW, Hallstrom A, and CAPS investigators (1987) Value of dose-titration in the cardiac arrhythmia pilot study (CAPS). J Am Coll Cardiol 9:70A

25. Bigger JT (1986) Long-term continuous electrocardiographic recordings and elec-trophysiologic testing to select patients with ventricular arrhythmias for drug trials and to determine antiarrhythmic drug efficacy. Am J Cardiol 58:58C–65C

26. Wellens HJJ, Brugada P, Stevenson WG (1985) Programmed electrical stimulation of the heart in patients with life-threatening ventricular arrhythmias: what is the significance of induced arrhythmias and what is the correct stimulation protocol? Circulation 72:1–7

27. Velebit V, Podrid PJ, Lown B, Cohen BH, Graboys TB (1982) Aggravation and provocation of ventricular arrhythmias by antiarrhythmic drugs. Circulation 65: 886–894

28. Poser RF, Podrid PJ, Lombardi F, Lown B (1985) Aggravation of arrhythmia induced with antiarrhythmic drugs during electrophysiologic testing. Am Heart J 110:9–16

29. Binder MJ, Rosove L (1952) Paroxysmal ventricular tachycardia and fibrillation due to quinidine. Am J Med 12:491–495

30. Meltzer RS, Robert EW, McMorrow M, Martin RP (1978) Atypical ventricular tachy-cardia as a manifestation of disopyramide toxicity. Am J Cardiol 42:1049–1053

31. McGovern B, Garan H, Kelly E, Ruskin JN (1983) Adverse reactions during treatment with amiodarone hydrochloride. Brit Med J 287:175–180

32. Morganroth J, Horowitz LN (1984) Flecainide: its proarrhythmic effect and expected changes on the surface electrocardiogram. Am J Cardiol 53:89B–94B

33. Nathan AW, Hellestrand KJ, Bexton RS, Banim SO, Spurrell RAJ, Camm AJ (1984) Proarrhythmic effects of the new antiarrhythmic agent flecainide acetate. Am Heart J 107:222–228

34. Winkle RA, Mason JW, Griffin JC, Ross D (1981) Malignant ventricular tachyarrhyth-mias associated with the use of encainide. Am Heart J 102:857–864

24. Thrombolytic agents

H. OSTERMANN & U. SCHMITZ-HUEBNER

Department of Internal Medicine, University of Münster, F.R.G.

Introduction

Thrombolytic agents have been in clinical use for about 30 years (Tillet et al. 1955). The classical thrombolytic drugs have been streptokinase and urokinase. Streptokinase has been used in several clinical conditions such as myocardial infarction, pulmonary embolism, deep venous thrombosis and peripheral arterial thrombosis. Its widespread use in the therapy of thrombotic events has been hampered by severe side effects, mainly bleeding and allergic complications. A significant improvement was the discovery and clinical application of urokinase (Hansen et al. 1961) which as a human protein lacked some of the drawbacks of streptokinase. Clot specificity however was still not thought of until the gain in knowledge concerning the fibrinolytic system led to the characterization, purification and clinical application of tissue plasminogen activator (t-PA) (Ranby 1982) and single-chain urokinase plasminogen activator (scu-PA) (Husain et al. 1983). But although these natural substances achieve much attention in clinical studies, interest in the classical substance streptokinase has been renewed recently by coupling it to plasminogen whose biological properties had been modified to improve the thrombolytic capabilities of the complex.

The first part of this chapter will deal with the physiology and pharmacology of the components of the fibrinolytic system, followed by an overview on therapeutic applications. In the third part new developments promising even better drugs for the future will be discussed.

The fibrinolytic system

Four protease cascade systems exist in mammalian blood, namely the coagulation, the complement, the kinin and the fibrinolytic system. These are responsible for the keeping of homeostasis in the circulation. Though

V. Hombach, H. H. Hilger and H. L. Kennedy (eds), Electrocardiography and Cardiac Drug Therapy. ISBN 978-94-010-6976-2
© 1989, Kluwer Academic Publishers, Dordrecht –

once considered separate entities, there is now increasing evidence for
several connections between these systems (Preissner and Müller-Berghaus
1986). Many of these proteins are serine proteases sharing a high degree of
homology to pancreatic proteases like trypsin in regard to their catalytic
center. They are however much larger and have acquired additional
functional domains in evolution that are responsible for their high substrate
specificity and for interactions with specific inhibitors (Patthy 1985).

Plasminogen

The fibrinolytic system acts as a counterbalance to the coagulation system
in the blood. Fibrin thrombi developing in the blood stream are cleared
from the circulation by the action of plasmin. Plasmin is generated from the
proenzyme plasminogen which is synthezised by the liver. Its molecular
weight is 90 kd and it occurs at a concentration of 2 μM in plasma. It is a
glycoprotein consisting of 760 amino acids (Castellino 1984). It has five
domains called kringles structures on which the binding sites for the
substrate fibrin and plasminogen's specific inhibitor alpha2-antiplasmin
reside. Conversion of plasminogen to plasmin is accomplished by proteolytic cleavage of a single peptide bond Arg560–Val561. This cleavage is
accomplished by all plasminogen activators and yields a two chain plasmin
molecule termed Glu-plasmin due to its N terminal glutamic acid. Glu-
plasmin is converted by plasmin itself to Lys-plasmin after cleavage of the
peptide bond Lys76–Lys77. Lys-plasmin has slightly different properties
than Glu-plasmin. The two chains of the plasmin molecule are called the
heavy or A chain and the light or B chain. The heavy chain contains the
kringle structures responsible for fibrin binding, the light chain contains the
catalytic center responsible for degradation of fibrin. The proteolytic action
of plasmin is directed not only against fibrin. Freely circulating plasmin has
access to fibrinogen which is cleaved as well leading to the generation of
fibrinogen split products. Several other proteins predominantly blood
coagulation factors V and VIII are degraded as well. Thus confining the
proteolytic action of plasmin to the fibrin surface is of great importance for
avoiding a systemic lytic state. This is accomplished under physiological
conditions by the action of alpha2-antiplasmin.

Alpha2-antiplasmin

The main plasmin inhibitor is a single-chain glycoprotein. Its molecular
weight is 67 kd (Moroi et al. 1976), plasma concentration is 1 uM. Alpha2-
antiplasmin forms a complex with plasmin in a very fast reversible reaction
followed by a slower irreversible one. The first reaction is dependent on the

existence of a free lysine binding site and an active center in the plasmin molecule. When plasmin is attached to the fibrin surface its lysine binding sites are occupied. Thus it is protected from the inhibiting action of alpha2-antiplasmin, which will only inhibit freely circulating plasmin at a very fast rate.

Plasminogen activators

Streptokinase. Streptokinase is a catalytically inert streptococcal protein of 47 kd. It forms an equimolar complex with plasminogen (Taylor et al. 1978). In this complex plasminogen undergoes a conformational change resulting in the exposition of the active center. The complex is thus able to act as a plasminogen activator and cleave plasminogen to plasmin. Being a streptococcal protein streptokinase antibodies are commonly prevalent in patients due to previous infections with streptococci. An initial loading dose can be given to neutralize these antibodies. Streptokinase itself is immunogenic and leads to the formation of anti-streptokinase antibodies. This prohibits the application of streptokinase if a second thrombolysis is necessary. As streptokinase possesses no fibrin affinity plasmin is generated in the circulation where most of it will rapidly complex with alpha2-antiplasmin. Only fibrin bound plasminogen will be available for clot lysis. After depletion of alpha2-antiplasmin however, a systemic lytic state ensues with circulating plasmin which will then bind to the fibrin clot and degrade it.

Urokinase. Urokinase was initially isolated from human urine (Williams 1951). It has subsequently been isolated from several cell lines and human plasma (Wun 1982). Urokinase is a two chain serin protease connected by a single disulfide bridge. Its molecular weight is 54 kd. The light chain shares features with other proteases, namely a kringle structure and a growth factor domain. The function of these is unknown. Urokinase does not bind to fibrin. The heavy chain contains the active center of the molecule. A single chain form of urokinase (scu-PA) has been isolated from urine (Husain et al. 1983), several cell lines (Nielsen et al. 1902, Skriver et al. 1982) and by recombinant DNA expression in E. coli (Holmes et al. 1982). There is an ongoing controversy whether the single-chain form of uro-kinase constitutes a proenzyme or an active enzyme. In many ways scu-PA behaves like a proenzyme: it does have no activity against low molecular substrates, and it can not be inhibited by active site titrants like DFP (Gurewich et al. 1984). Evidence from the work of one group, working with recombinant, unglycosylated scu-PA showed that it is an active enzyme, possessing a high affinity for plasminogen and thus being able to activate plasminogen directly (Lijnen et al. 1986a, Collen et al. 1986d).

Once small amounts of plasmin have been formed through this reaction plasmin is able to cleave single-chain urokinase plasminogen activator to two-chain urokinase, which in turn activates plasminogen. These experiments were done in a purified in vitro system. When performed in a plasma system no activation of plasminogen by scu-PA could be observed, unless fibrin was added. This led the authors to hypothesize that in plasma inhibition of scu-PA takes place as long as there is no fibrin, but in the presence of fibrin scu-PA acts as an active enzyme. For this reason the International Society on Thrombosis and Haemostasis chose the designation single-chain urokinase plasminogen activator (scu-PA) instead of pro-urokinase as it was called earlier (Collen 1985). Natural scu-PA was found to possess a 20 fold lower catalytic activity for the first reaction described above than does unglycosylated recombinant scu-PA (Lijnen et al. 1986b). Another view in this matter is held by the group of Gurewich. He and his coworkers claim that scu-PA is in fact an inactive proenzyme (Pannell and Gurewich 1987). According to this view small amounts of plasmin would be needed to start the conversion to two-chain urokinase. Plasmin could be generated by t-PA (Bando et al. 1987). A second controversy regarding scu-PA is its fibrin specificity. Fibrin binding has long been regarded to be a feature of scu-PA since the initial isolation from urine was performed by binding to a fibrin-celite column (Husain et al. 1982). Subsequent reports of substantial fibrin binding of scu-PA (Kasai et al. 1985a, 1985b) were published. These experiments were done by allowing plasma to be clotted by thrombin in the presence of scu-PA. The residual latent urokinase activity after incubation with plasmin was measured and found to be decreased suggesting fibrin-binding of scu-PA. These results were questioned by the finding that thrombin degrades scu-PA to a non catalytic two-chain form (Conforti and Loskutoff 1985), thus the proposed fibrin binding of scu-PA seemed to be a thrombin artefact. An experimental design where scu-PA was added to performed fibrin showed that there was no fibrin binding except when zinc ions were added at high concentrations (Gurewich and Pannell 1987). While the non fibrin-binding of scu-PA was found by other authors as well (Lijnen et al. 1986b), a fibrin effect on the activation of plasminogen by scu-PA is exerted by the reversion of the inhibition by plasma of this reaction.

APSAC. A reason for the complications associated with streptokinase therapy is its nonselectivity for the activation of plasminogen. Circulating plasminogen is activated as well as fibrin bound plasminogen. This causes plasminemia associated with a severe fibrinogenolysis. One way to make streptokinase more fibrinselective was to use a preformed streptokinase-plasminogen complex whose active site had been acetylated rendering the complex inactive (reviewed by Monk and Heel 1987). Upon infusion of the inert complex deacylation occurs in the plasma leading to a sustained activation of plasminogen over a long period of time. The complex can thus be injected as a bolus. It was thought that a certain degree of fibrin selectivity could be reached by allowing the inactive complex to be bound to the fibrin surface via the unoccupied lysine binding sites of plasminogen and thereafter become active and exerting its fibrinolytic effect on the fibrin surface. Half lives of the deacylation reaction are between minutes and several hours. One substance has so far been clinically tested and is available. This substance has a deacylation halflife of 105 minutes in human plasma (Ferres et al. 1987).

t-PA. Tissue type plasminogen activator (t-PA) was first isolated from uterine tissue (Rijken et al. 1979). It has since been found to be synthesized by many tissues and cell cultures (Bachmann and Kruithof 1984). The gene for t-PA has been cloned and expressed in E. coli (Pennica et al. 1983). T-PA is a glycoprotein of 70 kd, its plasma concentration is about 3 to 10 μg/l. It occurs in a one-chain and a two-chain form which is generated from the one chain form by proteolytic cleavage of a single peptide bond Arg275–Ile276. The two chain molecule is held together by a single disulfide bridge. The catalytic center is located on the light chain and bears homology to the catalytic center of trypsin. Thus t-PA is another member of the family of serine proteases. In the heavy chain several structural features can be distinguished. It contains two kringle regions, one region that is homologous to the epidermal growth factor and one region that is homologous to the finger structure of fibronectin. T-PA has a high affinity for fibrin and the fibrin binding structures have been identified to be in the finger and in the second kringle (Verheijen et al. 1986, Ichinose et al. 1986). The one-chain form of t-PA has very little activity towards low molecular synthetic substrates but the fibrinolytic properties of the one-chain and two-chain form are virtually the same (Rijken et al. 1982). T-PA's efficacy to activate plasminogen increases in the presence of fibrin (Ranby 1982) some 500 fold. This makes t-PA a fibrinspecific thrombolytic agent.

Inhibitors of plasminogen activators

Physiological regulation of the fibrinolytic system occurs not only at the level of plasmin but also at the level of the plasminogen activator. A fast acting inhibitor that inhibits t-PA (Chmielewska et al. 1983) as well as urokinase (Kruithof et al. 1986) has been described in 1983. It was subsequently called plasminogen activator inhibitor 1 (PAI1) (Collen 1986). This inhibitor is secreted by endothelial cells (Van Mourik et al.

1984), found in the supernatant of many cell cultures (Urden et al. 1987) and in platelets (Kruithof et al. 1986b). It inhibits one-chain and two-chain t-PA as well as two-chain urokinase at comparable rates (Colucci et al. 1986b). Its level was found to be increased in young survivors of myocardial infarction (Hamsten et al. 1985) and in patients with coronary artery disease (Paramo et al. 1985). A second inhibitor was characterized (Astedt et al. 1984) and appears to exist at very low levels in males and non pregnant women. During pregnancy it rises constantly and appears to be responsible for the impairment of the fibrinolytic system in pregnant women (Lecander and Astedt 1986). The influence of these inhibitors in therapeutic thrombolysis is negligible due to their very low concentrations in plasma (0–10 ng/ml). However PAI1 behaves as an acute phase reactant and in situations with an increase of PAI1 there might be an influence on therapeutical thrombolysis (Colucci et al. 1986).

Therapeutic properties

Venous thrombosis

The urge for therapeutic intervention in deep venous thrombosis (DVT) lies in its complications—pulmonary embolism and postthrombotic syndrome. Quite a few studies have been performed in order to evaluate the efficacy of thrombolytic treatment in DVT (reviewed by Samama 1987, Duckert 1984). Streptokinase has proven to be superior in the resolution of thrombi compared to heparin in several randomized trials (Robertson et al. 1968, Kakkar et al. 1969, Robertson et al. 1970, Tsapogas et al. 1973, Seaman et al. 1976, Marder et al. 1977, Arnesen et al. 1978, Elliot et al. 1979). Lysis rates with streptokinase ranged from 40 to 70%, those in patients treated with heparin from 10 to 25%. The dosage usually applied was a loading dose of 250.000 IU followed by an hourly dose of 100.000 IU. Recently an alternative approach has been published (Martin et al. 1983, Theiss et al. 1987) using ultra high dosages of streptokinase 1 500 000 IU/h, six hours daily. In these patients thrombolysis could be observed much earlier than in patients treated with a conventional dosage regimen. There seems to be no advantage of urokinase compared to streptokinase (Van de Loo et al. 1983). Bleeding complications however are about three times more often in association with thrombolytic treatment than with heparin only (Goldhaber et al. 1984). In regard to the prevention of postthrombotic syndrome some studies show favorable results in patients having received thrombolytic treatment (Arnesen et al. 1982, Common et al. 1976, Johanson et al. 1979), while another study could not detect differences (Kakkar and Lawrence 1985).

Peripheral arterial thrombosis

Systemic intravenous infusion of streptokinase in patients with recently (<3 days) obstructed arteries achieved patency rates of almost two thirds (Amery et al. 1970). In older occlusions it is more difficult to obtain lysis (Martin 1979). The incidence of major hemorrhage using a systemic thrombolytic approach is rather high, fatal bleeding complications occurring in about 1 to 3% of patients (Fiessinger et al. 1976). Due to this fact systemic thrombolysis in arterial obstruction has been used only rarely recently. An alternative method developed in the last 10 years is low-dose local thrombolysis (reviewed by Verhaeghe et al. 1987). Intraarterial infusion of 5000 IU streptokinase/h. is a common procedure. Local intraarterial lysis is usually applied to patients in whom surgery is difficult or contraindicated. Femoropoliteal occlusions are one example. A few studies on local thrombolysis in this condition have been done, yielding success rates of 50 to 80% (Graor et al. 1985, Hess et al. 1982, Lammer et al. 1985, Wilms et al. 1986). Data on long term success is only scarcely available. Bleeding complications are rare, but severe bleeds of gastrointestinal or intracranial origin have been reported. Data on the local use of urokinase or t-PA is very limited (Fiessinger 1981, Graor 1986). Though a promising approach prospective controlled studies have to be performed to evaluate the benefit from local thrombolysis in patients with arterial obstructions. The basis for thrombotic occlusions is an atherosclerotic vessel, so measures have to be taken after successful thrombolysis to retain patency of the vessel by either surgical or drug therapy.

Pulmonary embolism

The application of streptokinase and urokinase in acute pulmonary embolism has recently been reviewed (Cella et al. 1987). In two large, controlled studies (UPET 1973 and USPET 1974) a comparable degree of clot resolution and of hemodynamic improvement was found, using either streptokinase or urokinase. No difference was observed between a 12 or a 24 h infusion of urokinase, except in patients with massive pulmonary embolism who benefitted from the 24 h regimen. A wide variety of different doses of urokinase has been applied in many studies of thrombolysis in pulmonary embolism. Improvement as measured by pulmonary angiography is usually between 30 and 40%. A long term beneficial effect of thrombolysis in acute pulmonary embolism might be the reduced incidence of pulmonary hypertension which may be due to resolution of emboli from the pulmonary microcirculation (Sharma et al. 1980). In conclusion thrombolytic therapy has proven to be an efficient treatment in pulmonary embolism. The regimen to be applied could be streptokinase therapy in standard dosage. Urokinase may alternatively be given at a dosage of 4400 IU/kg for 12 hours. In patients with massive embolism, application of the same dosage for 24 h should be considered to achieve maximum resolution of the thrombi. T-PA has not yet been widely applied in the treatment of pulmonary embolism. From one ongoing, uncontrolled trial results are available. 43 patients have been treated with rt-PA, in 40 patients angiographic improvement was achieved after 2 or 6 h of therapy. Major bleedings were noted in 2 patients. Although this seems to indicate better results than could be obtained with streptokinase and urokinase, randomized studies will have to be performed to permit this conclusion to be drawn.

Acute myocardial infarction

The most rapid development of thrombolytic therapy in recent years has been in the field of acute myocardial infarction (AMI), reviewed by Acar et al. 1987. It is nowadays widely accepted that an occluding thrombus in a coronary artery is responsible for the development of AMI in the majority of patients (DeWood et al. 1980, Silver et al. 1980). Thrombolytic therapy is able to restore blood flow by lysing the thrombus, however a thrombus does not develop on intact endothelium but usually at the site of an atherosclerotic lesion (Roberts 1974). The persistant narrowing of the coronary artery favours early reocclusion (Harrison et al. 1984). This has led to an approach combining thrombolysis with percutaneous coronary angioplasty (PTCA) in recent studies, to improve the underlying stenosis and thus the long term results of thrombolytic therapy.

Streptokinase has been the first thrombolytic agent to be applied in AMI. Results of many studies performed since 1966 have been evaluated by Stampfer et al. (1982) and by Yusuf et al. (1985). These studies were performed using a 24 h infusion of 100 000 to 150 000 IU streptokinase/h. Pooled analysis of these trials showed a 21% reduction in mortality in 3110 patients in the weeks following the acute event. Severe bleeding complications were in the range of 2–3%. This approach to coronary thrombolysis has been left in recent years in favour of intracoronary or short term systemic lysis. Intracoronary thrombolysis was introduced by Rentrop et al. in 1979. The usual dosage was 2000 to 5000 IU/min for 60 to 90 minutes. Reperfusion rates with this regimen were in between 60 and 90%. In randomized controlled studies the effect of early coronary lysis on left ventricular function and infarct size was determined. It was repeatedly found that a reduction of hypokinetic zones occurred in patients in whom thrombolysis was successful (Serruys et al. 1986). An inverse correlation exists between the time from onset of symptoms to therapy and the benefit to the patient (Sheehan et al. 1985). Clinical outcome of patients with thrombolytic treatment seems to be superior to patients receiving conventional treatment (Kennedy et al. 1985, Simoons et al. 1986). Bleedings in patients treated with intracoronary streptokinase are usually limited to the puncture sites, however intracranial bleedings have been observed. Thus intracoronary thrombolysis provides an effective way for reopening an occluded artery, however it is limited to situations where there is immediate access to a catheter laboratory. The procedure does prolong the time to therapy by at least 1 hour. This time delay might be important in the salvage of jeopardized myocardium. A way to overcome these limitations has been the introduction of short term, high dosage intravenous lysis with streptokinase. The usual regimen consists of a dose of 1 500 000 U streptokinase administered in 60 min. Patency rates with streptokinase have been found to be between 44 and 60% (Neuhaus et al. 1983, Schröder et al. 1983, Rogers et al. 1983, Alderman et al. 1984). Two large studies have been published, the I.S.A.M. study (1986) with 1741 patients and G.I.S.S.I. study (1986) with 11806. Patients were treated with either streptokinase or placebo. The I.S.A.M. study could only show an improved left ventricular function and no improvement of hospital mortality. The G.I.S.S.I. study showed a beneficial effect on hospital mortality, predominantly for patients treated early after onset of symptoms (all patients 10.7% versus 13.0; <3 h; 9.2% versus 12.0%). At one year follow-up survival data were 74.0% in the streptokinase group and 72.1% in the control group (Mauri 1987).

The result of reopening of coronary vessels might not only be beneficial. One study showed that patients with early reopening are prone to a high risk for subsequent ischemic events, due to persistent narrowing of the reperfused artery (Koren et al. 1987). In conclusion, while there is no doubt that intravenous streptokinase is a relatively safe and efficient method to reopen thrombosed coronary vessels, the effect of long term survival and improvement seems to be less striking.

Urokinase has been applied in AMI in few studies only (Tennant et al. 1984; Mathey et al. 1985). Patency rates were comparable to those found in streptokinase treatment, while hemorrhagic complications seem to occur less often. The fibrinogenolytic effect is less pronounced.

Acylated streptokinase-plasminogen complex has been used in many small trials in acute MI. Only one study published was placebo controlled and randomized (Been et al. 1985). The small number of patients treated (16 in each group) makes analysis difficult. However it seems that with

intravenous APSAC comparable lysis rates as with intracoronary streptokinase can be achieved. Further randomized studies are necessary to
confirm these results.

Only one report on the application of scu-PA in coronary thrombolysis
has been published so far (Van de Werf et al. 1986). 40 mg of scu-PA
infused over 1 hour intravenously induced lysis in 4 out of 6 patients. In
two patients substantial systemic fibrinolysis was observed. More data on
the application of scu-PA in AMI is until now available in abstract form
only (Loascalzo 1987, Diefenbach et al. 1987, Welzel et al. 1987, Bode et
al. 1987).

For theoretical reasons t-PA was thought to induce clot specific lysis and
less systemic fibrinogenolysis. Several studies have been performed in
Europe and in the USA, comparing rt-PA to placebo (Collen et al. 1984,
Verstraete et al. 1985a, Topol et al. 1987), and to streptokinase (Verstraete
et al. 1985b, The TIMI study group 1985). Patency rates of t-PA are
between 60 and 85%, thus being highly superior to heparin or to intravenous streptokinase. Reocclusion after t-PA therapy was found
however in 20 to 37% of patients (Collen et al. 1984, Williams et al. 1986,
Gold et al. 1986). Two studies have been published trying to prevent the
high rate of reocclusions by a maintenance infusion of t-PA. While in one
study a decrease of reocclusions during hospital stay after a maintenance
infusion could be shown (Gold et al. 1986), this could not be validated by
the other study (Verstraete et al. 1987).

The fibrin selectivity of t-PA has been found to be a relative one. A dose
dependent systemic lytic state is induced by infusion of t-PA (Topol et al.
1985, Collen et al. 1986a). Bleeding complications in t-PA thrombolysis
are mostly from puncture sites. However gastrointestinal bleeding was
observed (Williams et al. 1986, TIMI 1985). So far there is no evidence
that t-PA reduces hospital mortality.

Another open question is the treatment after coronary lysis. It is
generally agreed that a severely obstructed vessel has a high incidence of
reocclusion. Thus percutaneous coronary angioplasty (PTCA) is considered
to be of worth after coronary lysis. Two studies on PTCA treatment after
thrombolysis have recently been published. The first (Topol et al. 1987a)
showed less postinfarction angina and reinfarction in a group of patients
receiving immediate PTCA after thrombolysis with t-PA compared to a
control group on conventional treatment. Infarct-zone regional movement
was improved too. In the other study (Topol 1987b) randomization was
done after thrombolysis into an immediate and an elective PTCA group.
No differences could be shown regarding clinical complications or ventricular function and wall motion regarding the time point of PTCA. Thus
immediate PTCA seems to offer no advantage compared to elective PTCA

after thrombolysis. Interestingly in the last mentioned study 14% of patients with a severely stenotic vessel after thrombolysis who were randomized to receive elective PTCA at 7 to 10 days were then found to have a stenotic lesion of less than 50%, obviating the need for PTCA. Despite the success of PTCA in restoring flow in a diseased vessel, restenosis after PTCA does occur in about 30% of the patients after at least six months (Satler et al. 1987). In conclusion t-PA seems to be able to reopen more vessels in AMI than does streptokinase when applied intravenously. Complications of therapy could be less in t-PA, while no data are available on the long term results.

Thrombolytic therapy in AMI seems to be of benefit to many patients. However patients should be treated early, preferably less than 4 hours after onset of pain. Angiography should be performed after thrombolysis to validate the residual stenosis and to decide whether PTCA should be performed. At the moment there is no way to prevent severe bleeding complications in some patients. Arrhythmias after reperfusion however rarely seem to produce clinical symptoms (Cercek et al. 1987).

Laboratory management of thrombolytic therapy

The problems in laboratory management of patients receiving therapy with thrombolytic agents has recently been reviewed (Conard and Samama 1987). In patients eligible for thrombolytic treatment screening tests (prothrombin time, partial thromboplastin time, fibrinogen) should be performed to exclude an underlying hemostatic defect. In patients receiving streptokinase the level of streptokinase antibodies might be of value in calculating a necessary loading dose. During treatment blood collection should be done under standardized conditions. It is advisable to collect blood on ice, centrifuge as soon as possible and freeze the plasma samples until determination commences. If fibrinogen determinations are being done, blood should be collected on citrate with additional aprotinin (100–500 KIU/ml). The usual fibrinogen determination according to Clauss might result in too low levels of fibrinogen due to high fibrin(ogen) degradation products. An alternative method is the one described by Rampling and Gaffney which measures besides intact fibrinogen the fragments X and Y, thus yielding higher values in patients with t-PA therapy (Verstraete 1985). During thrombolytic therapy it is advisable to perform determinations of fibrinogen and thrombin time as well as blood cell counts twice daily for longer thrombolytic treatments. For a short term treatment like in myocardial infarction it is sufficient to make these determinations after the end of infusion. Determinations of factors of the fibrinolytic system like plasminogen and alpha2-antiplasmin have to be done only for research purposes. There is no laboratory test available to measure the efficacy of thrombolytic treatment. A test newly available measuring D-Dimer, plasmin split product of fibrin, might correlate to resolution of thrombi. Preliminary results in patients with AMI under thrombolytic therapy with t-PA could not sustain this hypothesis (Soria et al. 1987). Bleeding associated with thrombolytic therapy is difficult to predict. At the moment there is no laboroatory test that identifies patients at risk. This is mainly due to the mechanisms involved in bleeding complications in thrombolytic therapy. Any fresh hemostatic plug in the circulation will be lysed by thrombolytic agents. Besides the one that should be eliminated, there can be other known or unknown sites of hemostatic plug formation. This is for example any venous or arterial puncture site, which are the most common bleeding sites under therapy. There may as well be unrecognized gastrointestinal ulcers that may bleed considerably, as well as small clinically silent cerebral hematomas or aneurysms. Even fibrin-specific drugs like t-PA are not able to differentiate between unwanted clots and hemostatic plugs.

Future developments

Synergism of plasminogen activators

The issue of synergism especially between t-PA and scu-PA has been a matter of controversy. A distinction has to be made between data obtained in in vitro and in in vivo systems. Working in vitro there was one group stating that no synergism could be found (Lijnen et al. 1986, Collen et al. 1986b), while another group deducted from their experiments a synergistic effect of both drugs (Gurewich and Pannell 1986). Despite new experimental evidence (Gurewich et al. 1987) this dispute has not been finally settled (Gurewich and Pannell 1987, Collen 1987). In vivo there seems to be concluding evidence that synergism exists, as could be shown in animal models and in patients with acute myocardial infarction (Collen et al. 1986c). The advantage of this approach would be the lacking of systemic fibrinogenolysis and a possible decrease in bleeding complications. Further controlled studies have to determine the place of this form of thrombolytic therapy.

Mutants of fibrinolytic drugs

Different features of fibrinolytic agents like t-PA are related to different regions on the molecule (Van Zonneveld et al. 1987). On the molecular level these domains are coded for by separate exons, flanked by introns (Ny et al. 1984). By constructing mutants containing structural domains in a different order and/or number than the natural molecule (Ehrlich et al. 1987), it could be envisaged that useful features of different agents could be combined in one molecule. For example additional fibrin binding sites could be coupled to a fibrinolytic agent, thus increasing its specificity. Another way would be that by altering the structures of the molecule its clearance could be impeded. As clearance rates from the circulation are very short for t-PA and scu-PA (Devries et al. 1987, Gurewich et al. 1984) structural changes might lead to diminished clearance rates, thus allowing for sustained thrombolytic action. Such alterations could be achieved by coupling molecules either chemically or by genetic engineering. Coupling of the plasmin heavy chain containing the fibrin binding sites to low molecular weight urokinase increased the thrombolytic properties of the new molecule in an animal model (Nakayama et al. 1986).

Fibrin specificity by immunological coupling

The idea behind this approach is to couple potent thrombolytic agents with no or limited fibrin-binding properties like urokinase to a fibrin specific antibody. This concept has been successfully applied to the coupling of a fibrin specific antibody to urokinase (Bode et al. 1985) and of a fibrin specific antibody FAB' to urokinase (Bode et al. 1987), resulting in increased thrombolytic activity of the complexes compared to urokinase alone.

References

Acar J, Vahahnian A, Michel P-L, Slama M, Cormier B, Roger V (1987) Thrombolytic treatment in acute myocardial infarction. Sem Thromb Haemost 13:186–200

Alderman EL, Jutzy KR, Berte LE, Miller RG, Friedman JP, Creger WP, Eliastman M (1984) Am J. Cardiol 54:14–19

Amery A, Deloof W, Vermylen J, Verstraete M (1970) Outcome of recent thromboembolic occlusions of limb arteries treated with streptokinase. Br Med J 4:639–644

Arnesen H, Heilo A, Jocobson E, Ly B, Skaga E (1978) A prospective study of streptokinase and heparin in the treatment of deep vein thrombosis. Acta Med Scand 203:457–463

Arnesen H, Hoiset A, Ly B, Godal HC (1982) Streptokinase or heparin in the treatment of deep vein thrombosis—follow up results of a prospective study. Acta Med Scand 211:65–68

Bachmann F, Kruithof EKO (1984) Tissue plasminogen activator: Chemical and physiological aspects. Sem Thromb Haemost 10:6–17

Bando H, Okada K, Matsuo O (1987) Thrombolytic effect of prourokinase in vitro. Fibrinolysis 1:169–176

Been M, de Bono DP, Muir AL, Boulton FE, Hillis WS, Hornung R (1985) Coronary thrombolysis with intravenous anisoylated plasminogen streptokinase complex BRL 26291. Br Heart J 53:253–259

Bode C, Matsueda GR, Hui KY, Haber E (1985) Antibody directed urokinase: a specific fibrinolytic agent. Science 222:1129–1132

Bode C, Runge MS, Newell JB, Matsueda GR, Haber E (1987) Thrombolysis by a fibrin-specific antibody Fab'-urokinase conjugate. J Mol Cell Cardiol 19:335–341

Bode C, Schwarz F, Schuler G, Zimmermann R, Kübler W (1987) Intravenous thrombolytic therapy with single-chain urokinase-type plasminogen activator in patients with myocardial infarction. Thromb Haemost 58:209

Castellino FJ (1984) Biochemistry of human plasminogen. Semin Thromb Haemost 10:18–23

Cella G, Palla A, Sasahara AA (1987) Controversies of different regimens of thrombolytic therapy in acute pulmonary embolism. Sem Thromb Haemost 13:163–169

Cercek B, Lew AS, Laramee P, Shah PK, Peter TC, Ganz W (1987) Time course and characteristics of ventricular arrhythmias after reperfusion in acute myocardial infarction. Am J Cardiol 60:214–218

Chmielewska J, Ranby M, Wiman B (1983) Evidence for a rapid inhibitor to tissue plasminogen activator in plasma. Thromb Res 31:427–436

Clauss A (1957) Gerinnungsphysiologische Schnellmethode zur Bestimmung des fibrinogens. Acta Haematol 17:237–246

Collen D (1986) Report of the subcommittee on fibrinolysis, Jerusalem, Israel, June 2, 1986. Thromb Haemost 56:415–416

Collen D, Bounameaux H, de Cock F, Lijnen HR, Verstraete M (1986a) Analysis of coagulation and fibrinolysis during intravenous infusion on recombinant human tissue-type plasminogen activator in patients with acute myocardial infarction. Circulation 73:511–517

Collen D, Topol EJ, Tiefenbrunn AJ, Gold HK, Weisfeldt ML, Sobel BE, Leinback RC, Brinker JA, Ludbrock PA, Yasuda T, Bulkey BH, Robison AK, Hutter AM, Bell WR, Spadoro JJ, Khaw BA, Grossbard ED (1984) Coronary thrombolysis with recombinant tissue type plasminogen activator: A prospective, randomized, placebo-controlled trial. Circulation 70:1012–1017

Collen D (1985) Report of the meeting of the subcommittee on fibrinolysis, San Diego, Ca, USA, July 13, 1985. Thromb Haemost 54:893

Collen D (1987) Molecular mechanisms of fibrinlysis and their application to fibrin-specific thrombolytic therapy. Journal of Cellular Biochemistry 33:77–86

Collen D (1987) Rebuttal. Synergism of tissue-type plasminogen activator (t-PA) and single-chain urokinase-type plasminogen activator (scu-PA) on clot lysis in vitro and a mechanism for this effect. Thromb Haemost 57:373

Collen D, de Cock F, Demarsin E, Lijnen HR, Stump DC (1986b) Absence of synergism between tissue-type plasminogen activator (t-PA), single-chain urokinase-type plasminogen activator (scu-PA) and urokinase on clot lysis in vitro. Thromb Haemost 56:35–39

Collen D, Stump DC, van de Werf F (1986c) Coronary thrombolysis in patients with acute myocardial infarction by intravenous infusion of synergic thrombolytic agents. Am Heart J 112:1083–1084

Collen D, Zamarron C, Lijnen HR, Hoylaerts M (1986d) Activation of plasminogen by pro-urokinase. II. Kinetics. J Biol Chem 261:1259–1266

Colucci M, Paramo JA, Stassen JM, Collen D (1986a) Influence of the fast-acting inhibitor of plasminogen activator on in vivo thrombolysis induced by tissue-type plasminogen activator in rabbits. J Clin Invest 78:138–144

Colucci M, Paramo JA, Collen D (1986b) Inhibition of one-chain and of two-chain forms of human tissue type plasminogen activator by the fast acting inhibitor of plasminogen activator in vitro and in vivo. J. Lab Clin Med 108:53–59

346

Common HH, Seaman AR, Rosch J, Porter JM, Dotter C (1976) A deep vein thrombosis treated with streptokinase or heparin: follow up of a randomized study. Angiology 27:645–654

Conard J, Samama MM (1987) Theoretic and practical considerations on laboratory monitoring of thrombolytic therapy. Sem Thromb Haemost 13:212–222

Conforti G, Loskutoff DJ (1985) Plasmin and thrombin modulate plasminogen activation by fibro-sarcoma cells. (Abstr.) Thromb Haemost 54:171

Devries SR, Fox KAA, Robison A, Rodriguez RU, Sobel BE (1987) Determinants of clearance of tissue-type plasminogen activator (t-PA) from the circulation. Fibrinolysis 1:17–21

DeWood MA, Spores J, Notske R, Mouser LT, Burroughs R, Golden MS, Lang HT (1980) Prevalence of total coronary occlusion during the early hours of transmural myocardial infarction. N Engl J Med 303:897–902

Diefenbach C, Erbel R, Meyer J, Hamm CW, Schofer J, Mathey DG (1987) Dose-finding study of thrombolysis in acute myocardial infarction by single-chain prourokinase. Thromb Haemost 58:208

Duckert F (1984) Thrombolytic therapy. Sem Thromb Haemost 10:87–103

Ehrlich HJ, Bang NU, Little SP, Jaskunas SR, Weigel BJ, Mattler LE, Harms CS Biological properties of a kringleless tissue plasminogen activator (t-PA) mutant. Fibrinolysis 1:75–81

Elliot MS, Immelman EJ, Jeffery P, Benatar SR, Funston MR, Smith JA (1979) A comparative randomized trial of heparin versus streptokinase in the treatment of acute proximal venous thrombosis, an interim report of prospective trial. Br J Surg 66:806–810

Ferres H, Hibbs M, Standring R (1987) Deacylation studies in vitro on anisoylated plasminogen streptokinase activator complex. Drugs 33(Suppl. 3) (In press)

Fiessinger JN, Aiach M, Capron L, Devanlay M, Vayssairat M, Juillet Y (1981) Effect of local urokinase on arterial occlusions of lower limbs. Thromb Haemost 45:230–232

Fiessinger JN, Aiach M, Lagneau P, Husson JM, Cormier JM, Housset E (1976) Indications de la streptokinase dans les oblitérations arteriélles des membres. Cœur Méd Interne 15:453–459

Gold HK, Leinbach RC, Garabedian HD, Yasuda T, Johns JA, Grossbard EB, Palacios I, Collen D (1986) Acute coronary reocclucion after thrombolysis with recombinant human tissue-type plasminogen activator: prevention by a maintenance infusion. Circulation 73:347–352

Goldhaber SZ, Buring JE, Lipnick RJ, Hennekens CH (1984) Pooled analysis of randomized trials of streptokinase and heparin in phlebographically documented acute deep venous thrombosis. Am J Med 76:393

Goldhaber SZ, Markis JE, Kessler CM, Meyerovitz MF, Kim D, Vauchan DE, Selwyn AP, Loscalzo J, Dawley DL, Sharma GVRK, Sasahara A, Grossbard EB, Braunwald E (1987) Perspectives on treatment of acute pulmonary embolism with tissue plasminogen activator. Sem Thromb Haemost 13:171–176

Graor RA, Risius B, Denny KM, Young JR, Beven EG, Hertzer HR, Ruschhaupt WF, O'Hara PJ, Geisinger MA, Zelch MG (1985) Local thrombolysis in the treatment of thrombosed arteries, bypass grafts and arteriovenous fistulas. J Vasc Surg 2:406–414

Graor RA, Risius B, Young JR, Denny K, Beven E.G., Geisinger MA, Hertzer NR, Krajewski LP, Lucas VF, O'Hara PJ, Ruschhaupt WF, Winton S, Zelch MG, Grossbard EB (1986) J Vasc Surg 3:115–124

Gruppo Italiano per lo Studio della Streptochinasi nell'Infarto Miocardico (GISSI) (1986) Effectiveness of intravenous thrombolytic treatment in acute myocardial infarction. Lancet I:397–401

Gurewich V, Black J, Pannell R (1987) A mechanism for the potentiating effect of urokinase

(UK) or tissue plasminogen activator (t-PA) on clot lysis by pro-urokinase (pro-uk). Thromb Haemost 58:439

Gurewich V, Pannell R. (1986) A comparative study of the efficacy and specificity of tissue-plasminogen activator and pro-urokinase: demonstration of synergism and of different thresholds of non-selectivity. Thromb Res 44:217–228

Gurewich V, Pannell R (1987) Fibrin binding and zymogenic properties of single-chain urokinase (pro-urokinase). Sem Thromb Haemost 13:146–151

Gurewich V, Pannell R, Louie S, Kelley P, Suddith RL, Greenlee R (1984) Effective and fibrin-specific clot lysis by a zymogen precursor form of urokinase (pro-urokinase). A study in vitro and in two animal species. J. Clin Invest 73:1731–1739

Gurewich V, Pannell W (1987) Synergism of tissue-type plasminogen activator (t-PA) and single-chain urokinase-type plasminogen activator (scu-PA) on clot lysis in vitro and a mechanism for this effect. Thromb Haemost 57:372

Hamsten A, Wiman B, DeFaire U, Blombäck M (1985) Increased plasma levels of a rapid inhibitor of tissue plasminogen activator in young survivors of myocardial infarction. N Engl J Med 313:1557–1563

Harrison DG, Ferguson DW, Collins SM, Skorton DK, Ericksen EE, Kioschos JM, Marcus ML, White CW (1984) Rethrombosis after reperfusion with streptokinase: Importance of geometry of residual lesions. Circulation 69:991–999

Hess H, Ingrisch H, Mietaschk A, Rath H (1982) Local low-dose thrombolytic therapy of peripheral arterial occlusions. N Engl J Med 307:1627–1630

Holmes WE, Pennica D, Blaber, M, Rey MW, Günzler WA, Steffens GJ, Heynecker HL (1982) Cloning and expression of the gene for pro-urokinase in escherichia coli. Biotechnology 3:923–929

Husain SS, Gurewich V, Lipinski B (1983) Purification and partial characterization of a single-chain high-molecular-weight form of urokinase from human urine. Arch Biochem Biophys 220:31–38

Ichinose A, Takio K, Fujikawa K (1986) Localization of the binding site of tissue-type plasminogen activator to fibrin. J Clin Invest 78:163–169

Johanson L, Nylander G, Hedner U, Nilsson IM (1979) Comparison of streptokinase with heparin: Late results in the treatment of deep vein thrombosis. Acta Med Scand 206:93–98

Kakkar VV, Flanc C, Howe CT, O'Shea M (1969) Treatment of deep vein thrombosis. A trial of heparin streptokinase and arvin. Br Med J 1:806–810

Kakkar VV, Lawrence D (1985) Hemodynamic and clinical assessment after therapy for acute deep vein thrombosis. Am J Surg 10:54–63

Kasai S, Arimura H, Nishida M, Suyama T (1985a) Proteolytic cleavage of single-chain pro-urokinase induces conformational change which follow activation of the zymogen and reduction of its high affinity for fibrin. J Biol Chem 260:2377–2381

Kasai S, Arimura H, Nishida M, Suyama T (1985b) Thrombolytic properties of an inactive proenzyme form of human urokinase secreted from human kidney cells. Cell Struct Funct 10:151–159

Kennedy JW, Ritchie JL, Davis KB, Stadius ML, Maynar C, Fritz JK (1985) The Western Washington randomized trial of intracoronary streptokinase in acute myocardial infarction. A 12 months follow-up report. N. Engl J Med 312:1073–1077

Koren G, Luria MH, Weiss, AT, Kriwisky M, Mosseri M, Lotan C, Applebaum D, Welber S, Sapoznikov D, Ben-David Y, Hasin Y, Gotsman MS (1987) Early treatment of acute myocardial infarction with intravenous streptokinase. A high risk syndrome. Arch Intern Med 147:237–240

Kruithof EKO, Tran-Thang C, Bachmann F (1986b) Studies on the release of a plasminogen activator inhibitor by human platelets. Thromb Haemost 55:201–205

Lammer J, Pilger E, Justich E, Neumayer K, Schreyer H. (1985) Fibrinolysis in chronic arteriosclerotic occlusions: Intrathrombotic injections of streptokinase. Radiology 157:45–50

Lecander I, Astedt B (1986) Isolation of a new specific plasminogen activator inhibitor from pregnancy plasma. Brit J Haematol 62:221–228

Lijnen HR, van Hoef B, Collen D (1986a) Comparative kinetic analysis of the activation of human plasminogen by natural and recombinant single-chain urokinase-type plasminogen activator. Biochim Biophys Acta 884:402–408

Lijnen HR, Zamarron C, Blabert M, Winkler ME, Collen D (1986b) Activation of plasminogen by pro-urokinase. I. Mechanism. J Biol Chem 261:1253–1258

Loscalzo J (1987) The efficacy and relative fibrin-selectivity of prourokinase in patients with acute myocardial infarction. Thromb Haemost 58:209

Marder VJ, Soulen RL, Atichartakarn V, Budzynski AZ, Parelukar S, Kim JR, Edward N, Zahavi J, Algazyk KM (1977) Quantitative venographic assessment of deep vein thrombosis in the evaluation of streptokinase and heparin therapy. J Lab Clin Med 89:1018–1029

Martin M, Fiebach BJO, Feldkamp M (1983) Ultrahohe Streptokinase-Infusionsbehandlung bei peripheren Gefäßverschlüssen. DMW 108:167

Martin M, Schoop W, Zeitler E (1970) Streptokinase in chronic arterial occlusive disease. JAMA 211:1169–1173

Mathey DG, Schofer J, Sheehan FH, Becher H, Tilsner V, Dodge HT (1985) Intravenous urokinase in acute myocardial infarction. Am J Cardiol 55:878–882

Mauri F (1987) Effectiveness of intravenous thrombolytic treatment in acute myocardial infarction: short and medium term prognosis. Thromb Haemost 58:224

Monk JP, Heel RC (1987) Anisoylated plasminogen streptokinase activator complex (APSAC). Drugs 34:25–49

Moroi M, Aoki N (1976) Isolation and characterization of alpha-plasmin inhibitor from human plasma. A novel proteinase inhibitor which inhibits activator-induced clot lysis. J. Biol Chem 251:5050

Nakayama Y, Shinohara M, Tani T, Kawaguchi T, Furuta T, Izawa T, Kaise H, Miyazaki W (1986) The plasmin heavy chain-urokinase conjugate: A specific thrombolytic agent. Thromb Haemost 56:364–370

Neuhaus KL, Tebbe U, Sauer G, Kreuze H, Köstering H (1983) High dose intravenous streptokinase in acute myocardial infarction. Clin Cardiol 6:426–434

Nielsen LS, Hansen JG, Skriver L, Wilson EL, Kaltoft K, Zeuthen J, Dano K (1982) Purification of zymogen to plasminogen activator from human glioblastoma cells by affinity chromatography with monoclonal antibody. Biochemistry 24:6410–6415

Pannell R, Gurewich V (1987) Activation of plasminogen by single-chain urokinase or by two-chain urokinase—A demonstration that single-chain urokinase has a low catalytic activity (prourokinase). Blood 69:22–26

Pathy L (1985) Evolution of the proteases of blood coagulation and fibrinolysis by assembly from modules. Cell 41:657–663

Pennica D, Holmes WE, Kohr WJ, Harkins RN, Vehar GA, Ward CA, Bennet WF, Yelverton E, Seeburg PH, Heyneker HL, Goeddel DV, Collen D (1983) Cloning and expression of human tissue-type plasminogen activator cDNA in E. coli. Nature 201:214–221

Preissner KT, Müller-Berghaus G (1986) Molekulare Wechselwirkungen zwischen Komplement-, Gerinnungs- und Fibrinolysesystem. Hämostaseologie 6:67–81

Rampling MW, Gaffney PJ (1976) The sulfite precipitation method for fibrinogen measurement: its use on small samples in the presence of fibrinogen degradation products. Clin Chim Acta 67:43–52

Ranby M (1982) Studies on the kinetics of plasminogen activation by tissue plasminogen activator. Biochem Biophys Acta 704:461–469

Rentrop KP, Blanke H, Köstering K, Barsch KR (1979) acute myocardial infarction: intracoronary application of nitroglycerin and streptokinase in combination with transluminal recanalisation. Clin Cardiol 2:354–363

Rijken DC, Wijngaards G, Zaal de Jong M, Welbergen J (1979) Purification and partial characterization of plasminogen activator from human uterine tissue. Biochim Biophys Acta 580:140–153

Rijken DC, Hoylaerts M, Collen D (1982) Fibrinolytic properties of one-chain and two-chain human extrinsic (tissue-type) plasminogen activator. J. Biol Chem 257:2920–2925

Roberts WC (1974) Coronary thrombosis and fatal myocardial ischemia. Circulation 49:1–3

Robertson BR, Nilsson IM, Nylander G (1968) Value of streptokinase and heparin in treatment of acute deep vein thrombosis. Acta Chir Scand 134:203–208

Robertson BR, Nilsson IM, Nylander G (1970) Thrombolytic effect of streptokinase as evaluated by phlebography of deep vein thrombosis of the leg. Acta Chir Scand 136: 173–180

Rogers WJ, Mantle JA, Hood JP, Baxley WA, Whitlow PI, Reeves RC, Soto B (1983) Prospective randomized trial of intravenous and intracoronary streptokinase in acute myocardial infarction. Circulation 68:1051–1061

Samama M, Verdy E, Conard J, Vahanian A, Michel P, van Dreden P, Nguyen G, Horellou MH, Combrisson A, Acar J (1986) Activateur tissulaire du plasminogene (t-PA) dans l'infarctus du myocarde: aspects biologiques. Arch Mal Cœur 11:618–624

Samama MM (1987) Deep vein thrombosis of inferior limbs; Are thrombolytic agents superior to heparin? Sem Thromb Haemost 13:178–180

Satler LF, Green CE, McNamara NM, Lavelle JP, Pallas RS, Pearle DL, Kent KM, Rackley CE (1987) Late angiographic follow-up after successful coronary arterial thrombolysis and angioplasty during acute myocardial infarction. Am J Cardiol 60:210–213

Schröder R, Biamino G, von Leitner ER, Linderer T, Brüggemann T, Heitz J, Voehringer HF, Wegscheider K (1983) Intravenous short term infusion of streptokinase in acute myocardial infarction. Circulation 67:536–548

Seaman AJ, Common HH, Rosch J, Dotter CT, Porter JM, Lindell TD, Lawler WL, Schlueter WJ (1976) Deep vein thrombosis treated with streptokinase or heparin. A randomized study. Angiology 27:549–553

Serruys PW, Simoons ML, Suryapranata H, Vermeer F, Wijns W, van den Brand M, Bär F, Zwaan C, Krauss XH, Remme WJ, Res J, Verheugt FWA, van Domburg R, Lubsen J, Hugfenholtz PG (1986) Preservation of global and regional left ventricular function after early thrombolysis in acute myocardial infarction. J Am Coll Cardiol 7:729–742

Sheehan FH, Mathey DG, Schofer J, Dodge HT, Bolson EL (1985) Factors that determine recovery of left ventricular function after thrombolysis in patients with acute myocardial infarction. Circulation 6:1121–1128

Silver MD, Baroldi G, Mariani F (1980) The relationship between acute occlusive coronary thrombi and myocardial infarction studied in 100 consecutive patients. Circulation 61:219–227

Simoons ML, Serruys PW, van den Brand M, Res J, Verheugt FWA, Krauss XH, Remme WJ, Bär F, de Zwaan C, van der Laarse A, Vermeer F, Lubsen J (1986) Early thrombolysis in acute myocardial infarction: Limitation of infarct size and improved survival. J Am Coll Cardiol 7:717–728

Skriver L, Nielsen LS, Stephens R, Dano K (1982) Plasminogen activator released as inactive proenzyme from murine cells transformed by sarcoma virus. Eur J Biochem 124:409–414

Soria J, Soria C, Mirshahi M, Xi M, Mirshahi M, Samama MM, Caen JP (1987) Sem Thromb Haemost 13:223–227

Stampfer MJ, Goldhaber SZ, Yusuf S, Peto R, Hennekens CH (1982) Effect of intravenous streptokinase on acute myocardial infarction. Pooled results from randomized trials. N Engl J Med 307:1180–1182

Taylor FB Jr, Comp PC (1978) Biochemistry of streptokinase. In: Markwardt F (ed.) Fibrinolytics and antifibrinolytics. Berlin: Springer-Verlag, pp 137–149

Tennant SN, Dixon J, Venable TC, Page HL, Roach A, Kaiser AB, Fredericksen R, Tacogue L, Kaplan P, Babu NS, Anderson EE, Wooten E, Jennings HS, Breinig J, Campbell WB (1984) Intracoronary thrombolysis in patients with acute myocardial infarction: Comparison of the efficacy of urokinase with streptokinase. Circulation 69:756–760

The I.S.A.M. Study Group (1986) A prospective trial of intravenous streptokinase in acute myocardial infarction (I.S.A.M.). N Engl J Med 314:1465–1471

The TIMI Study Group (1985) The thrombolysis in myocardial infarction (TIMI) trial: phase I findings. N Engl J Med 312:932–936

The Urokinase Pulmonary Embolism Trial (1973) A national cooperative study. Circulation 47(Suppl. II):1–108

Theiss W, Baumann G, Klein G (1987) Fibrinolytische Behandlung tiefer Venenthrombosen mit Streptokinase in ultrahoher Dosierung. DMW 112:668–674

Topol EJ, Bell WR, Weisfeldt ML (1985) Coronary thrombolysis with recombinant tissue-type plasminogen activator. Ann Int Med 103:837–843

Topol EJ, Califf RM, George BS, Kereiakes DJ, Abbottsmith CW, Candela RJ, Lee KL, Pitt B, Stack RS, O'Neill WW, and the TAMI Group (1987) A randomized trial of immediate versus delayed elective angioplasty after intravenous tissue plasminogen activator in acute myocardial infarction. N Engl J Med 317:581–588

Topol EJ, O'Neill WW, Langburd AB, Walton JA, Bourdillon PDV, Bates ER, Grines CL, Schork AM, Kline E, Pitt B (1987) A randomized placebo controlled trial of intravenous recombinant tissue-type plasminogen activator and emergency coronary angioplasty patients with acute myocardial infarction. Circulation 75:420–428

Tsapogas MJ, Peabody RA, Wu KT, Karmdy AM, Devaraj KT, Erkert C (1973) Controlled study of thrombolytic therapy in DVT. Surgery 74:973–984

Urden G, Chmielweska J, Carlsson T, Wiman B (1987) Immunological relationship between plasminogen activator inhibitors from different sources. Thromb Haemost 57:29–34

Urokinase-Streptokinase Pulmonary Embolism Trial. Phase 2 results. (1974) JAMA 229:1606–1613

Van de Loo JCW, Kriessmann A, Trübestein G, Knoch K, de Swart CAM, Asbeck F, Marbet GA, Schmidt HE, Sewell AF, Duckert F, Theiss W, Ritz R (1983) Controlled multicenter pilot study of urokinase-heparin and streptokinase in deep vein thrombosis. Thromb Haemost 50:660–663

Van de Werf F, Nobuhara M, Collen D (1986) Coronary thrombolysis with human single-chain, urokinase-type plasminogen activator (pro-urokinase) in patients with acute myocardial infarction. Ann Int Med 104:345–348

Van Mourik JA, Lawrence DA, Loskutoff DJ (1984) Purification of an inhibitor of plasminogen activator (antiactivator) synthesized by endothelial cells. J Biol Chem 259:14914–14921

Van Zonneveld A-J, Veerman H, Brakenhoff JPJ, Aarden LA, Cajot J-F, Pannekoek H (1987) Mapping of epitopes on human tissue-type plasminogen activator with recombinant deletion mutant proteins. Thromb Haemost 57:82–86

Verhaghe R, Wilms G, Vermylen J (1987) Local low-dose thrombolysis in arterial disease of the limbs. Sem Thromb Haemost 13:206–211

Verheijen JH, Caspers MPM, Chang GTG, de Munk GAW, Pouwels PH, Enger-Valk BE (1986) Involvement of finger domain and kringle 2 domain of tissue-type plasminogen activator in fibrin binding and stimulation of activity by fibrin. EMBO J 5:3525–3530

Verstraete M, Arnold AER, Brower RW, Collen D, de Bono DP, de Zwaan C, Erbel R, Hillis S, Lennane RJ, Lubsen J, Mathey D, Reid DS, Rutsch W, Schartl M, Schofer J, Serruys PW, Simoons ML, Uebis R, Vahanian A, Verheugt FWA, von Essen R (1987) Acute coronary thrombolysis with recombinant human tissue-type plasminogen activator: Initial patency and influence of maintained infusion on reocclusion rate. Am J Cardiol 60:231–237

Verstraete M, Bleifeld W, Brower RW, Charbonnier B, Collen D, de Bono DP, Dunning AJ, Lennane RJ, Lubsen J, Mathey DG, Michel PL, Raynaud P, Schofer J, Vahanian A, Vahhaecke J, van de Kley GA, van de Werf F, von Essen R (1985) Double blind randomized trial of intravenous tissue type plasminogen activator versus placebo in acute myocardial infarction. Lancet II:965–969

Verstraete M, Bernard R, Bory M, Brower RW, Collen D, de Bono DP, Erbel R, Huhmann W, Lennane RJ, Lübsen J, Mathey D, Meyer J, Michels HR, Rutsch W, Scharl M, Schmidt W, Uebis R, von Essen R (1985) Randomized trial of intravenous recombinant tissue-type plasminogen activator versus intravenous streptokinase in acute myocardial infarction. Lancet I:842–847

Walker ID, Davidson JF (1987) Acyl enzymes for thrombolytic therapy. Sem Thromb Haemost 13:139–145

Welzel D, Wolf H (1987) Clinical research on single-chain urokinase-type plasminogen activator (scu-PA) in Germany. Results in patients with acute myocardial infarction. Thromb Haemost 58:47

Williams DO, Borer J, Braunwald E, Chesebro J, Cohen LS, Dalen J, Dodge HT, Francis CK, Knatterud G, Ludbrook P, Markis JE, Mueller H, Desvigne-Nickens P, Passamani ER, Powers ER, Sobel BE, Winniford M, Zaret B (1986) Intravenous recombinant tissue-type plasminogen activator in patients with acute myocardial infarction: a report from the NHLBI thrombolysis in myocardial trial. Circulation 73:338–346

Williams JRB (1951) The fibrinolytic activity of urine. Brit J Exp Pathol 32:530–537

Wilms GE, Verhaeghe RH, Pouillon MM, Dewaele D, Baert AJ, Vermylen J, Verstraete M Local thrombolysis in fermoropopliteal occlusions; Early and late results. Cardiovasc Intervent Radiol (In press)

Wun TC, Schleuning WD, Reich E (1982) Isolation and characterization of urokinase from human plasma. J Biol Chem 257:3276–3283

Yusuf S, Collins R, Peto R, Furberg C, Stampfer MJ, Goldhaber SZ, Hennekens CH (1985) Intravenous and intracoronary fibrinolytic treatment in acute myocardial infarction: Overview of results on mortality, reinfarction, and side effects from 33 randomized controlled trials. Eur Heart J 6:556–585

25. Treatment of familial hypocholesterolemia by means of specific immunadsorption

H. BORBERG[1], A. GACZKOWSKI[1], V. HOMBACH[2], K. OETTE[3] &
W. STOFFEL[4]

[1] Haemapheresis Unit, Department of Medicine, University of Köln, F.R.G.; [2] Cardiology, Department of Medicine, University of Köln, F.R.G.; [3] Division of Clinical Chemistry, University of Köln, F.R.G.; [4] Department of Physiological Chemistry, University of Köln, F.R.G.

Introduction

Low density lipoprotein (LDL) is considered to be the major risk factor for the development of atherosclerosis and thus cardiovascular diseases. Familial hypercholesterolemia is an inherited, autosomal, dominant disease with massively elevated LDL levels due to an LDL receptor defect. 0.2% of the total population suffers from this disease, characterized from early atherosclerosis, mainly of the coronary arteries. The majority of these patients is heterozygous with total cholesterol levels ranging from 300–500 mg/dl. They die from myocardial infarction mainly between their 40–55th year of life. Homozygous patients are rare with a frequency of $1:1\,000\,000$, with total cholesterol levels beyond 500 mg/dl and myocardial infarction occurring generally not later than at an age of 25–30 years, often much earlier. Both groups of patients suffer much earlier from coronary heart disease for many years.

Conventional therapy with diet and drugs is ineffective in approximately 20% of the heterozygous patients with FH and virtually all homozygotes. Thus extracorporeal LDL-elimination may be considered to be an alternative. In contrast to plasmaexchange, which is entirely unspecific, removing all plasma proteins, and selective procedures, like differential plasma filtration or precipitation, still eliminating considerable amounts of normal or even protective plasma constituents, LDL-apheresis is characterized from the immune specific removal of LDL (immunadsorption, therapeutic affinity chromatography) [5]. It was introduced into clinical medicine in 1981 [6] and is since then in routine application of 16 patients by now in Cologne.

V. Hombach, H. H. Hilger and H. L. Kennedy (eds), Electrocardiography and Cardiac Drug Therapy. ISBN 978-94-010-6976-2
© 1989, Kluwer Academic Publishers, Dordrecht –

Method

As the procedure is published in detail [1, 2, 3, 6] and the technical equipment is commercially available, the principle shall be summarized just briefly.

Heparin-citrate anticoagulated plasma, continuously separated in a blood cell separator, is permitted to pass through a pair of columns alternatively loaded and desorbed at a flow rate of 30–45 ml/min corresponding to a whole blood flow rate of 50–80 ml/min (Table 1). The columns contain 300–400 ml of Sepharose 4b carrying an anti apoprotein B antibody. Both columns stay with the same patient until they are worn out after an average of 50 treatments (Table 2). The loading and desorption is performed under the control of an automated device, especially developed in our laboratory for this purpose and is generally repeated twice during the course of each treatment lasting between three to four hours (Figure 1). The features of the adsorption-desorption automate are summarized in Table 3. We strongly suggest to apply only those plasma separation devices, which can be used on a veno-venous flow basis from one arm to the other, except for unusual working conditions. The character and the rate of complication as well as its

Table 1. LDL-Apheresis: technical system

Plasma separation	
Blood removal and -return	Cubital veins (no artificial access necessary)
Whole blood flow rate	50–80 ml/min
Separation	1. Continuous flow blood cell separators (IBM-COBE 2997, FENWAL Celltrifuge II)
	2. Flat sheet membrane filtration (COBE-TPE)
Plasma flow	30–50 ml/min
Extracorporeal volume (incl. AD-system)	450–550 ml

Table 2. LDL-Apheresis: immunoadsorption columns

Number/patient	2 columns
Cycles/treatment	2/column
Livespan	Approx. 50 treatments = 1 year (Range: 40–140 treatments)
Flowrates	
– Loading (plasma)	30–45 ml/min
– Desorption (aqueous solutions)	80–90 ml/min

354

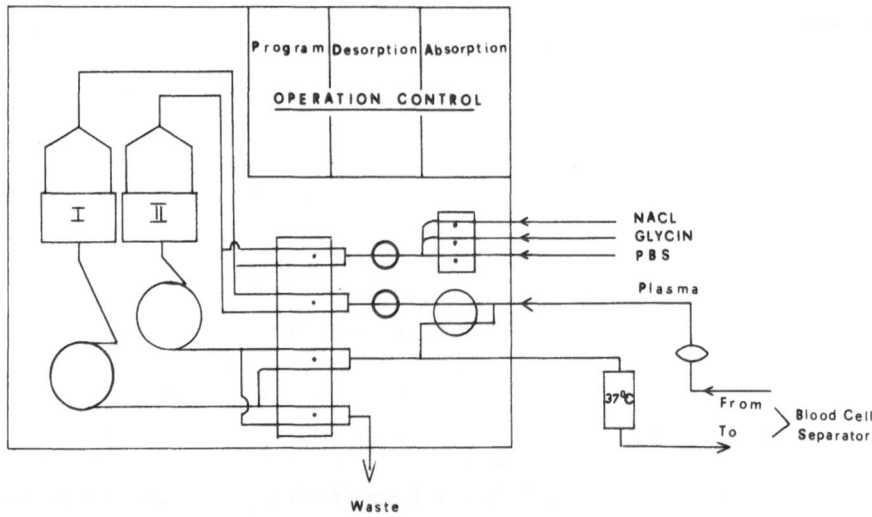

Waste

Figure 1. Flow diagram of an automated adsorption-desorption system developed for the clinical application of affinity chromatography.

life expectancy, renders an artificial access to the circulation, using shunts or central venous approaches, often applied with hollow fiber devices, clearly unethical for these patients. Also technical (mainly relatively high plasma flow rates due to the application of high g-forces) and economical reasons stimulated us to prefer blood cell separators against other technologies. The application of high g-forces also virtually eliminates the

Table 3. Essentials of a completely automated, volume controlled system with electronic operation for the selective and specific plasma absorption therapy*

---

1. Universal application due to a free selection of volumes and flow rates for an alternate use of plasma and desorption fluids

Loading volumes	1–9990 ml/cycle	Loading flowrates	0– 75 ml/min
Desorption volumes	1–9990 ml/cycle	Desorption flowrates	0–150 ml/min
(separate for 3 different fluids)		Number of cycles	9

2. Safety system with electronic operation
   - separate air detectors for plasma and elution buffers
   - mechanical valves with electronic control
   - digital display of accomplished plasma- and desorption volumes
   - volume constant pumps
   - prefixed program preventing operational mistakes during therapy
3. Free choice of manual or automated operation
4. Separate operational program for the preparation of disposables and for priming

---

* (Developed in cooperation with Medicap, Medizinische Spezialgeräte, D-6314 Ulrichstein, Germany.

Table 4. Safety of LDL-Apheresis

A. Safety of the columns (Stoffel, Borberg 1981) by exclusion of

    1. complement activation
    2. antibody leakage
    3. particle leakage
    4. bacterial contamination during production, handling and storage
    5. pyrogenicity during production, handling and storage

B. Development and application of an automated, electronically controlled adsorbtion-desorbtion system (Borberg, 1983)

---

potential problem of platelet loss. The safety of the procedure was investigated with the tests, listed in Table 4. No side effects attributable to the adsorption–desorption have been observed within more than 3000 treatments performed so far.

The capacity of the system permits to remove up to 48 gm LDL-cholesterol per treatment (Table 5). The length of the treatments is individualized according to the pre-treatment level of total-cholesterol to obtain the post-treatment values wanted. The treatments are performed once per week. The receptor status of all patients was evaluated from fibroblast cultures prior to the initiation of the therapy.

The clinical evaluation included a detailed history of the patient and his family, physical examination, documentation of visible or measurable lipo-protein deposits of the skin and tendons by either photography or x-ray, clinical chemistry and cardiological examinations like ECG, exercise ECG, myocardial scintigraphy, and coronary angiography under standardized conditions. Angina pectoris was graded according to the recommendations of the Canadian Cardiovascular Society into 4 grades, coronary athero-

Table 5. Capacity of the immunosorbtion columns for LDL-Apheresis

---

Capacity (LDL-Cholesterol)

1981	2 gm/column	×4	=	8 gm/therapy
1983	4 gm/column	×4	=	16 gm/therapy
1985	8 gm/column	×4	=	32 gm/therapy
1986	up to 12 gm/column	×4	=	48 gm/therapy

Volume

Approximately   400 ml

356

sclerosis was evaluated according to the recommendations of the American Heart Association with the coronary artery disease reporting system. The coronary angiograms were evaluated applying the criteria of percutaneous transluminal coronary angioplasty (PTCA) by calculating the stenosis area of the vessel, using the data obtained from measuring the diameters with calipers in a standardized fashion. A change was considered to be significant, if the stenosis area changed for more than 20%. Further details may be seen from our previous work already published [4].

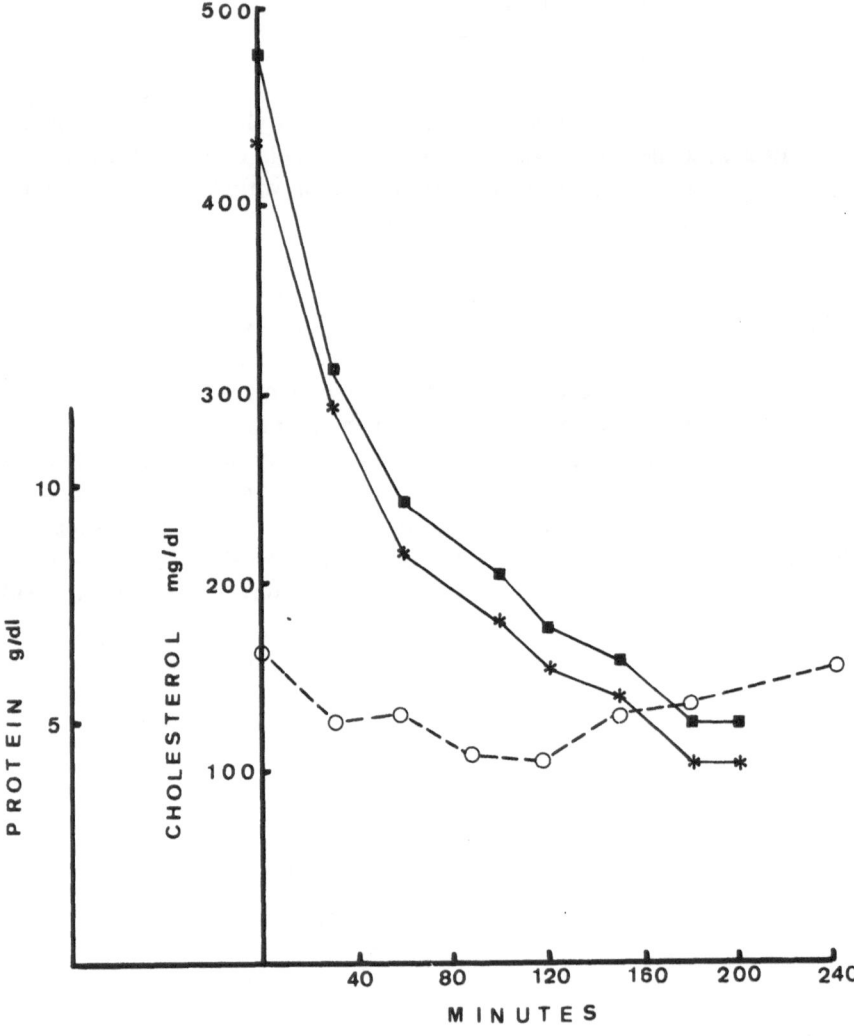

Figure 2. Decrease of lipid and protein during LDL-apheresis: ■———■ = total cholesterol; *———* = LDL plus VLDL; O----O = plasma protein.

Results

1) *Efficacy of the single treatment*

As Figure 2 demonstrates, the LDL level can be lowered to normal or subnormal levels during the course of each treatment. It is important to know, that this is independent from the initial LDL-titer or other substrates like fibrinogen for instance lost, when selective LDL-elimination is applied. The extent of the removal naturally correlates with the length of the individual treatment, which must not exceed 4 hours. This means that the treating physician can adapt the treatment time to predictive post-treatment values meeting the requirements of regression of each individual patient. After the treatment one observes a rapid increase (Figure 3) within the next 24 hours subsequently diminishing over time. We explain the first reaction with the reflux from the extravascular compartment, whereas the subsequent slow increase may represent the rate of production

THE INCREASE OF TOTAL CHOLESTEROL AFTER LDL-APHERESIS

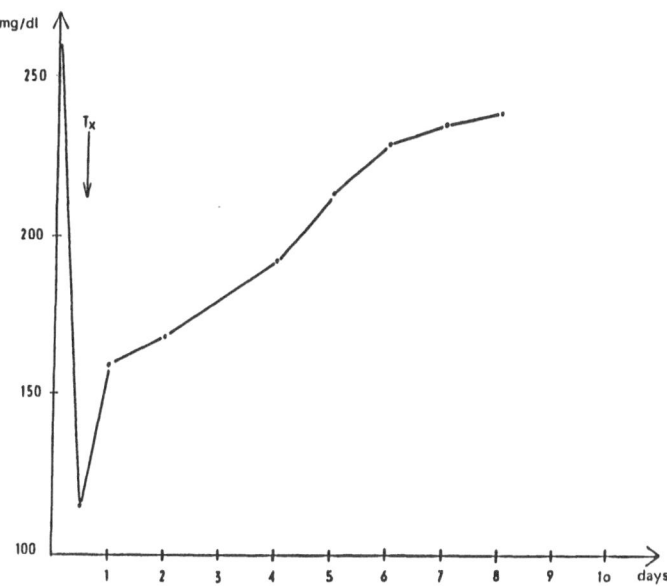

Figure 3. The increase of total cholesterol after LDL-Apheresis.

Results of Long Term LDL-Apheresis

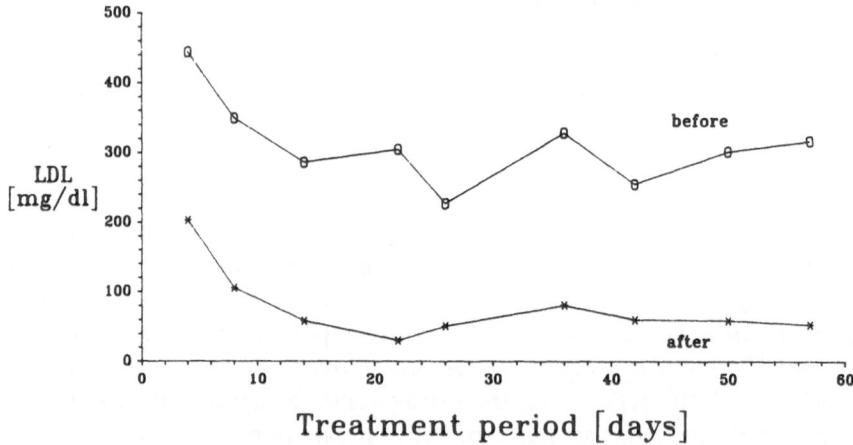

Figure 4. Results of long term LDL-Apheresis. Decrease of LDL during continuous therapy.

Table 6. Average cholesterol levels under longterm LDL-Apheresis therapy

Patient		1981	1982	1983	1984	1985	1986
W.R.	Total Chol. (mg/dl)	–	–	193	207	222	200
	LDL-Chol. (mg/dl)	–	–	148	171	180	159
	HDL-Chol (mg/dl)	–	–	36	33	42	42
H.W.	Total Chol. (mg/dl)	–	–	217	204	283*	291*
	LDL-Chol. (mg/dl)	–	–	143	152	247*	261*
	HDL-Chol. (mg/dl)	–	–	25	27	30*	35*
B.Th.	Total Chol. (mg/dl)	–	–	–	245	261	227
	LDL-Chol. (mg/dl)	–	–	–	202	223	180
	HDL-Chol. (mg/dl)	–	–	–	37	38	41
S.A.	Total Chol. (mg/dl)	–	–	–	417	339	281
	LDL-Chol. (mg/dl)	–	–	–	389	312	250
	HDL-Chol. (mg/dl)	–	–	–	20	17	25
G.N.	Total Chol. (mg/dl)	–	–	–	248	232	207
	LDL-Chol. (mg/dl)	–	–	–	192	195	178
	HDL-Chol. (mg/dl)	–	–	–	17	28	22

* Bi-weekly treatments.

Results of Long Term LDL-Apheresis

Increase of HDL during continuous therapy

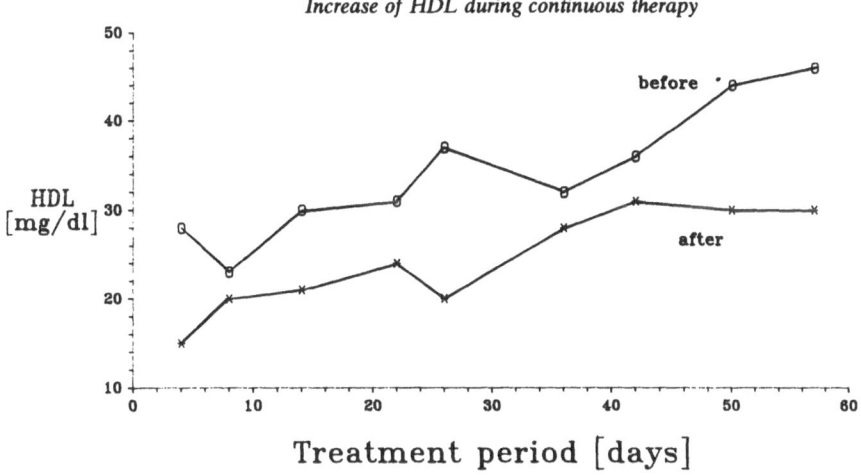

Treatment period [days]

Figure 5. Results of long term LDL-Apheresis. Increase of HDL during continuous therapy.

2) *Long term efficacy*

The picture of long term treatments is given in the next figures. After an initial period with decreasing total and LDL cholesterol levels, a steady state between elimination and production appears to exist (Figure 4). We consider the average of the post- and pre-treatment values to be representative for the patient values between treatment. These values could already be maintained in the normal range during our phase 1 trial, which tended to establish post-treatment values of 150 mg/dl total cholesterol (Table 6) and are even lower in our phase 2 trial started last year aiming at post-treatment values of 100 md/dl without additional drug therapy. If we look at the HDL-level, it increases in at least 50% of the patients, improving the LDL/HDL ratio favourably (Figure 5). The following slide summarizes the

Table 7. Advantages of specific extracorporeal LDL-elimination using LDL-Apheresis

1. *Specificity* of elimination
   (no loss of non-pathogenic or protective plasma components)

2. *Capacity* of the system
   (Patient treatments can be 'tailored' according to the needs of the patient)

3. *Versatility* of the technical device
   (Applicable to all kinds of selective or specific sorption columns)

advantages of LDL-apheresis drawn from our experience of the last 6 years (Table 7).

3) *Clinical results*

The clinical data presented here derived from our first trial on 10 patients (Table 8). 4 of the 10 patients are homozygous and 6 heterozygous. It is obvious, that the homozygous patients with an average of 17.5 years at the

Table 8. Longterm LDL-Apheresis in familial hypercholesterolaemia: general patient data

	Patient	Age	Sex	Genotype	Total cholesterol without therapy (mg/dl)	First Apheresis
1.	K.H.	40 Y	F	heterozygous	477	I/1981
2.	Pe.Dr.	14 Y	M	homozygous	644	XI/1981
3.	Pa.Dr.	16 Y	F	homozygous	660	XI/1981
4.	Z.S.	29 Y	M	heterozygous	532	III/1982
5.	K.W.	56 Y	M	heterozygous	459	VI/1982
6.	B.Sch.	19 Y	F	homozygous	924	XII/1982
7.	A.T.	29 Y	F	homozygous	764	XII/1982
8.	B.T.	21 Y	F	heterozygous	518	III/1984
9.	W.R.	41 Y	F	heterozygous	363	VII/1984
10.	G.N.	38 Y	F	heterozygous	491	IV/1984

Table 9. Radiological size determinations of xanthomata of the achilles tendons*

	Tendon thickness	RIGHT/LEFT (In mm)	
Patient	Initial values[+]	Observation period (months)	Extent of reduction
1. K.H.	12/ 8	39	−1.5/ 0
2. Pe.Dr.[++]	10/ 9	48	0 / 0
3. Pa.Dr.[++]	16/20	48	−7.0/−4.0
4. Z.S.	7/ 8	45	−0.5/−0.1
5. K.W.	19/18	41	− 1.0/−1.2
6. Br.Sch.[++]	17/18	36	−2.5/−2.0
7. A.T.[++]	24/24	36	−4.0/−3.0
8. B.T.	12/14	21	−1.5/−0.5
9. G.N.	21/21	20	−2.0/−1.5
10. W.R.	26/25	15	−2.0/−1.2

* Until December 1985; [+] Normal value: up to 10 mm; [++] Homozygous patients.

Table 10. Follow-up* of coronary status in patients with familial hypercholesterolaemia under long-term LDL-Aphersis

Progression of stenosis:	1/23 (6%)
Unchanged:	11/23 (48%)
Regression of stenosis:	10/23 (46%)
Progression of sclerosis:	2/79 (3%)
Unchanged:	56/79 (70%)
Regression of sclerosis:	21/79 (27%)

* Follow-up: 35.7 ± 17.4 months.

start of therapy (range from 12–27 years) are considerably younger as compared to the heterozygous patients with a medium of 38 years (range from 21–54 years). All homozygous patients are receptor defective.

Xanthomata of the tendons or the skin were reduced or completely resolved, as can be seen from Table 9 and Figure 6. Cardiac symptoms generally disappeared or were considerably reduced in relation to the variables influencing the efficacy of the treatment. The grading of the angina pectoris was reduced from an average of 1.8 to 0.8. Patients suffering from dyspnoe reported a disappearance of the symptom.

This correlated with improvements of the exercise ECG: the initial average values of 90 Watt increased to 100 Watt and more impressingly over time from an average of 322.5 ± 250 Watt × min to an average of 478 ± 251 Watt × min. None of the parameters mentioned so far, deteriorated. The initial coronary morphology demonstrated 23 stenoses in 22 coronary segments (Table 10). 1 stenosis appeared to progress, 11 remained constant and 10 regressed. The average stenosis degree was $76.6 \pm 19.8\%$ prior to LDL-apheresis therapy and 57% at the date of evaluation.

The extent of sclerosis determined according to the suggestions of the international nomenclature commission was generally grade 1 in 79 major and minor segments. A progress appeared to occur in 2 segments, 56 segments remained unchanged and regression was seen in 21 segments.

Discussion

For the discussion of the results one has to keep in mind, that the data did not derive from a predictive well planned, controlled clinical investigation, but represent a phase I trial, supposed to establish safety, efficacy and economy of the procedure. However beyond the scope of this study trends

362

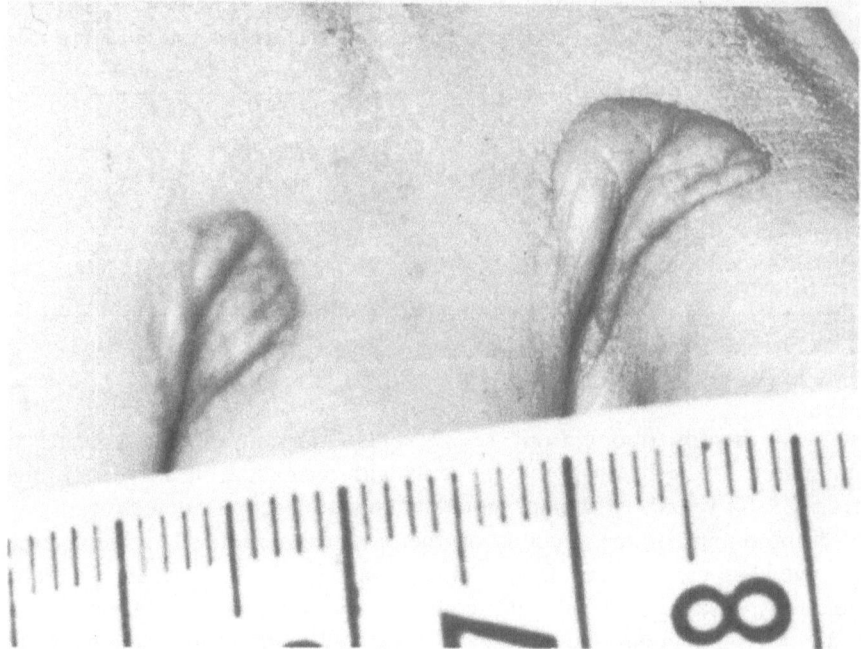

Figure 6a. Interdigital space of the left hand 1981.

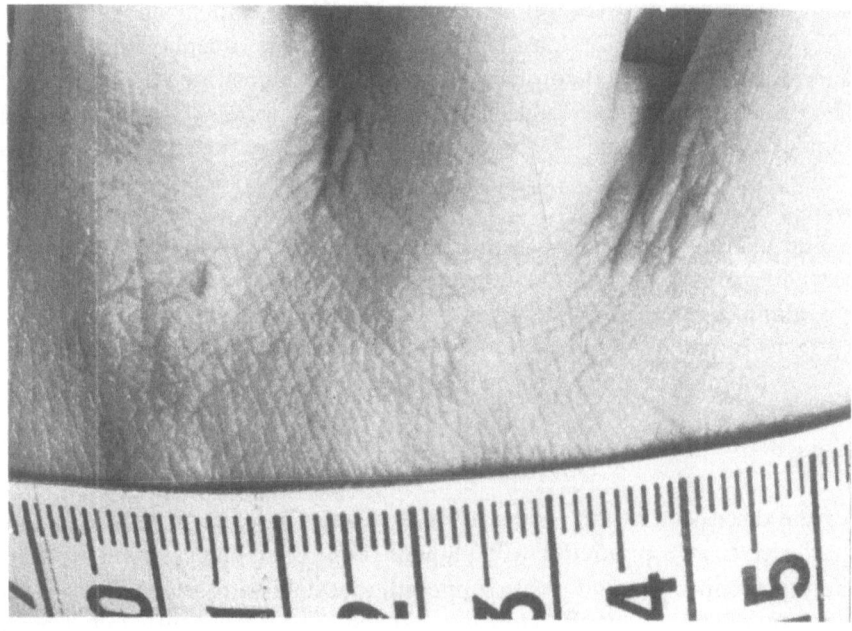

Figure 6b. The same location after 4 years of regular therapy.

363

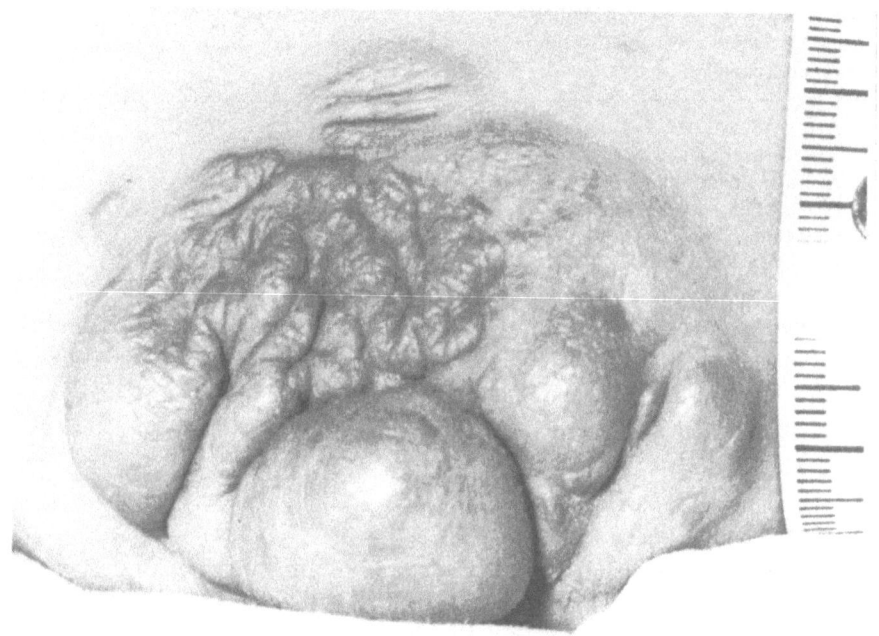

Figure 6c. Right elbow 1981.

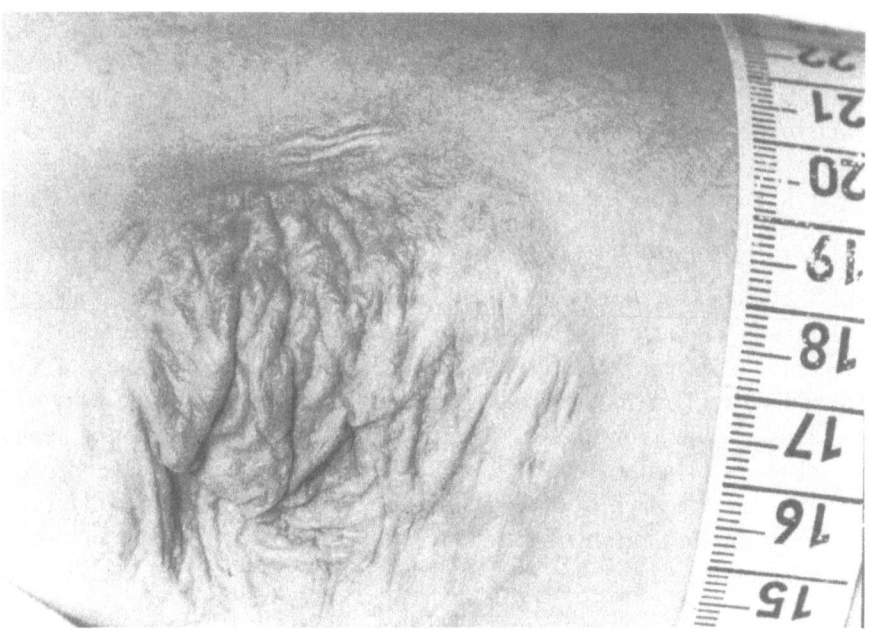

Figure 6d. The same location after 4 years of regular therapy.

Figure 6. Disappearance of xanthomas under LDL-apheresis in a homozygous 12 years old girl.

Table 11. Obvious variables for regression of atherosclerosis in patients with familial hyper-cholesterolaemia

---

1. Age
2. Genetic background
3. Average cholesterol level between treatments
4. Length of the treatment period
5. Initial clinical status prior to the first LDL-Apheresis (skin, tendens, coronary system)

---

for the recognition of variables determining the process of regression in atherosclerosis may be recognized (Table 11). The regression observed in our patients seems to correlate with:

1. the age of the patients;
2. their genetic background;
3. the average cholesterol level in between treatments;
4. the length of the treatment period and
5. the initial clinical status prior to the first LDL-apheresis, referring to both, the extent of lipoprotein deposits in the skin and the tendons and the status of the coronary system.

Considering the regression of xanthomata, it appears that younger patients regress quicker than older patients. However, one has to keep in mind that homozygous patients are generally diagnosed earlier as compared to heterozygous patients. This may lead to the conclusion that the extent of the genetic defect may also play a role. We do not know, how far apheresis may influence the receptor function in these patients. If an assumed correlation between genetic background and regression obtained does not exist or is indirect only, depending on the number or the functional status of the receptors, homozygous receptor negative patients suffering from extremely high LDL-levels would regress less quickly as compared to receptor defective patients, provided a constant identical amount of LDL would always be removed from both groups of patients.

This consideration hints to the importance of the post-treatment cholesterol levels or, alternatively, to the average cholesterol level in between treatments. We have to keep in mind that we have no sufficiently precise information on the rate of the LDL production under the influence of the elimination therapy. We assume that after an initial phase of disequilibrium removing more than being produced, we enter into a phase of equilibrium between removal and production, but we do not know, on what level this equilibrium is established.

The recognition of the importance of the post-treatment or intermediate cholesterol level led us to question, whether our earlier post-treatment aim of 150 mg/ml total cholesterol was optimal. This question is associated with a rather complex number of problems, which cannot immediately be solved. The paucity of information on the production rate was already mentioned. We have no or little knowledge on the mechanism and the speed of lipoprotein mobilization from the deposits. There is no information on the pool sizes of LDL under elimination therapy. Presuming however, that these factors are of secondary importance, we concluded from the length of time needed to obtain a complete regression that a further decrease to a post-treatment level of 100 mg/dl total cholesterol was desirable to accelerate the process of regression. It is obvious that these questions just mentioned need further evaluation.

The period a patient is under therapy appears to be another variable. It seems logical that the process of regression is more impressive, the longer the treatment lasts. However, this has to be seen in relation to the initial clinical status of the patient. The wider xanthomas are expressed, the more time appears to be necessary for resolution, even if the other variables are maintained at an optimal level. Calcification appears to be hardly or not regressable at all. This observation may restrict the goal of treatment of patients beyond a certain age for instance of approximately 45–50 years to achieve prevention of the progress of the disease rather than regression.

The discussion referred so far to the regression of xanthomata. Though we assume that basically the same variables are valid for the regression of coronary stenoses, this issue may be even more difficult to discuss, as local factors like blood pressure, lipoprotein uptake or removal through the intima, calcification and metabolic differences may play an additional role. It appears from our data that the process of regression in the coronaries takes longer than that of deposits in the skin and tendons. This may be explained with the higher frequency of coronary alterations in our heterozygous patients as compared to the homozygous. It has also to be kept in mind that the procedures to measure regression of coronary heart disease are rather of qualitative or semiquantitative nature only, rendering evaluation more difficult.

Drawing from our current experience it may be worthwhile to summarize the indication for applying LDL-apheresis in patients with familial hypercholesterolaemia: Receptor negative homozygoty appears to be an absolute indication at any age to prevent the establishment of atherosclerosis, whereas receptor defectiveness may allow to begin the therapy at an age, when the blood volume permits the on-line treatment. However, as regression can be obtained, these patients should be treated at the earliest possible age.

Heterozygous patients should generally not be treated by apheresis, unless conventional means like diet, exercise and drug treatment are exhausted. If it is ascertained that these therapies cannot normalize the LDL-level, the patients should also be treated as early as possible with apheresis. At an age of less than 30–40 years, regression may be achieved, eventually permitting the termination or a decrease of the frequency of aphereses.

Patients with symptomatic coronary heart disease may also not need extracorporeal LDL-elimination, if their cholesterol levels can be normalized by drugs, but naturally, cardiosurgery or PTCA are necessary. If critical stenoses are present and the LDL-level cannot be normalized by conventional therapy, they should first be treated either with bypass surgery or PTCA. The subsequent long-term LDL-apheresis is then at least able to prevent the establishment or reestablishment of stenoses in older patients, whereas younger patients may finally regress to complete normalcy after years.

Summary

In summary we conclude that LDL-apheresis permits at least to prevent the progress of atherosclerosis in patients with familial hypercholesterolaemia. Regression occurs in correlation to certain variables, which need to be investigated furthermore. This is the aim of a multicenter trial initiated last year.

References

1. Borberg H, Stoffel W, Oette K (1983) Plasma Ther Transfus Technol 4,4:459–466
2. Borberg H (1983) Europ J Clin Invest 13,11:A 39
3. Borberg H, Gaczkowski A, Hombach V, Oette K, Stoffel W (1986) Ärztl Lab 32,3:57–62
4. Hombach V, Borberg H, Gaczkowski A, Oette K, Stoffel W (1986) Dtsch med Wschr 111,45:1709–1715
5. Stoffel W (1981) Th Demant: Proc Natl Acad Sci (USA) 78:611–615
6. Stoffel W, Borberg H, Greve V (1981) The Lancet ii:1005–1007

Index of Subjects

DEVELOPMENTS IN CARDIOVASCULAR MEDICINE

Recent volumes

Heintzen, P.H., Bürsch, J.H., eds.: Progress in digital angiocardiography. 1988.
ISBN 0-89838-965-8.

Scheinman, M.A., ed.: Catheter ablation of cardiac arrhythmias. 1988.
ISBN 0-89838-967-4.

Spaan, J.A.E., Bruschke, A.V.G., Gittenberger-de Groot, A.C., eds.: Coronary circulation. 1987. ISBN 0-89838-978-X.

Visser, C., Kan, G., Meltzer, R., eds.: Echocardiography in coronary artery disease. 1988.
ISBN 0-89838-979-8.

Bayés de Luna, A., Betriu, A., Permanyer, G., eds.: Therapeutics in cardiology. 1988.
ISBN 0-89838-981-X.

Mirvis, D.M., ed.: Body surface electrocardiographic mapping. 1988.
ISBN 0-89838-983-6.

Konstam, M.A., Isner, J.M., eds.: The right ventricle. 1988. ISBN 0-89838-987-9.

Kappagoda, C.T., Greenwood, P.V., eds.: Long-term management of patients after myocardial infarction. 1988. ISBN 0-89838-352-8.

Gaasch, W.H., Levine, H.J., eds.: Chronic aortic regurgitation. 1988.
ISBN 0-89838-364-1.

Singal, P.K., ed.: Oxygen radicals in the pathophysiology of heart disease. 1988.
ISBN 0-89838-375-7.

Reiber, J.H.C., Serruys, P.W., eds.: New developments in quantitative coronary arteriography. 1988. ISBN 0-89838-377-3.

Morganroth, J., Moore, E.N., eds.: Silent myocardial ischemia. 1988.
ISBN 0-89838-380-3.

Ter Keurs, H.E.D.J., Noble, M.I.M., eds.: Starling's law of the heart revisited. 1988.
ISBN 0-89838-382-X.

Sperelakis, N., ed.: Physiology and pathophysiology of the heart. 1988.
ISBN 0-89838-388-9

De Jong, J.W., ed.: Myocardial energy metabolism. 1988. ISBN 0-89838-394-3.

Hombach, V., Hilger, H.H., Kennedy, H.L., eds.: Electrocardiography and cardiac drug therapy. 1988. ISBN 0-89838-395-1.

Iwata, H., Lombardini, J.B., Segawa, T., eds.: Taurine and the heart. 1988.
ISBN 0-89838-396-X.

Rosen, M.R., Palti, Y., eds.: Lethal arrhythmias resulting from myocardial ischemia and infarction. 1988. ISBN 0-89838-401-X.

Kluwer Academic Publishers
DORDRECHT / BOSTON / LONDON